Manual of Neonatal and Paediatric
Heart Disease

Manual of Neonatal and Paediatric Heart Disease

FIONA S HORROX BSc(Hons) RGN RSCN

Clinical Development Coordinator, Paediatric Intensive Care Unit,
Royal Liverpool Children's NHS Trust at Alder Hey Hospital

Illustrations **Guy Heaton**

W
WHURR PUBLISHERS
LONDON AND PHILADELPHIA

© 2002 Whurr Publishers

First published 2002 by
Whurr Publishers Ltd
19b Compton Terrace, London N1 2UN, England
325 Chestnut Street, Philadelphia PA19106, USA

British Library Cataloguing in Publication Data

A catalogue record for this book is available from the British Library.

ISBN 1 86156 244 6

Printed and bound in the UK by Athenaeum Press Limited, Gateshead, Tyne & Wear.

Contents

Acknowledgements

I would like to thank the following people for their patience, encouragement and help in preparing this book:

Guy Heaton, who produced the illustrations, and all those who reviewed the material:

Steve Gilroy, BSc(Hons), PGDL
Jan Taylor, Sister PICU, RLCH
Andy Darbyshire, Nurse Consultant, PICU, RLCH
Pam Harris, Cardiac Liaison Nurse, RLCH
Denise Kitchiner, Paediatric Cardiologist, RLCH
Marco Pozzi, Paediatric Cardiac Surgeon, RLCH
Roger Franks, Paediatric Thoracic Surgeon, RLCH
Nicky Reilly, Pharmacist, PICU, RLCH
Paul Daly, Perfusionist, RLCH
Karen McDonald, Datascope UK
Steve McGlaughlin, PICU, Manchester Children's Trust

In addition I wish to thank Douglas and Sandra Stenhouse, parents of Edward, who kindly allowed reproduction of the diary they kept on discovering that their son had a congenital heart defect.

Dedication

This book is dedicated to my godchildren: Timmy, Caitlin, Max and Molly.

I would like to express my gratitude to my parents Joyce and John, brother and sister Ian and Kate, and other close family and friends for their kind help and support over the last few years.

Glossary of terms and common abbreviations

ABG	Arterial blood gas
ACE	Angiotensin converting enzyme
ACT	Activated clotting time
ACTH	Adrenocorticotrophic hormone
ADH	Antidiuretic hormone
AE	Atrial ectopics
AF	Atrial fibrillation
Afterload	Resistance against which vessels must eject their contents
AIDS	Acquired immune deficiency syndrome
ANS	Autonomic nervous system
Ao	Aorta
Aortic Root Replacement	Dissection of the aorta and annulus below the coronary arteries
AP	Aortopulmonary
APTT	Activated partial prothrombin time
AR	Aortic regurgitation
ARDS	Acute respiratory distress syndrome
AS	Aortic stenosis
ASD	Atrial septal defect
AV	Atrioventricular
AVN	Atrioventricular node
AVSD	Atrioventricular septal defect
AVV	Atrioventricular valve
BP	Blood pressure
BSA	Body surface area

BT shunt	Blalock–Taussig shunt — right or left pulmonary artery connected to the corresponding subclavian artery
CAS	Critical aortic stenosis
CAVSD	Complete atrioventricular septal defect
Central shunt	Main pulmonary artery connected to the aorta
CHB	Congenital heart block
CHD	Congenital heart disease
CHF	Congestive heart failure
CI	Cardiac index — cardiac output divided by BSA. Accurate value assessing cardiac output related to the size of patient
CJD	Creutzfeld-Jakob disease
CMV	Cytomegalovirus
CO	Cardiac output = stroke volume + heart rate
CoAo	Coarctation of the aorta
Concordant	"In the right position" — the relationship between the atria and ventricles is normal, for example, if the morphological left atrium is connected to a morphological left ventricle, it is concordant
Coronary sinus	Where the cardiac veins terminate. Blood then flows into the right atrium
CP	Cavopulmonary
CP anastomosis	Connection of the superior vena cava to the right pulmonary artery
CPAP	Continuous positive airway pressure
CPB	Cardiopulmonary bypass
CPR	Cardiopulmonary resuscitation
CRP	C-reactive protein
CT	Computed tomography
CTGA	Corrected transposition of the great arteries
CVA	Cerebrovascular accident
CVP	Central venous pressure
Damas-Kaye-Stansel	The main pulmonary artery is transected. Proximal end is connected to the ascending aorta which forms the left ventricular outflow tract for the systemic circulation. A valved conduit from the right ventricle to the distal pulmonary artery forms the right ventricular outflow tract for the pulmonary circulation

Dextrocardia	The heart is on the right side of the chest
DIC	Disseminated intravascular coagulation
DILV	Double inlet left ventricle
Discordant	The relationship between the atria and ventricles is abnormal so if the morphological left atrium is connected to the morphological right ventricle/ anatomical right ventricle, it is discordant
DORV	Double outlet right ventricle
ECG	Electrocardiogram
EDRF	Endothelium derived relaxing factor
EDV	End diastolic volume – the volume of blood in the ventricle at the beginning of systole
Eisenmenger's complex	The pulmonary vascular resistance exceeds the systemic vascular resistance so the shunt becomes permanently right to left
Ejection fraction	How much of the total volume of the ventricles is ejected during contraction. The normal left ventricle ejection fraction is 60–75%, the right, 50–60%
ESR	Erythrocyte sedimentation rate
ESV	End systolic volume – the volume of blood in the ventricle at the end of systole, before the valves open
ETT	Endotracheal tube
FBC	Full blood count
FFP	Fresh frozen plasma
FiO_2	Fraction of inspired oxygen
Fontan (modified)	Following a CP anastomosis, the SVC is connected to the IVC by means of either an intra-aortic baffle or extra cardiac conduit
Gradient	The pressure differential across two areas
HAS	Human albumin solution
HCT	Haematocrit
HLHS	Hypoplastic left heart syndrome
HOCM	Hypertrophic obstructive cardiomyopathy
HR	Heart rate
IAA	Interrupted aortic arch
IABP	Intra-aortic balloon pump
ICP	Integrated care pathway
INR	International ratio of prothrombin time

Isomerism	Mirroring sides (bilateral one sidedness) — Usually occurs on the right side. For example, both the atrial appendages resemble the morphological right atria. Commonly there are two right lungs and asplenia
IVC	Inferior vena cava
IVH	Intraventricular haemorrhage
IVS	Intact ventricular septum
Konno operation	Surgery performed for extensive narrowing within the LVOT. The aortic root is enlarged
LA	Left atrium
LADCA	Left anterior descending coronary artery
LAP	Left atrial pressure
LBBB	Left bundle branch block
LCA	Left coronary artery
LFT	Liver function tests
LPA	Left pulmonary artery
LSA	Left subclavian artery
LV	Left ventricle
LVH	Left ventricular hypertrophy
LVOT	Left ventricular outflow tract
LVOTO	Left ventricular outflow tract obstruction
MAP	Mean arterial pressure
MAPCA	Major aortopulmonary collateral arteries
MBTS	Modified Blalock–Taussig Shunt — the right or left pulmonary artery is connected to the corresponding subclavian artery by means of a Gortex connection
MCT	Medium chain triglyceride
MDT	Multidisciplinary team
Mesocardia	The heart has a midline position
MPA	Main pulmonary artery
MR	Mitral regurgitation
MRI	Magnetic resonance imaging
NBM	Nil by mouth
NEC	Nectrotising enterocolitis
Norwood procedure	The MPA is transected. The distal pulmonary artery is patched. An incision is made into the aorta. The pulmonary artery is anastomosed to the aortic arch using an aortic allograft. A modified Blalock–Taussig shunt or central shunt is performed to enhance pulmonary blood flow

PA	Pulmonary atresia
	Pulmonary artery
PA IVS	Pulmonary atresia with intact ventricular septum
PAP	Pulmonary artery pressure
PAPVD	Partial anomalous pulmonary venous drainage
PA VSD	Pulmonary atresia with ventricular septal defect
PBF	Pulmonary blood flow
PCV	Packed cell volume
PD	Peritoneal dialysis
PDA	Patent ductus arteriosus
PEEP	Positive end expiratory pressure
PFO	Patent foramen ovale
PPHN	Persistent pulmonary hypertension of the newborn
Preload	Filling pressure
PS	Pulmonary stenosis
PVOD	Pulmonary vascular obstructive disease
PVR	Pulmonary vascular resistance — the elastic recoil of the vessels. The recoil creates resistance in the vessel against which pressure the RV is pumping. It is calculated by PAP minus LAP divided by the PBF
Qp	Pulmonary blood flow
Qs	Systemic blood flow
RA	Right atrium
RAP	Right atrial pressure
Rastelli procedure	The MPA is divided and the LV end oversewn. An intra-cardiac tunnel is placed between the VSD and aorta. RV is connected to the PA with an aortic homograft or valved conduit
RBBB	Right bundle branch block
RCA	Right coronary artery
Ross procedure	The patient's pulmonary valve is sewn in place of the aortic valve. A pulmonary homograft replaces the patient's pulmonary valve. The coronary arteries are reimplanted
RPA	Right pulmonary artery
RSA	Right subclavian artery
RV	Right ventricle
RVH	Right ventricular hypertrophy
RVOT	Right ventricular outflow tract
RVOTO	Right ventricular outflow tract obstruction

SAGM	Saline adenine glucose and mannitol
SAN	Sinoatrial node
SB	Sinus bradycardia
SBE	Subacute bacterial endocarditis
Scimitar syndrome	Total or partial anomalous pulmonary venous connection of the right lung to the IVC. It is associated with hypoplasia of the lung and pulmonary artery
Shöne syndrome	Four left sided obstructions, e.g., subaortic stenosis, supravalvular stenosis, parachute mitral valve, coarctation of the aorta. Not all four have to be present
Situs	Normal
Situs ambiguus	Ambiguous position
Situs inversus	Opposite position to the normal position
Situs solitus	Normal position
SP shunt	Systemic pulmonary shunt, e.g., modified BT shunt
SR	Sinus rhythm
ST	Sinus tachycardia
Stroke volume (SV)	Cardiac output × heart rate
SVC	Superior vena cava
SVR	Systemic vascular resistance — the elastic recoil of the vessels. The recoil creates resistance in the vessel against which pressure the left ventricle is pumping. It is calculated by aortic pressure minus RAP divided by the systemic blood flow
SVT	Supra ventricular tachycardia
Syncope	Loss of consciousness due to reduced cardiac output or metabolic or neurological causes
TA	Tricuspid atresia
	Truncus arteriosus
TAPVD	Total anomalous pulmonary venous drainage
Taussig–Bing anomaly	DORV which resembles TGA and VSD
TENS	Transcutaneous electrical nerve stimulation
TGA	Transposition of the great arteries
THAM	Trihydroxymethyl-amino-methane
TOF	Tetralogy of Fallot
TORCH	A viral screen for toxoplasma, rubella, CMV and herpes
TPN	Total parenteral nutrition

TR	Tricuspid regurgitation
TSH	Thyroid stimulating hormone
TV	Tricuspid valve
U&E	Urea and electrolytes
VA	Ventriculoarterial
VF	Ventricular fibrillation
VSD	Ventricular septal defect
VT	Ventricular tachycardia
WPW syndrome	Wolff–Parkinson–White syndrome

Preface

Purpose

A number of books have been written relating to congenital heart disease, but in the main they reflect individualised medical management of local practice and philosophies.

Although this book assumes a prior working knowledge of congenital heart disease, it aims to provide the reader with a reference guide to be utilised at the bedside. It is not designed to be an exhaustive text on congenital heart disease.

For whom it is intended

The main aim of this book is to provide a comprehensive, affordable guide for paediatric, neonatal and adult nurses of young people with congenital heart disease. Currently, there are no books on the market written for nurses that are both affordable and easily used at the bedside. What appear to be available, however, are chapters in paediatric nursing texts which do not allow for adequate knowledge to be gained for nurses caring for these infants, children and adolescents.

Although this book is primarily written for nursing staff, a multidisciplinary team approach to managing this group of children is vital. When discussing the management of the children, the words "nursing care" are not used, rather "key management issues", as all team members have a role to play. Other professions which will find the book of interest are community staff (district nurses, health visitors, GPs, midwives), dietitians, doctors, neonatal staff, perfusionists, pharmacists, physiological measurement technicians, physiotherapists, psychologists, social workers, theatre staff and other personnel coming into contact with this group of children.

Contents

Starting with the introduction to congenital heart disease, the normal heart, anatomy and physiology, fetal circulation and the changes that occur at birth are covered. This appropriately leads on to cardiac procedures and investigations for patients with congenital heart disease. Subsequent chapters are divided into acyanotic defects, obstructive defects, cyanotic defects, mixed defects and acquired defects. Each defect is subdivided into the aetiology, definition, classification, anatomy and related pathophysiology, signs and symptoms, diagnosis, specific preoperative management, medical and surgical management, specific postoperative management and long-term follow-up. A diagram for each defect and complex surgical procedure is included.

Chapters on cardiopulmonary bypass, elective admission with reference to the psychological and physical care, the preparation in intensive care and receiving a patient postoperatively are discussed. Specific complications related to the cardiovascular, respiratory, haematological, neurological, renal and gastrointestinal systems, drug therapy, the dying child, integrated care pathways and discharge planning are also included. There is also a contribution from the father of a child with a congenital heart defect to give a psychological perspective. Appendices include normal blood and haemodynamic parameters, blood group compatibility, and an example of an integrated care pathway.

Using the book

The book aims to be a practical guide. For example, a nurse expecting the admission of a baby with an interrupted aortic arch could review the section on fetal circulation and the subsection on an interrupted aortic arch, taking particular note of the specific preoperative key management issues. Once the baby arrives on the ward, during initial assessment, the book could be used to guide the nurse through any specific complications that may have arisen. When the baby is stable enough for theatre, usually within the first couple of days of life, the book could be consulted on how to prepare for a postoperative patient and the specific postoperative management, for example management of low cardiac output.

Every attempt has been made to ensure all material is accurate and up-to-date. However, it is up to practitioners to assess their patients on an individual basis and manage them according to policies and procedures relevant to their place of work. Therefore, no responsibility can be taken by the author for interventions undertaken as a result of information provided by this book.

Fiona S Horrox
February 2002

Chapter 1
The normal heart

Introduction

Congenital abnormalities are responsible for the hospitalisation of many sick neonates, infants and children. Thirty per cent of abnormalities can be attributed to congenital heart disease, this being the largest individual group of congenital abnormalities[1–3]. The incidence per live birth is around 0.8% [1,3,4].

Heart defects can be put into two categories. The first group is responsible for 80% of all defects and includes ventricular septal defects (VSD), atrial septal defects (ASD), patent ductus arteriosus (PDA), tetralogy of Fallot (TOF), pulmonary stenosis, coarctation of the aorta, aortic stenosis and transposition of the great arteries (TGA). The remaining 20% are rare or complex and include interrupted aortic arch (IAA) and aortic atresia[3].

Currently in the UK, it is considered preferable to repair and reconstruct the heart with a congenital defect as opposed to cardiac transplantation. Transplantation may be surgically less challenging than some of the complex heart reconstructions, but the availability of hearts, the aftercare and the average three year survival in 50% of patients[3] normally influences the team's decision to repair the abnormal heart. Transplantation will therefore not be discussed further in this book.

Factors associated with congenital heart disease (CHD)

The causative factors in the development of CHD are poorly understood and generally are thought to be idiopathic in nature. However, certain situations predispose to its development and include the following:

Environmental

- Drugs: The anticonvulsant phenytoin is linked to pulmonary and aortic stenosis; amphetamines to ASD and VSD; warfarin to VSD; lithium to Ebstein's anomaly; oestrogen and progesterone to TGA, VSD and TOF.
- Alcohol: Fetal alcohol syndrome predisposes to VSD, TGA, TOF and ASD.
- Infection: Rubella is associated with PDA and pulmonary stenosis. Cytomegalovirus is not associated with a specific defect.
- Maternal disease: Diabetes mellitus predisposes the fetus to CHD (5%), namely transposition of the great arteries (TGA), VSD and cardiomyopathy; systemic lupus erythematosus is connected with congenital complete heart block; maternal CHD raises the risk of the fetus having a CHD from 5% to 10%[1,4].

Genetic

Chromosomal abnormalities

Of newborns with a chromosomal defect, approximately 30% will have a CHD:

- Trisomy 13:   90% – VSD, PDA.
- Trisomy 18:   85% – VSD, PDA, pulmonary stenosis (PS).
- Trisomy 21:   40% – atrioventricular septal defect (AVSD).
- Turner's syndrome: 35% – coarctation of the aorta, ASD.
- Klinefelter's syndrome: 15% – PDA, ASD.
- Di George syndrome: 10% – interrupted aortic arch, truncus arteriosus, less commonly, pulmonary atresia with VSD and tetralogy of Fallot[1, 4–7].

Other diseases associated with CHD

- Apert syndrome: VSD, TOF.
- Charge association: TOF, truncus arteriosus, IAA.
- Crouzen association: PDA, coarctation of the aorta.
- Diaphragmatic hernia: Various defects.
- Imperforate anus: TOF, VSD.
- Marfan's disease: Aortic root dilatation and aneurysm.
- Mucopolysaccharidosis: Aortic and mitral regurgitation.
- Noonan's syndrome: Pulmonary stenosis.
- Tracheoesophageal fistula: VSD, ASD, TOF[4–6, 8].

Embryological development of the heart

The heart is the first organ to function within the embryo and begins to develop from the mesoderm within the first month of fetal life, being complete at eight weeks' gestation.

During this period, only a small percentage of women will know that they are pregnant. If a preconception plan is in place, it may help in the prevention of exposure to teratogenic agents such as drugs, alcohol and other environmental issues discussed previously. Despite this, in 90% of cases of CHD no cause is identified.

The heart initially develops when the mesoderm splits into two — the somatic mesoderm and the splanchnic mesoderm. The splanchnic mesoderm forms paired endocardial tubes which fuse to form a single tube — the primitive heart tube. This folds over on itself into an "S"-shaped structure that subsequently develops into a "U"-shaped structure. In subsequent weeks, the single tubular heart enlarges and twists. Five further areas develop off this "U"-shaped structure, namely the ventricle, bulbus cordis, atrium, sinus venosus and truncus arteriosus.

Landmarks in the development of the heart

- Days 14–49: Formation of the five areas of the "U" letter — four heart chambers develop.
- Days 20–24: The fetus is 1.5–3 mm long. Formation of the heart tube takes place.
- Days 23–25: The fetus is 2.5–3.2 mm long. Formation of the cardiac loop takes place. Abnormalities occurring at this time include TGA, congenitally corrected TGA and double outlet right ventricle (DORV).
- Day 28: The heart beats for the first time.
- Days 27–37: The fetus is 4–16 mm long. Septation occurs in both the atrium and ventricles. Septation is a complex developmental stage in heart formation, so defects of the septum are particularly common.
- Day 29: Septation of the bulbus cordis divides the truncus into an aortic and pulmonary channel.
- Day 56: Heart development is complete at 8 weeks.

Fetal circulation

Whilst in utero, the fetus with a congenital heart defect will usually tolerate the condition well. However, once born, the same condition can render the neonate critically ill. This may be attributed to the fetal circulation and the changes that occur at birth and shortly afterwards. Therefore, in order to understand the pathophysiology and haemodynamic effects of CHD, fetal circulation and the changes which occur at birth must be understood.

The fetus relies on the placenta to receive nutrients, oxygen and water from its mother, via the umbilical cord. Arterial blood is oxygenated in the placenta and leaves via the umbilical vein, which branches and delivers blood to the inferior vena cava (IVC) by either:

- Directly emptying into the IVC through the ductus venosus.
- Receiving blood directly from the branches of the umbilical vein into the liver and out via the hepatic veins.
- Passing through the liver, mixing with portal venous blood and leaving via the hepatic veins.

IVC blood thus contains umbilical, portal venous and lower body blood accounting for 65–70% of systemic venous return to the right atrium[9]. One-quarter of IVC blood passes from the right atrium through one of the fetal ducts, the foramen ovale, into the left atrium. A small amount of blood from the pulmonary veins is mixed with blood from the IVC. Blood then passes into the left ventricle and leaves through the aorta perfusing the coronary arteries, head, brain and upper extremities. Only a small proportion enters the descending aorta.

Blood from the head and neck returns to the right atrium via the superior vena cava (SVC), goes through the tricuspid valve to the right ventricle and up into the pulmonary artery. The left and right branches of the pulmonary artery divert 15% of their contents to the lungs which do not expand as they contain no air and thus the pulmonary vascular resistance (PVR) is very high. Conversely, the systemic vascular resistance (SVR) is low. The remaining 85% flows through the ductus arteriosus into the descending aorta where perfusion of the lower extremities and abdominal viscera occurs. The abdomen supplies the two arteries which feed the blood back into the placenta. The ductus arteriosus has the same diameter as the aorta.

Changes in the fetal circulation after birth

Changes are obviously necessary to allow the neonate to oxygenate his or her own blood, the placenta now being redundant. The physiological changes which occur are profound.

Systemic and pulmonary circulations

- As the umbilical cord is clamped, the SVR increases due to the increased blood volume in the placenta.
- Fluid which is present in the alveoli moves to the interstitial compartments where it is absorbed by the pulmonary capillaries and the lymphatic vessels. The baby takes a breath to expand the lungs and replace the fetal lung fluid. Passage through the birth canal squeezes the thorax so further fluid is pushed out of the lungs into the nose and mouth. This relieves alveolar hypoxia and subsequent vasodilation occurs[10].

Factors stimulating the first breath have a chemical element in which a low percentage of oxygen, increasing carbon dioxide and low pH, stimulate the respiratory centre in the medulla oblongata. Furthermore, a thermal component stimulates the medulla as the baby has left a warm environment for a cooler one[11].

The first breath results in a decrease in PVR as a response to an increase in pO_2. There is an increase in pulmonary blood flow as the pulmonary arteries dilate. The muscle layer of the pulmonary arteries continues to thin out. Over the next few days the pulmonary artery pressure continues to fall but ultimately takes about a month to fall to a mean level of one-third of mean systolic pressure.

Fetal shunts

- The ductus arteriosus begins to constrict due to the increase in pO_2, lowering levels of placental prostaglandin E_2[9] and the decreasing blood supply through it. In a normal gestation heart, the duct fibroses and closes within two to three weeks of birth and is then known as the ligamentum arteriosus. Duct closure is delayed in cyanotic infants where saturations of oxygen (SaO_2) are low, therefore the stimulus for closure, that is, oxygen, is reduced.
- The ductus venosus closes to become the ligamentum venosum which passes through the liver, from the portal vein to the IVC.
- Once the cord is clamped, the umbilical vein constricts and obliterates, becoming the ligamentum teres, and the umbilical arteries become the medial umbilical ligament.
- The flapped atrial opening, the foramen ovale becomes the fossa ovalis when left atrial pressure supersedes right atrial pressure.

Other changes

- Both ventricles are similar in size and mass at birth but during the first month the wall of the right ventricle becomes proportionately thinner due to the rapid growth of the left ventricle.
- There is a gradual change from fetal haemoglobin to adult haemoglobin.

The normal heart

The heart is a muscular, hollow, cone-shaped organ 10 cm long in the adult, 255–350 g in weight and the approximate size of the owner's fist. It is situated in the thoracic cavity, between the lungs in a mass of tissue known as the mediastinum. Approximately two-thirds of the heart mass is on the left side of the midline and at the level of the fifth intercostal space. In the adult, the apex or tip of the left ventricle is about 9 cm from the midline (Figure 1.1).

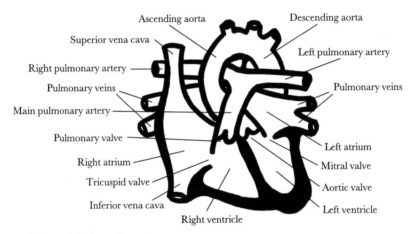

Figure 1.1 Normal heart

General structure of the heart

The heart is composed of three layers of tissue.

Pericardium

The pericardium is a double-layered sac. The outer pericardium is made from fibrous connective tissue which is adherent to the diaphragm and coats the great vessels, maintaining their position within the mediastinum. It protects and prevents the organ from over-distension. The inner serous pericardial sac is a double layer with fluid between. It is on the outside of the heart and is reflected back onto the inside of the fibrous layer. This tissue secretes a substance known as pericardial fluid which prevents friction between the layers of the heart. It can, however, become inflamed predisposing to pericarditis or cardiac tamponade if a build-up of fluid occurs.

Myocardium

The myocardium is composed of specialised striated, involuntary muscle tissue, which is branched in appearance. It is called cardiac muscle and is only found in the heart. This muscle is responsible for contraction of the heart and ejection of blood into both the pulmonary and systemic circulations.

Endocardium

The endocardium is a thin single layer of endothelium lining the myocardium on the inside.

The chambers

The normal heart consists of four chambers, two on the left and two on the right. They are divided by a muscular and fibrous tissue known as the septum. The superior chambers or atria are smaller and are receiving chambers. The left and right atria are separated by septum which contains the foramen ovale in the fetus and the fossa ovalis in the postnatal infant. The inferior chambers or ventricles are pumping chambers, the left ejects blood into the aorta for systemic circulation, the right into the pulmonary artery and onwards to the lungs.

The valves

There are four main valves within the heart to prevent blood flowing backwards.

Atrioventricular valves

The atrioventricular valves separate the atria from the ventricles. The right valve is known as the tricuspid valve and has three cusps or leaflets, consisting of endocardium and fibrous tissue. These flaps are attached to chordae tendineae, originating in the papillary muscle and stop the inversion of the valves from the ventricle to the atrium during contraction[12]. The left valve is named the mitral or bicuspid valve, having two cusps. When blood flows from the atrium to the ventricle, the atrioventricular valve is opened by the pressure difference across the valves, relaxing the papillary muscles and chordae tendineae.

Semilunar valves

There are left and right semilunar valves, each having three cusps which are half-moon shaped in appearance. They are fixed by their curved edges into the arterial wall. On the right side, the pulmonary valve separates the right ventricle from the pulmonary artery. On the left side, the aortic valve separates the left ventricle from the aorta.

Blood supply to the heart

The arterial supply of blood to the heart is by the right and left coronary arteries which deliver oxygen and nutrients to the myocardium. They derive their supply from the aorta. The left coronary artery travels in the atrioventricular groove and divides into the circumflex and anterior interventricular branches, supplying most of the left ventricle. The right coronary artery flows beneath the right atrium and divides into the posterior interventricular and marginal branches. Venous drainage is from the myocardial veins — the great cardiac and middle cardiac veins — which empty into the coronary sinus.

Blood flow through the heart

The flow of blood through the heart is controlled by the opening and closing of the four valves which in turn is controlled by the blood pressure (Figure 1.2) and by the contraction and relaxation of the myocardium stimulated by the conduction tissue.

Venous drainage from the inferior vena cava, superior vena cava and the coronary sinus, empties into the right atrium. From here it passes into the right ventricle via the tricuspid valve. Blood leaves the right ventricle via the pulmonary valve into the left and right pulmonary arteries and flows into the lungs where gaseous exchange occurs — oxygen is absorbed and carbon dioxide diffuses out. Oxygenated blood (Figure 1.2) returns from both lungs via the four pulmonary veins which empty their contents into

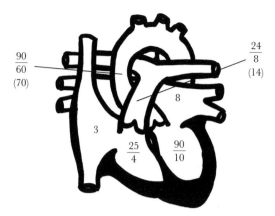

Figure 1.2 Normal saturations and pressures within the heart
Saturations: Right side of heart = 70%; Left side of heart = 96–100%
Pressures: in mmHg

the left atrium. The mitral valve opens and blood flows into the left ventricle. It enters the aorta, via the aortic valve and into the systemic circulation.

Conduction system of the heart

Specialised cardiac muscle can contract independently of any nerve supply. However, this intrinsic system is usually controlled by the autonomic nervous system or chemicals such as adrenaline or thyroxine. The electrical impulse which stimulates contraction arises in the sinoatrial node (SAN) or the natural pacemaker of the heart. It is found in the wall of the right atrium near to the superior vena cava. The impulse discharges across both atria resulting in contraction and depolarisation of the atrioventricular node (AVN). This is situated in the wall of the atrial septum near the atrioventricular valves. From here, the impulse passes down the conduction fibres called the bundle of His which divides at the top of the intraventricular septum into the left and right branches continuing down each side of the septum. The bundle branches terminate in a complex array of filaments known as Purkinje fibres which cause the impulse to spread rapidly through the inner surface of both ventricles resulting in ventricular contraction.

Nerve supply to the heart

The heart is innervated by the autonomic nervous system (ANS), originating in the cardiac centre of the medulla oblongata. The following arise from the ANS.

Sympathetic nerves (stimulatory)

The sympathetic nerves are partially responsible for innervation of the sinoatrial node and myocardium. They release adrenaline from the adrenal medulla which speeds up the heart rate, conduction via the atrioventricular node and the force of contraction.

Parasympathetic nerves (inhibitory)

The vagus nerve (10th cranial nerve) innervates the sinoatrial muscle and the atrioventricular node. It releases acetylcholine, transmitting the nerve impulse to the cardiac receptor resulting in a slower heart rate and decreased power of contraction. The sympathetic and parasympathetic nerves have opposing actions. Reflex mechanisms also control the heart rate.

Baroreceptors

Baroreceptors are receptive to changes in blood pressure. They are sensitive to the stretch of the vessel wall and are situated in the aortic arch and carotid arteries. Stimulation of the baroreceptors by increased blood pressure, will inhibit sympathetic nerves, slowing the heart rate and helping to lower the blood pressure. Conversely a drop in blood pressure will stimulate cardiac activity, speeding up the heart and increasing contractility.

Chemoreceptors

Chemoreceptors are also situated in the aortic arch and carotid arteries. They are sensitive to changes in oxygen and carbon dioxide, particularly a decrease in oxygen, increase in carbon dioxide and low pH. These factors relay a message to the cardiac centre of the medulla oblongata, resulting in an increase in heart rate and subsequently an increased supply of oxygen to the tissues.

The cardiac cycle

The cardiac cycle comprises atrial systole completing filling of the ventricles from the atria, followed by ventricular systole ejecting blood from the ventricles into the great vessels. Each systolic phase is followed by a diastolic (relaxation) phase.

Phases of the cardiac cycle

Atrial diastole (relaxation)

Blood flows into the right atrium from the IVC, SVC and coronary sinus and from the pulmonary veins into the left atrium. During this period of atrial filling, the atrial pressure gradually rises to the ventricular pressure causing the atrioventricular valves (AVVs) to open. Seventy per cent of the blood flows passively through the AVV into the ventricle — the period of rapid ventricular filling. The mean right atrial pressure is the same as the ventricular end diastolic pressure[10].

Atrial systole (contraction)

The remaining 30% of ventricular filling — period of slow ventricular filling — is reliant upon the sinoatrial node discharging an impulse so atrial depolarisation and subsequent contraction and reopening of the AVVs can take place. The timing of this is towards the end of ventricular diastole. It is represented on the electrocardiogram (ECG) trace as the P wave.

Ventricular systole (contraction)

The first phase of ventricular contraction is marked only by the rapidly rising ventricular pressure which causes the AVVs to close. There is no ejection of blood so the ventricular volume is constant as the semilunar valves remain closed. This is referred to as isovolumic contraction. The second phase of ventricular systole is the ejection period and occurs once ventricular pressure exceeds arterial pressure. This results in the semilunar valves opening, ejecting blood into the pulmonary artery from the right ventricle and the aorta from the left ventricle. The amount of blood ejected is approximately half the ventricular content, further known as the stroke volume. It follows the QRS on the ECG and is represented by the heart sound, S1 — lub — as the AVVs close.

Ventricular diastole (relaxation)

This has a biphasic component:

• Initially there is isovolumic relaxation where the ventricle begins to relax. The ventricular pressure falls when contraction ceases, but the volume remains unchanged. When the ventricular pressure falls below that in the arteries, the AVVs close.

- The ventricular pressure continues to fall below that in the atria, allowing opening of the AVVs and repeating the whole cycle again. It is represented on the ECG tracing as the T wave (repolarisation), by the second heart sound, S2 — dub — as the aortic valve closes and by the dicrotic notch on the arterial trace as there is a brief rise in the arterial pressure after closure of the aortic valve.

Cardiac output

The amount of blood ejected from a ventricle per minute is referred to as cardiac output. This is ruled by two factors, the first being the quantity of blood pumped by either ventricle during each beat and second, the heart rate per minute. The amount of blood ejected by either ventricle during contraction is the stroke volume thus:

cardiac output = stroke volume × heart rate

The normal cardiac output is dependent upon age and weight (Table 1.1).

Table 1.1 Normal cardiac output

Age	Output (ml/kg/min)
Infant	200
Child	150
Adolescent	100

However, cardiac index is a more accurate measurement and is calculated by:

$$\text{cardiac index} = \frac{\text{cardiac output}}{\text{body surface area (m}^2)}$$

Cardiac output also varies according to the demands for oxygen and nutrients as when exercising or pyrexial.

Stroke volume

Stroke volume (SV) is the difference between end diastolic volume (EDV) — the amount of blood remaining in the ventricle at the end of diastole

— and the end systolic volume (ESV) — the amount of blood remaining in the ventricle at the end of systole.

$$SV = EDV - ESV$$

EDV is the volume determined by:

- The length of ventricular diastole. A faster rate causes the length of diastole to be reduced and a shorter filling time, resulting in a lower EDV.
- The venous pressure. An increase in venous pressure results in an increase in blood volume being forced into the ventricle. This results in a higher EDV and more forceful contraction of the ventricle[12].

ESV is determined by:

- The arterial pressure in the aorta and pulmonary arteries before ventricular systole.
- The force of the ventricular contraction.

To summarise, cardiac output is dependent on four factors:

- Preload.
- Contractility.
- Afterload.
- Heart rate and rhythm.

Preload

This is described as the amount of stretching of myocardial muscle fibres in response to the variation in EDV before any contraction. In a child or adolescent, preload can be increased by manipulating the fibre length with intravenous infusions of colloid preparations and thus increasing the stroke volume. Increasing venous return increases preload. This results in increased ventricle filling from higher atrial pressures and the muscle fibres lengthening at the start of each contraction. It can be measured by the left and right atrial pressures and pulmonary capillary wedge pressure. However, the neonate has a limited ability to increase stroke volume due to lower ventricular diastolic compliance. This may be attributed to the ventricular mass ratio where there is less contractile muscle than non-contractile muscle.

Contractility

Contractility is how efficiently the myocardial muscle fibres shorten. The force of the ventricular contraction is reliant upon the length of the muscle fibres — the longer the fibre, the more forceful the contraction. This theory is known as Frank-Starling's Law and has been described as similar to stretching elastic — the more it is stretched, the harder it contracts. This causes an increase in the strength of contractility of the muscle fibres allowing for greater ventricular ejection as seen by a lower EDV, the ventricular systolic pressure rises quickly and there is an increase in stroke volume. However, this "elastic" recoil can reach a maximum; if preload is excessive, the fibres will become overstretched, the contraction becomes less forceful, effectively resulting in reduced cardiac output.

Afterload

This can be defined as the resistance to ventricular ejection[13]. The left ventricle must generate sufficient force to overcome the SVR, and the right ventricle must generate sufficient for it to overcome the PVR. Any pulmonary or aortic valve narrowing must also be overcome. For example, if the SVR is too high, the blood pressure may be high resulting in an increase in afterload, delaying the ventricle from emptying; a decrease in stroke volume; and a reduction in cardiac output. Manipulating the afterload to achieve the desired result of an increase in ventricular function usually means reduction of afterload. This can be achieved by vasodilatory drugs or, in the case of a ventricular outlet tract problem, by surgical intervention. Conversely, a significant decrease in afterload can be a major problem. In septic shock the SVR falls so blood pressure falls due to severe vasodilation. Cardiac output subsequently decreases. The intravascular volume is inadequate and needs to be refilled with colloid infusion.

Heart rate and rhythm

Cardiac output is dependent on a sinus heart rate in addition to stroke volume. Factors affecting the heart rate include:

- The autonomic nervous system: If there is a reduction in stroke volume, the sympathetic nervous system will affect the heart chronotropically, speeding up the heart rate to maintain cardiac output, and inotropically to increase contractility. Arrhythmias can result in a reduction in cardiac output. Atrial arrhythmias may reduce atrial contractility. Tachycardias predispose to a reduction in diastolic filling time, reduce coronary blood flow and increase oxygen consumption.

- Chemicals such as epinephrine, dobutamine, sodium, potassium, calcium and magnesium all affect heart rate and rhythm.
- Temperature: Pyrexia increases heart rate, hypothermia decreases heart rate.
- Sex and age of the patient: Females have higher heart rates and the heart rate becomes slower with age.

Chapter 2
Cardiovascular assessment and investigation

The young patient presenting with suspected congenital heart disease needs to undergo an array of tests to confirm the diagnosis and provide the multidisciplinary team with the relevant information with which to treat the child.

Cardiovascular assessment

Cardiovascular assessment should include the following:

- Psychological preparation of the child and family for the tests.
- Family, antenatal and postnatal history.
- Vital signs.
- General appearance of the patient.
- Palpation.
- Heart sounds on auscultation.
- Investigations necessary to diagnose a congenital heart disorder.
- Examination of the chest, abdomen and central nervous system.

Psychological preparation

Whether the patient presents as an emergency or electively, the trauma for the patient and family can be immense. The psychological care of the patient and family is discussed in Chapter 9 which includes a father's description of his feelings on discovering his son has a congenital heart defect.

History taking

- The family history must be taken with special regard to any congenital abnormalities, especially that of congenital heart disease.

- Any relevant antenatal history must be obtained, particularly maternal drug taking, alcohol consumption, illness or infection.
- The postnatal history and course of the illness need to be established. Each system should be evaluated for signs of disease. See Table 2.1.

Table 2.1 Assessment

System	Assessment
Respiratory system	Is there a history of chest infection, respiratory distress, cyanosis, haemoptysis, exercise intolerance?
Cardiovascular system	Are the vital signs normal for the age of the patient? Is there any oedema, chest pain, murmurs or clubbing of the fingers and toes?
Gastrointestinal system	Are the feeding habits poor with failure to thrive? Are the liver and spleen enlarged? Is jaundice present?
Neurological signs	Is there a history of headache, cerebral vascular accident, or fainting due to spelling?
Other	Presence of lymphadenopathy
Drug therapy	What medication is the patient on and what has he or she had in the past?

Vital Signs

Pulse

The pulse is caused by distension followed by elastic recoil in the artery wall, related to systole and diastole of the left ventricle. The left ventricle forces blood into the aorta which is already full. This distension causes a wave within the artery which can be felt, usually against an adjacent bone.

The following should be considered when taking the pulse:

- Site: In the neonate and infant, the apical pulse taken with a stethoscope is more accurate than palpation of a peripheral pulse. Over the age of two years, radial pulse can be measured accurately with experience. Comparison of the brachial or axillary pulse with femoral pulses should be undertaken if coarctation of the aorta is suspected, as the femoral pulse can be severely reduced or absent.

- Rate: This can be affected by numerous variables, namely,
    1. Age — it is faster in children than adults.
    2. Sex — females have a slightly faster rate than males.
    3. Exercise.
    4. Emotions — especially in a child who is upset and frightened by hospitalisation.
    5. Disease — for example, congenital heart disease, hyper/hypothyroidism, pyrexia.

The pulse should be taken over at least 30 seconds, or for a full minute should it be irregular.

- Rhythm: The regularity of the pulse should be assessed. The interval between each pulse should be the same. However, if the pulse feels irregular, does the irregularity occur at regular or irregular intervals?
- Volume: The pulse volume can be described as the amplitude of pulse pressure, or rather, the difference between systolic and diastolic blood pressure. The volume is assessed as either normal, small or large. Patients with a large pulse volume may have a patent ductus arteriosus, aortic regurgitation or be anaemic. Patients with a small pulse volume may be shocked or in heart failure[14].

Blood pressure

The blood pressure may be defined as the cardiac output × peripheral resistance and can be measured by noninvasive or invasive methods, in millimetres of mercury (mmHg). The three pressures used are the systolic, mean and diastolic blood pressures. Systolic pressure reflects the force of contraction of the heart and the injection of blood into the arterial vessels. Diastole represents the elastic recoil of the artery or relaxation of the heart and the aortic valve opening. The mean arterial pressure (MAP) is an indication of coronary artery perfusion and may be calculated by using the formula:

MAP = 1/3 systolic BP + 2/3 diastolic BP

Non-invasive taking of blood pressure is possible by either a cuff with a sphygmomanometer or a cuff with an oscillometric machine such as the Dinamap. Several considerations are necessary to avoid error in taking blood pressure manually.

- Selecting a cuff: Due to the diverse age range, the appropriate sized cuff is paramount. The width should cover two-thirds of the upper arm or thigh and the bladder or length of the cuff must completely encircle the arm.
- Positioning of the patient: Blood pressure should always be taken in the right arm. The young patient should be prepared for the investigation with a thorough explanation appropriate to age. Encouraging toddlers and younger children to sit on their parents' lap may allay some of their fears as will allowing them to explore the pieces of equipment to be used. Older children and adolescents may wish to either sit up or lie down.
- Positioning of the arm: The arm should be at the level of the heart as if it is allowed to dangle below, gravity will distort the reading adding pressure to the brachial artery[11].
- Measuring the pressure by auscultation: Jowett[14] describes this in several steps:
  1. Palpate the brachial pulse.
  2. Inflate the cuff slowly until the pulse disappears. This will indicate the systolic pressure.
  3. Fully deflate the cuff, allowing the veins to empty.
  4. Place the stethoscope over the palpated pulse. Do not press.
  5. Reinflate the cuff 30 mmHg higher than the previously ascertained systolic pressure.
  6. Ensure that the mercury column is at eye level and allow it to fall at 2–3 mm/second.
  7. The first sound to be heard represents the systolic blood pressure or phase one of the Korotkoff sounds.
  8. Once the first sound disappears, there is a silence. This is phase 2.
  9. Sounds are heard again — phase 3.
  10. Sounds become faint — phase 4.
  11. Sounds disappear, representing the diastolic pressure — phase 5.

Summary of the Korotkoff sounds and their representations

- Phase 1 = systolic blood pressure.
- Phase 2 = silence.
- Phase 3 = the sound returns.
- Phase 4 = sound becomes distant which represents diastole in children under 12 years.
- Phase 5 = sound completely disappears again. This represents diastolic blood pressure in children over 12 years.

Points to consider when taking blood pressure

- Equipment: The cuff size must be appropriate — too narrow a cuff will over-read the blood pressure, a wide cuff will under-read. Care is needed when choosing a cuff for an obese child. The equipment must be checked regularly for perished rubber tubing, worn cuffs and valves, all of which will contribute to inaccurate readings.
- Practitioners: Leaving the cuff inflated for a prolonged period of time results in venous congestion raising the systolic pressure by 30 mmHg or lowering it by 15 mmHg below the actual systolic pressure[14]. If the patient is upset or stressed, blood pressure will be affected. Taking blood pressure prior to any stress-provoking tests or procedures will ensure a more realistic reading. This applies not only to neonates but equally to adolescents. Taking a thigh blood pressure in children over one year of age will give higher readings 10–20 mmHg higher than taking it in the right arm. Atrial fibrillation or flutter may allow for an inaccurate blood pressure reading.
- Invasive blood pressure monitoring: See cardiovascular management.

Respiration

The respiratory system is closely linked to the cardiovascular system so assessment of respiratory effort is important.

- Rate: This must be taken over 1 minute. Tachypnoea can cause respiratory alkalosis and may be present in anxiety, pyrexia, metabolic acidosis, pain, respiratory distress and heart failure. A slow respiratory rate may indicate central nervous system disease or hypercarbia.
- Regularity: Newborn infants do not breathe regularly and can go for long periods without a breath. However, in older children, this is an abnormal finding and could proceed to apnoea.
- Depth: Deep breathing is found in fever, metabolic and respiratory acidosis. Shallow breathing is associated with metabolic alkalosis and pain.
- Other characteristics:
  1. Recession: Intercostal and subcostal recession are present in respiratory disease and distress. Suprasternal and supraclavicular recession are present in severe respiratory disease.
  2. Accessory muscles: To aid ventilation in respiratory distress, extra muscles to supplement those of the respiratory system are utilised, particularly those of the shoulder, head and abdomen. Nasal flaring is also seen.

3. Colour changes: Discussed in the next section.
4. Chest symmetry: The chest should be examined for equal movement.
5. Auscultation: A wheeze indicates narrowing of the bronchioles on expiration. Rhonchi indicate an obstruction of the larger airways and rales are secretion related. Additionally, inspiratory stridor may indicate some form of inspiratory obstruction or croup. Grunting is present in respiratory distress and increases the end expiratory pressure which prolongs gaseous exchange in the lungs.

The general appearance of the patient

Clinical assessment by the practitioner is vital as much information can be ascertained by examination of the patient.

The skin

Several considerations are necessary:

- Colour: Assessment of colour needs to be divided into central colour of the head, trunk and mucous membranes, and peripheral colouring, assessing limbs, fingers and toes.
  The patient should be examined for changes in colour:
  1. Cyanosis — central and peripheral cyanosis is manifested as a bluish tinge in light-skinned people and an ashen appearance in dark-skinned people. If cyanosis is present, the patient should be examined for clubbing of the fingers and toes which will indicate whether the cyanosis is a chronic problem.
  2. Jaundice — This may be found in the sclera of the eyes, and in skin, palms and soles.
  3. Pallor — There is loss of the pinky tone in light skin, an ashen tone in dark skin and a yellow/brown tone in brown skin. This may indicate low cardiac output if associated with cool skin.
  4. Mottling — This has the appearance of 'corned-beef', initially over the extremities but can develop over the trunk if left untreated. It is a serious sign indicative of poor systemic perfusion. There is reduced tissue oxygenation. Capillary refill is prolonged.
  5. High colouring — If cyanosed, this may indicate venous congestion in patients with complex cardiac disease and high central venous pressure. If red, pyrexia is probably the cause. However, vasodilators will cause a flushed appearance and the use of vancomycin which can cause 'red-man syndrome', needs to be considered.

- Temperature: Comparison of central and peripheral temperatures indicate the effectiveness of cardiac output. If the patient has cold extremeties, a degree of vasoconstriction may be present, thus ensuring vital organs are perfused but output remains inadequate to sustain the peripheries.
- Texture: Additionally, the skin can be assessed for clamminess, reflecting heart failure, or dryness, indicative of dehydration or shock.
- Turgor: This refers to the amount of elasticity in the skin. Elastic skin recoils immediately when pinched. In dehydrated patients, the skin may remain suspended for extended periods. Equally, in oedematous patients the skin may indent when a finger is pressed onto the swollen area. As oedema worsens, ascites and pleural effusions develop[14]. Oedema may be present in heart failure, hyponatraemia, hypoalbuminaemia and conditions in which right atrial pressure is elevated.

Neurological signs

If the patient is seriously ill, his or her level of responsiveness may be reduced. In hypoxaemia, the child may appear confused, irritable and drowsy progressing to unconsciousness. A well child, on the other hand, will be alert to his or her surroundings, responsive but can be easily distracted with play and other diversional activities.

Palpation

Palpation of pulses can relay vital information — see earlier. The area over the heart, the precordium, can be hyperdynamic indicating volume overload in conditions such as left to right shunts and valve regurgitation. A thrill, or tremor, felt over the heart, is suggestive of many congenital heart defects: pulmonary and aortic stenosis, ventricular septal defects and coarctation of the aorta, to name a few. Lateral displacement of the apex suggests cardiomegaly.

Heart sounds and auscultation

Normal heart sounds are heard in relation to the cardiac cycle. There are four normal heart sounds in total reflecting the following events.

- First sound (S1): This is representative of the mitral and tricuspid valves closing. The two components cannot normally be heard separately.

- Second sound (S2): This is produced by closure of the aortic and pulmonary valves. The two components can be heard separately during inspiration, in the presence of an ASD or in right bundle branch block.
- Third sound (S3): This is produced by the rapid filling of the ventricles in diastole. A loud third sound is usually normal in children and adolescents. In later life, it is indicative of left ventricular failure.
- Fourth sound (S4): This is also attributed to ventricular filling caused by atrial contraction. A loud fourth sound is an abnormal finding and is heard when blood fills a ventricle in which the compliance is reduced. This may occur with a hypertrophied ventricle as in hypertension.

Other sounds reflecting events occurring in systole or diastole:

- Ejection clicks: The click is related to the mobility of the cusps. If the click is heard near to S1, it indicates sounds of either the aortic or pulmonary valves. It is also found when the aorta is dilated in coarctation of the aorta, tetralogy of Fallot and truncus arteriosus[3].
- Mid diastolic clicks: These represent the mitral or tricuspid valve cusps prolapsing in systole[3]. An opening snap is present in early diastole and can occur in mitral or tricuspid stenosis.

Heart murmurs may be classified as either innocent (functional) or organic:

- Innocent murmurs: An innocent murmur can only be said to be innocent by the exclusion of all other causes. It may be heard when there is a structurally normal heart, for example in an asymptomatic child with no evidence of congenital heart disease, normal heart sounds, normal pulses, ECG (electrocardiograph) and chest x-ray. They may be present when the child is excited, pyrexial, on inspiration and expiration, and they may occur in up to 80% of children[4]. The child and parents must be reassured that everything is normal and a full life can be lived.
- Functional murmurs: A functional murmur is present in a structurally normal heart combined with the presence of a physiological process such as anaemia or increased cardiac output.
- Organic murmurs: An organic murmur may be heard in a structurally abnormal heart representing blood passing through an abnormal opening or valve. The cardiologist must decide: (1) the location, and (2) the intensity, graded one to six, one being barely audible, six being heard without the aid of a stethoscope.

Investigations

Chest x-ray

The chest x-ray provides vital information about the child with a suspected or confirmed congenital heart defect.

- Heart size: This may be assessed in the child and adolescent by measuring the cardiothoracic diameter. A ratio over 0.5 is indicative of cardiomegaly[4].
- Heart chambers: Individual enlargement of each chamber can be assessed fully if a lateral or anterior posterior exposure is taken.
- Great arteries: Enlarged arteries can be indicative of problems such as aortic stenosis or pulmonary hypertension.
- Lung vascularity: Increased pulmonary vascular markings are related to lesions with excessive pulmonary blood flow such as atrial septal defects, ventricular septal defects or patent ductus arteriosus. Decreased vascular markings are related to lesions with decreased pulmonary blood flow, for example, critical pulmonary stenosis, tetralogy of Fallot in the cyanosed infant[4].
- Analysis of other organs: This may be possible with a chest x-ray. The liver and stomach can be seen in the neonate and infant. Vertebrae and ribs can be seen in most instances.

Echocardiography

Since its introduction in the 1950s, echocardiography is undoubtedly the most frequently used diagnostic tool for assessment of congenital heart disease. A summary of the functions of echocardiography is shown in Table 2.2. The major benefit of this investigation is that in the majority of cases, a diagnosis can be made without invasive techniques, such as cardiac catheterisation and angiography. A transducer is placed on the chest transmitting high frequency sound waves. The returned waves or echoes are reflected back to the transducer at different speeds depending

Table 2.2 A summary of the functions of echocardiography

Pressure monitoring of individual chambers and great vessels

Diagnostic uses — cardiac tamponade, pericardial effusion

Structural abnormalities — congenital heart lesions

Assessing the effectiveness of cardiac function

on the type of tissue from which it is reflected. Currently there are three modes of echocardiography:

- M-mode echocardiography: This was the first type of echocardiography. It is used in a single dimension, with a crystal to transmit the sound waves. It provides a view of the heart at one point and still has its uses in the analysis of valve movement and left ventricular function.
- Two dimensional (2D) or cross-sectional echo: This provides detailed anatomical information in 2D, using numerous crystals to transmit high frequency sound waves thus allowing the cardiologist to diagnose defects with ease.
- Doppler echocardiography: Doppler's principle stipulated that moving objects changed the wavelength of sound waves that are reflected from them[3]. In relation to the heart, the object moving is the blood velocity and the direction of the flow. It is used to assess blood flow and cardiac output and analyse the degree of stenosis, obstruction and shunting. Colour Doppler echocardiography was introduced in the 1980s in conjunction with 2D echocardiography. It provides a qualitative assessment of blood flow. Specific colour coding demonstrates blood flow direction.

Electrocardiography

Electrocardiography (ECG) involves the interpretation of electrical changes within the heart muscle associated with muscular contraction. Electrodes are placed on the skin to transmit electrical impulses back to a recording machine[11]. Numerous texts pertaining to ECG are available[15,16]. Therefore, for the purpose of this book, a simple outline of ECG will be given here and common arrhythmias will be covered in cardiovascular management in Chapter 11.

Rates and intervals

Usual paper speed recordings are at 25 mm/second. Therefore, each horizontal box is consistent with a time of 0.04 seconds, five boxes being 0.2 seconds. The chart in Table 2.3 can be used to give a quick assessment of a patient's heart rate.

Bipolar three-lead ECGs

A bipolar ECG (any two of three leads) is acceptable for continuous monitoring and arrhythmia study in the accident and emergency department,

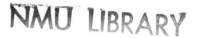

Table 2.3 Chart to assess a patient's heart rate

Heart rate	Number of occupied boxes (R–R interval)	Number of seconds
300	1	0.2
150	2	0.4
100	3	0.6
75	4	0.8
60	5	1
50	6	1.2

intensive care unit or ward. However, should a more complex study be required then a 12-lead ECG will be necessary — refer to specialised texts for information. Most patients will have a 12-lead ECG performed on admission to hospital and prior to discharge, followed by intermittent recordings when attending the outpatient department.

Table 2.4 Jowett's five recommendations for electrode placement to improve skin contact and enhance the signal[14]

The skin should be shaved — rarely necessary in paediatrics unless an adolescent

The skin should be rubbed with dry gauze to remove loose, dry skin

If the patient is oily, such as in a newborn baby covered in vernix, or a patient in heart failure who is sweaty or clammy, the skin should be cleaned and dried frequently. It often requires numerous attachments of new electrodes

Ensure that the electrode is in date and the gel is moist

Use only one make of electrode to prevent distortion of the trace

Analysis of the ECG

Normal conduction of the electrical impulse was covered in Chapter 1. The ECG represents the direction of amplitude of the electrical forces of the heart and consists of five successive waves designated by the characters P, Q, R, S and T. See Figure 2.1.

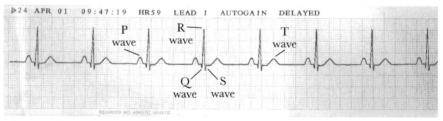

Figure 2.1 PQRST complex

- P wave (atrial depolarisation): This represents the passage of electrical impulses from the sinoatrial node across both atria. The P wave in infants and children has a shorter duration than in adults[3]. In infants it is 0.04–0.07 seconds and in adults it is 0.06–1.00 second. Tall P waves indicate right atrial hypertrophy.
- P–R interval: This is the interval from the start of the P wave to the beginning of the QRS complex, therefore the time taken from atrial depolarisation to ventricular depolarisation. It varies according to age and heart rate; the slower the heart rate, the longer the P–R interval. A long P–R interval can indicate first degree heart block, a short interval is found in Wolff–Parkinson–White syndrome.
- QRS complex (ventricular depolarisation): This represents the passage of the electrical impulse from the atrioventricular node, down branch bundles in the interventricular septum and across both ventricles. The Q wave is depicted as depolarisation of the ventricular septum. The height of the R and S waves depends on the thickness of the ventricular wall. The duration of the QRS complex is 0.06–0.08 seconds in infants, 0.1 seconds in children and 0.12 seconds in adolescents. If prolonged, it may indicate bundle branch block.
- Q–T interval: This is the time taken from the start of the QRS complex to the end of the T wave. It represents ventricular depolarisation and ventricular repolarisation. Again, the duration is dependent on the age and heart rate of the patient; the faster the rate, the shorter the Q–T interval. A prolonged Q–T interval may indicate hypercalcaemia, hypokalaemia or hypomagnesaemia. A shortened Q–T interval reflects hypercalcaemia or hyperkalaemia.
- S–T interval: This is normally a flat line, i.e. isoelectric, measuring the interval between the start of the S wave and the beginning of the T wave. There is no electrical activity at this point. An elevated interval is indicative of ischaemic changes (e.g., post-myocardial infarction, reimplantation of coronary arteries in TGA).
- T wave: This represents ventricular repolarisation. If flat, a diagnosis of myocarditis or hypothyroidism can be suspected[3]. Tall T waves may indicate hyperkalaemia, myocardial infarction or ischaemic changes in the heart[14].

Magnetic resonance imaging (MRI)

MRI is a fairly new technique in the assessment of cardiac disease. It depicts soft tissues in a way not possible with any other technique. The advantages of MRI scanning are the accuracy of the image using a non-invasive technique with no radiation. Disadvantages include the expense, the young patient having to be anaesthetised for the procedure, and problems in critically ill patients with electrical and mechanical equipment as the magnetic field may interfere with the function of many mechanical devices.

Cardiac catheterisation and angiography

Cardiac catheterisation was, until recently, the definitive procedure for the diagnosis of congenital heart disease. It is now reserved for obtaining specific information. The procedure involves feeding a radio-opaque catheter, normally via the femoral vein or artery in a child, or the umbilical vessels in a neonate, up into the heart. It is usually performed in conjunction with angiography where radio-opaque contrast is injected through the catheter, outlining the cardiac chambers and vessels.

Table 2.5 Indications for cardiac catheterisation

Diagnostic indications	Interventional indications
To assess oxygen saturations in the four chambers and great vessels	Balloon septostomy
	Balloon angioplasty
Assessment of pressures within the chambers and great vessels	Balloon valvuloplasty
To assess complex anatomical lesions and their circulations	Radio frequency ablation for arrhythmias
	Stenting of structures
Assessment of cardiac output	Occlusion of structures, e.g., PDA, ASD
	Electrophysiological studies

Preparation for cardiac catheterisation

See Appendix 4 for preparation of the patient for cardiac catheterisation.

Procedure

The heart can be catheterised in two main ways: right heart (venous) or left heart (arterial).

- Right heart catheterisation: The catheter is fed into the right side of the heart via the peripheral vein. From here the catheter can pass into the lung vessels to assess changes in the saturations and the pressure within these structures. Abnormal communications and cardiac output can be assessed.

- Left heart catheterisation: Left-sided catheterisation may provide the most information about pressures and saturations if a septal defect is present. An artery is catheterised but there are risks so it should only be performed if deemed essential.

Nursing and medical care post-catheterisation

See Appendix 4.

Complications:

- Arrhythmias are the most common complication and include atrial and ventricular ectopics, atrial and ventricular fibrillation and heart block. Full resuscitation equipment should be available at all times.
- Perforation of the heart can occur. The catheter is removed and the patient observed for cardiac tamponade if bleeding into the pericardium occurs.
- Air or blood particulate emboli are a rare complication resulting in cerebral vascular accident.
- Localised vascular complications include thrombosis, phlebitis, infection, haematoma, and haemorrhage from the catheter site.
- Neonatal problems include necrotising enterocolitis due to hypoperfusion of the gut, hypothermia, hypoglycaemia, hypotension and respiratory depression.
- Allergic reactions to the contrast medium.
- Renal failure from the dye in patients with marked renal impairment.

Chapter 3
Acyanotic defects

Atrial septal defect (ASD)

Aetiology

This defect accounts for 5–10% of congenital heart disease[3,4]. It may be associated with partial anomolous pulmonary venous drainage (PAPVD), atrioventricular septal defect (AVSD), and complex heart defects. Atrial septal defects (ASD) present more commonly in females than males — a 2:1 ratio.

Definition

ASD is defined as communication or communications across the atrial septum. See Figure 3.1.

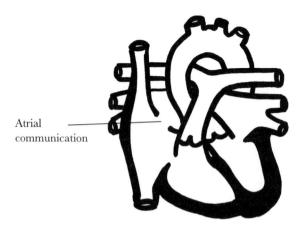

Atrial
communication

Figure 3.1 Atrial septal defect

Classification

ASD is an acyanotic defect with left to right shunting. The anatomy of the atrial septum is complex. A basic overview shows it is divided into two parts; the septum primum, which is a thin mobile tissue, developing first followed by the septum secundum, which is thick and muscular in nature[9]. The septum secundum has a naturally occurring defect which forms the fossa ovalis.

There are several types of ASD depending on their anatomical positioning:

- Sinus venosus ASD: This accounts for approximately 10% of cases of ASD[4] and occurs at the entrance to the superior vena cava or inferior vena cava, close to the opening of the right atrium. In approximately 90% of cases this type of ASD is associated with PAPVD[9].
- Coronary sinus ASD: This is a very rare type of ASD in which unroofing of the coronary sinus causes right to left shunting of blood from the coronary sinus into the left atrium. This results in cyanosis. Left to right shunting also occurs at atrial level.
- Ostium secundum ASD (fossa ovalis defect): A total of 50–80% of ASDs fall into this category[4,9]. It occurs from a deficiency in the fossa ovalis and is located in the centre of the atrial septum. If the septum primum is normal, the defect may be classified as a patent foramen ovale (PFO). Abnormality of the septum primum accounts for a genuine ostium secundum, varying from a fenestration to a total absence. It is infrequently associated with other defects.
- Ostium primum ASD: This accounts for approximately 30% of ASDs[4]. It is located in the bottom end of the septum, adjacent to the atrioventricular valves. It is considered to be part of the spectrum of atrioventricular septal defects which will be discussed in the AVSD section.

Anatomy and pathophysiology

In the neonate, the atrial pressures are the same and the walls of both ventricles are of similar thickness so little shunting across the defect will occur. When the pulmonary vascular bed matures the pulmonary vascular resistance falls so the right ventricle becomes much less thick. This lowers its filling pressures so blood flows from left to right across the defect, leading to an increase in right ventricular volume work. The amount of shunting is relatively dependent on the compliance of left and right ventricles. Under normal circumstances an infant's left atrial pressure is greater than the right atrial pressure. This pressure gradient is responsible for closing the PFO. Conversely, if it does not close — usually due to a deficiency of tissue — the patient will present with an ostium secundum type defect. If an ASD goes undetected the right atrium and ventricle will dilate and hypertrophy. Atrial arrhythmias, congestive cardiac failure and paradoxic emboli can result. Pulmonary hypertension can occur late but is rare. If the child has a complex congenital heart disease the presence of an ASD may be life-saving, providing a shunt to mix oxygenated and deoxygenated blood at atrial level[10].

Signs and symptoms

Most ASDs do not produce symptoms in childhood. The most common presentation is an asymptomatic murmur, even if the ASD is large[17], and pulmonary congestion, which can predispose to repeated respiratory infections. Classical symptoms are often not present in the patient with a large secundum ASD[18]. ASDs may be diagnosed antenatally, despite previously being notoriously difficult. This is due to advances in fetal echocardiography and in particular, the use of M-mode echocardiography rather than Doppler sonography[19].

Cardiac signs and symptoms

- Congestive cardiac failure rarely occurs in infants.
- Pulses are of normal volume.
- There is right atrial dilatation.
- Arrhythmias are present if ASD is left untreated.

Respiratory signs and symptoms

- The patient is pink unless a coronary sinus ASD is present in which case the child may exhibit the complications of polycythaemia and cyanosis.
- There is a history of chest infections.
- Shortness of breath is present on exertion.
- Respiratory rate is normal.
- The patient has slight fatigue.
- Pulmonary hypertension in adult life is a rare complication if ASD is left untreated.

Other signs and symptoms

- The patient is often below average weight.
- Very rarely, paradoxical emboli may occur if ASD is left untreated.

Diagnosis

- Auscultation: There is a pulmonary systolic ejection murmur resulting from the excessive blood flow across the pulmonary valve[20]. The second heart sound is split. This is normally the first clinical sign as the child is usually asymptomatic prior to this point.
- ECG: Mild right ventricular hypertrophy and incomplete right bundle branch block is present in approximately 95% of patients. This is useful when the child presents with nothing other than a murmur[21].
- Chest x-ray: Shows enlargement of the heart depending on the degree of shunt. The right atrium and pulmonary arteries are enlarged.
- Echocardiography: 2D and Doppler studies will show the position of the defect and demonstrate the shunt respectively.
- Cardiac catheterisation: Unnecessary unless another accompanying defect is present. However, if performed, it will show higher oxygen saturations in the right atrium than in the left atrium.

The spontaneous closure of medium-sized defects may occur in up to 40% of patients before the age of four[4]. In small ASDs the closure rate is much higher, around 80% before 18 months of age[4].

Key preoperative management issues

The key preoperative management issues are shown in Table 3.1.

Table 3.1 Assessment and management of potential preoperative problems in ASDs (for detailed management of individual problems, see Chapter 9)

Alleviate the anxiety of the child and parents pertaining to the elective surgery:

- See Chapter 9 on elective admission for detailed care
- Of all the cardiac defects, an ASD is potentially considered to be a straightforward procedure by the multidisciplinary team. However, the nurse must be aware of parental concerns. Children with an ASD are generally "healthy" so parents consenting to their "well" child undergoing a potentially risky procedure will be faced with a most worrying dilemma
- As the child is often pre-school aged, the importance of play in preparing the child for procedures, investigations and the operation is vital. How do parents explain to a well 4-year-old that they need an operation and subsequent management requiring lots of tubes and wires? The use of a play specialist in the preparation is advisable

Medical management

ASDs can sometimes be closed in the catheter laboratory. Transoesophageal 2D echocardiography can help in the determination of size and position of the lesion adjacent to other cardiac structures when considering interventional closure[22,23]. Various devices are available: The double umbrella device places an umbrella-like structure on the left and right sides of the defect attached to each other, thus closing the defect[24]. More recently, an Amplatzer device consisting of a mesh structure can be used for small to medium ASDs, which have good margins and are central in position[25]. There is a very small risk of embolisation but in general, the risks are much less than with operative techniques.

Surgical management

The indications for surgery fall into three main categories:

- The symptomatic infant whose symptoms are related to the degree of shunting.
- The asymptomatic/mildly symptomatic child. Elective surgery around the age of 2–4 years is preferred as evidence has indicated that the child will not suffer any untoward consequences[9]. However, from a psychological perspective, it may be preferable to offer the operation as a young toddler. Both physical and psychological aspects should be addressed to optimise the appropriate age for operation.
- Surgery should be carried out on any patient with a pulmonary to systemic flow ratio (Qp:Qs) of 1.5:1 at age 2 years[26]. Closure of smaller defects because of the risk of embolisation and cerebral vascular accident may also be carried out[4].

Surgical principles

The risk of surgery is around 1% risk of mortality[20]. The main principle of treatment is to correct the left to right shunt while avoiding damage to the conduction tissue and avoiding obstructing pulmonary and systemic venous drainage.

The operation to close an ASD involves:

- A midline sternotomy or, rarely, a right thoracotomy.
- Cardiopulmonary bypass at 32°C.

- Opening of the right atrium to close the hole either by direct suturing or by patch repair if large.

Recently, a minimally invasive method has been described: mini-sternotomy reduces length of incision, endotracheal intubation, postoperative bleeding, analgesia requirement and hospital stay[27]. The procedure may, however, place the patient under higher risk should a complication arise, as the incision may be too small to treat the child in an emergency situation.

Key postoperative management issues

The key postoperative management issues are shown in Table 3.2.

Table 3.2 Assessment and management of potential postoperative problems in ASDs (for detailed management of individual problems, see Chapters 10 and 11)

Pericardial and pleural effusions due to post pericardiotomy syndrome
Arrhythmias (if the ASD is an ostium primum type) due to the septal surgery undertaken

The child having had an ASD repair usually recovers swiftly requiring no or little inotropic support.

Long-term follow-up

The child and parents can be assured that a normal life can be enjoyed.
- No restrictions in activity are necessary unless complications of surgery have arisen.
- Antibiotic prophylaxis for dental extraction and other surgical procedures is considered essential for a specified length of time after the repair, the duration of which depends on the cardiologist's preference.
- Outpatient attendance is normally for one year.

Ventricular septal defect (VSD)

Aetiology

VSD is the most common form of congenital heart disease accounting for approximately 33%[3, 28]. It is associated with Down's syndrome in approximately 11% of patients[28], pulmonary stenosis, RVOTO and subaortic stenosis. Additionally, it is linked with parental use of marijuana and cocaine[29].

Definition

VSD is one or more communications between the left and right ventricles. The communication may vary in size and be part of a complex lesion, such as pulmonary atresia with VSD and TOF[30]. See Figure 3.2.

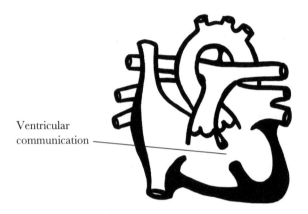

Ventricular communication —

Figure 3.2. Ventricular septal defect

Classification

VSD is an acyanotic lesion with left to right shunting. A VSD can occur in several places along the ventricular septum which is made up of two parts: a small membranous septum and a larger muscular septum consisting of the muscular, inlet and outlet portions[4]. The classifications are as follows:

- Perimembranous VSD (membranous, conoventricular VSD): Located within the membranous septum extending towards the muscular septum[9]. The majority (80–90%) of VSDs are classified in this group[20]. It is commonly associated with interrupted aortic arch if the septum is posteriorly malaligned or with tetralogy of Fallot if malaligned anteriorly[9].
- Muscular VSD (trabecular VSD): Located anywhere in the muscular or trabecular portion of the ventricular septum. The rim is totally made up of muscle[9]. It can be single or multiple resembling Swiss cheese. Of all VSDs, approximately 33% are classified as muscular[10].

- Inlet VSD (AV canal type VSD): In this variety of VSD, all or part of the atrial-ventricular septum is absent[9]. It lies beneath the atrioventricular valves and is associated with complete atrioventricular septal defect.
- Outlet VSD (infundibular, supracristal, conal VSD): Located within the infundibular septum and limited by the pulmonary valve[9].
- Doubly committed VSD: This is a VSD close to both semilunar valves.

Anatomy and pathophysiology

The majority of VSDs present in infancy at six to eight weeks of age[31]. Symptoms occur as the pulmonary vascular resistance falls. If the defect is unrestrictive, blood passes from the area of high pressure to the lower pressure right ventricle and up to the pulmonary vascular bed[20]. This is termed left to right shunting. At this time, the infant's pulmonary vascular resistance is falling and a large left to right shunt will cause increasing symptoms.

The size of the defect determines the initial pathophysiology:

- Small VSD: The small diameter of the defect provides a resistance which only allows a small left to right shunt and a small increase in right ventricular and pulmonary artery pressure and flow. Pulmonary hypertension is rare and growth and development may be normal. Of all small VSDs approximately 75% will have closed by 10 years[32]. These children are considered at low risk except for the chance of sub-acute bacterial endocarditis. The maximum pulmonary to systemic flow ratio (Qp/Qs) is less than 2 — that is, the amount of blood flowing through the lungs compared with flow to the rest of the body.
- Medium VSD: This will usually generate a Qp:Qs ratio greater than 2. Despite this ratio of pulmonary blood flow to systemic flow, it is restrictive enough only to cause minimal problems for the infant. Right ventricular pressure may or may not be elevated.
- Large VSD: This can be defined as the VSD being the same size as the aortic valve opening[9]. This causes a large left to right shunt. If there is no resistance to flow, the high systemic pressure will be directed to the pulmonary artery. This results in high pulmonary blood flow under high pressure causing an increased PAP and pulmonary hypertension. Pulmonary resistance will rise protecting the lungs from being flooded with blood, but subsequently, changes occur in the pulmonary artery vasculature which become irreversible. If surgical intervention is not undertaken before this stage, the pulmonary vascular resistance will

continue to rise until it becomes higher than the systemic vascular resistance. The shunt consequently reverses and the patient becomes cyanosed. This is termed Eisenmenger's complex[3]. Symptoms are dependent on lung blood flow. If this is reduced by pulmonary stenosis, the symptoms will be less severe and the lungs protected.

Small VSD

Signs and symptoms

There are usually no symptoms or signs as a neonate. However, once the pulmonary vascular resistance decreases, a systolic murmur can be heard.

Diagnosis

- Auscultation: Systolic murmur present after 6 weeks.
- ECG: Normal.
- Chest x-ray: Normal.
- Echocardiography: Diagnostic and shows the size and position of the VSD[33]. Some defects may not be detected. Doppler studies will show normal right ventricular pressures.

Medium VSDs

Signs and symptoms

Symptoms are present in infancy and include the following.

Cardiac signs and symptoms:

- Heart failure manifested as breathlessness on feeding, varying degrees of sweating, and dyspnoea at rest. This occurs approximately 4 weeks after birth.

Respiratory signs and symptoms:

- Chest infections.
- Normal or moderately high pulmonary artery pressures.

Other signs and symptoms:

- Slow to feed and gain weight. Once weaned, weight gain is better as feeding with a spoon is less tiring than sucking a bottle.

- Subsequently, the hole becomes smaller, but the baby still has less energy than a well baby[3].

Diagnosis

- Auscultation: Pan systolic murmur indicating a moderate left to right shunt through the defect[3].
- ECG: Left atrial and biventricular hypertrophy.
- Chest x-ray: Moderate heart enlargement with an enlarged pulmonary artery and increased vascularity of the lungs[3].
- Echocardiogram: Shows the size and position of the VSD and Doppler studies show the blood flow across the defect. The gradient across the hole will indicate right ventricular pressure.

Large VSD

Signs and symptoms

The patient presents at two to three weeks of life as a result of pulmonary vascular resistance falling. Commonly, parents report that their baby is not feeding well. The infant deteriorates and presents with the following signs and symptoms.

Cardiac signs and symptoms:

- Congestive cardiac failure.
- Tachycardia.

Respiratory signs and symptoms:

- Pulmonary hypertension in severe, untreated cases.
- Chest infections.

Other signs and symptoms:

- Greyish colouring of the infant.
- Failure to thrive.
- Weight gain may be related to fluid retention.

Diagnosis

- Auscultation: Pansystolic and mid diastolic murmur[3].

- ECG: Biventricular hypertrophy and left atrial hypertrophy. If there is significant pulmonary hypertension, the right ventricular hypertrophy will be marked.
- Chest x-ray: Cardiomegaly and a large pulmonary artery. Congested lung fields until severe pulmonary hypertension develops.
- Echocardiogram: Size and position of the VSD. Doppler studies can assess the pressure in the pulmonary artery by measuring the pressure difference across the septum[20].
- Cardiac catheterisation: Not routinely performed for VSDs but will indicate the pulmonary artery pressure and the degree of pulmonary vascular resistance. If the reversibility of the pulmonary resistance is in doubt, catheterisation may be performed.

Key preoperative management issues

The key preoperative management issues are shown in Table 3.3.

Table 3.3 Assessment and management of potential preoperative problems in VSDs (for detailed management of individual problems, see Chapters 10, 11 and 13)

Congestive heart failure
Chest infection
Low cardiac output
Failure to thrive

Surgical management

Surgical repair greatly improves the long-term morbidity and mortality outcome[34, 35]. The indications for operation are symptoms in the infant not controlled by medication, continuing rise in the pulmonary artery pressures after six months of age and small VSDs which have shown no indication of closing, thus predisposing to endocarditis.

- Small VSDs: It is recommended that small defects are not surgically closed as most will spontaneously close in childhood. Antibiotics to prevent bacterial endocarditis are a necessity.
- Medium VSDs: Normally surgically closed before six months of age especially if pulmonary hypertension is present. A Qp:Qs ratio greater than 2:1 and the absence of signs that the defect is becoming smaller is an indication for surgery. Again, antibiotic prophylaxis is essential.

Treatment of heart failure and chest infections must be prompt to prevent the baby from deteriorating before surgery. Research has indicated that early surgical intervention is recommended in patients with non-restricted VSDs and failure to thrive[36].

- Large VSDs: Infants with a history of congestive cardiac failure, increasing pulmonary vascular resistance, low cardiac output, failure to thrive and those who are unresponsive to medical treatment should be operated on from an early age, trying to ensure the infant is in the best condition for the surgical procedure. Improving symptoms can be a misleading sign as it indicates a rising resistance.

Palliative procedure

Pulmonary artery banding reduces lung flow but is rarely undertaken unless the patient has multiple VSDs, a complex lesion with VSD or intractable pulmonary symptoms. Primary closure of the VSD is performed in preference.

Surgical procedure

The aim of the operation is to correct the left to right shunt by closing the defect(s)[20, 37].

- A midline sternotomy is performed.
- Cardiopulmonary bypass is initiated. Infants below 3 kg undergo circulatory arrest. Above 3 kg, bicaval cannulation is undertaken and the infant is cooled to between 25 and 28°C.
- There are two main surgical approaches — transatrial or transpulmonary — depending on the position of the VSD. Most simple VSD repairs are completed via right atrial incision, through the tricuspid valve. When this method is not appropriate a transventricular incision is considered but will cause a degree of right ventricular dysfunction and the need for inotropic support postoperatively[38].
- A patch repair is used for holes of all sizes as the ventricle is under higher pressure making a suture repair less reliable.

Key postoperative management issues

The postoperative care is determined by the pre-existing condition of the patient preoperatively and the type of surgery undertaken. See Table 3.4.

Table 3.4 Assessment and management of potential postoperative problems in VSDs (for detailed management of individual problems, see Chapters 10 and 11)

Heart block and bradycardia due to damage of the conduction tissue during the septal repair

Pulmonary hypertension and hyper-reactive pulmonary vasculature due to the left to right shunt preoperatively. This most commonly occurs in the infant operated on after six months of age

Low cardiac output related to:
- A large VSD in the presence of pre-existing heart failure and high pulmonary artery pressures
- Ventriculotomy

Chest infection

Long-term follow-up

The team should reassure the child and parents that:

- No restrictions in activity are necessary unless complications of surgery have arisen.
- Antibiotic prophylaxis for dental extraction and other surgical procedures is considered essential for a specified length of time after the repair, the duration depends on the cardiologist's preference. The presence of a residual VSD entails prophylactic antibiotic cover for life.
- Outpatient follow-up is required for approximately one year. In the presence of a residual VSD, it will be for life or until the defect closes.

Atrioventricular septal defect (AVSD)

Aetiology

This defect accounts for 2–5% of all congenital heart defects[4, 10]. Approximately 30% of children with Down's syndrome have a congenital heart defect[3, 4], most commonly an AVSD[3, 4]. This defect may be isolated, or be in association with other lesions such as tetralogy of Fallot, total anomalous pulmonary venous drainage, patent ductus arteriosus, aortic arch anomalies, double outlet right ventricle or transposition of the great arteries[9, 39].

Definition

An AVSD, endocardial cushion defect or atrioventricular canal defect is an acyanotic left to right lesion, in which incomplete fusion of the endocardial cushions occurs[11]. This results in a septal defect above or below the atrioventricular valves and abnormal construction of these valves. See Figure 3.3.

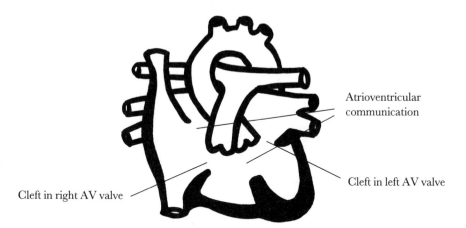

Atrioventricular communication

Cleft in left AV valve

Cleft in right AV valve

Figure 3.3 Atrioventricular septal defect (AVSD)

Classification

This is a group of defects varying greatly in severity, the most common classifications being partial, complete and intermediate:

- Partial AVSD (ostium primum ASD): This defect is discussed briefly in the section on ASD and accounts for 1–2% of congenital heart defects[4]. It is a partial form of AVSD in which ostium primum ASD is present accompanied by a cleft in the left atrioventricular valve. The ventricular septum is however intact.
- Complete AVSD: This also comprises an ostium primum ASD with the addition of a VSD. The left and right atrioventricular valves have clefts, the severe form resulting in a common atrioventricular valve or gap between the anterior and posterior leaflets which themselves straddle both orifices.
- Intermediate AVSD: Fibrous tissue from both valves adheres to the rim of ventricular tissue, giving the appearance of two separate valves[3, 10].

Anatomy and pathophysiology

The ventricular septum from below and the atrial septum from above fail to meet the common atrioventricular valve which itself develops abnormally.

The result is a semicircular VSD below, a semicircular ASD above and incompletely separated left and right atrioventricular valves.

Where VSD and ASD are both present, the defect is usually termed complete. Where the VSD does meet the atrioventricular valves, those valves usually remain incomplete but only an ASD remains; the defect is usually termed partial.

Other intermediate stages are possible and include asymmetric (unbalanced) division of the ventricles.

The physiological effect and symptoms will depend on:

- The degree of interatrial shunt[9].
- The degree of interventricular shunt[9].
- The competence of the atrioventricular valves.
- The systemic and pulmonary vascular resistances.
- Right ventricular compliance.
- The adequacy of both ventricles.
- Other cardiac defects.

Initially at birth, when the pulmonary vascular resistance is high, there is a small shunt across the septal defect. As pulmonary resistance falls a left to right shunt develops. In the partial defect, this shunt is interatrial.

The large left to right interventricular shunt increases flow and pressure in the pulmonary artery. Within 6–12 months, pulmonary hypertension and pulmonary vascular obstructive disease may develop, especially in patients with Down's syndrome who tend to be more susceptible to respiratory complications[40]. The pulmonary congestion and associated valve incompetence predisposes the patient to congestive heart failure and/or right ventricular overload due to the overall left to right shunt.

Signs and symptoms

Symptoms depend on the classification of AVSD:

- Partial AVSD: Symptoms associated with the ostium primum ASD and mild left AV valve incompetence are usually mild or absent during childhood and are similar to those of an ostium secundum ASD. The only notable difference being a pansystolic murmur in the presence of left AV valve incompetence. Bacterial endocarditis of the atrioventricular valve may occur[4].
- Complete AVSD: Symptoms present in early infancy. Babies with Down's syndrome should be routinely scanned due to the high probability of such a defect or other related cardiac defects.

Cardiovascular signs and symptoms

- Congestive cardiac failure is present only when the pulmonary vascular resistance is low.

Respiratory signs and symptoms

- Chest infection.
- Pulmonary hypertension, pulmonary vascular obstructive disease.
- Shortness of breath on exertion and rest.
- Mild cyanosis if the pulmonary vascular resistance is high.
- The Down's infant may have an upper airway obstruction which will exacerbate respiratory symptoms.

Other signs and symptoms

Failure to thrive and history of poor feeding.

Diagnosis

- Auscultation: Pulmonary ejection murmur and systolic regurgitant murmur due to atrioventricular valve regurgitation.
- ECG: First degree heart block, right and left ventricular hypertrophy.
- Chest x-ray: Cardiomegaly, increased pulmonary vascular markings and enlarged pulmonary arteries.
- Echocardiography: Diagnostic, identifying presence of an ASD, VSD, and valve abnormalities. Elongation of the left ventricular outflow tract due to displacement of the aorta — gooseneck deformity of the left ventricular outflow can be identified. The direction and degree of shunting and atrioventricular regurgitation can be measured.
- Cardiac catheterisation: Catheterisation may be needed to assess the degree of pulmonary hypertension and pulmonary vascular obstructive disease which may occur if the infant is diagnosed when older than six months .

Key preoperative management issues

The key preoperative management issues are shown in Table 3.5.

Surgical management

Partial AVSD

The timing of the operation is usually around 2–3 years of age.

Table 3.5 Assessment and management of potential preoperative problems in AVSDs (for detailed management of individual problems, see Chapters 10, 11 and 13)

Congestive heart failure

Chest infection

Pulmonary hypertension and pulmonary vascular obstructive disease

Failure to thrive

- A median sternotomy is performed.
- Cardiopulmonary bypass initiated.
- The ostium primum ASD is repaired with a patch.
- The cleft in the left atrioventricular valve is sutured.
- A valvuloplasty of the left atrioventricular valve may be required.

Complete AVSD

Surgery is undertaken electively at 2–4 months of age to prevent pulmonary hypertension.

The surgical indications are:

- The presence of a complete or unbalanced defect.
- Unresponsive congestive cardiac failure.
- Reversible pulmonary hypertension.
- Failure to thrive.
- A Qp:Qs ratio of more than 1.5:1.

The principles of treatment are:

- To correct the left to right shunt.
- Provision of competent atrioventricular valves.
- Closure of the septal defects without damage to the conduction tissue.
- Prevention of pulmonary vascular obstructive disease[20].

Ideally the operation should be performed at around three months of age, that is, in early infancy[41, 42]. After six months, pulmonary hypertension predisposes the patient to irreversible pulmonary vascular obstructive disease, and intractable heart failure occurs. If left untreated, premature death is inevitable, however many sufferers live until their teenage years.

Palliative surgery involving a pulmonary artery band to reduce pulmonary blood flow and pressure is only indicated for patients with intractable heart failure with constant respiratory infections — a contraindication to cardiopulmonary bypass[9] — or in unbalanced AVSD requiring a Fontan type operation in later life — see Chapter 6 for details of the Fontan procedure[43]. Banding of the pulmonary artery in a patient with severe left atrioventricular valve regurgitation will increase the left to right shunt and increase the degree of mitral regurgitation.

Corrective surgery has a mortality risk of 5–13%[4, 20, 44, 45]. The risk increases in the presence of pulmonary vascular obstructive disease, previous pulmonary artery banding and severe left atrioventricular valve incompetence[10].

- A median sternotomy is performed.
- Cardiopulmonary bypass initiated.
- Infants may have deep hypothermic circulatory arrest if under 3 kg or undergo low temperature bypass.
- The right atrium is incised.
- The septal defects are closed with two separate patches[46].
- Clefts in the left atrioventricular valve are sutured.
- A valvuloplasty of the left and right atrioventricular valves is performed.

Key postoperative management issues

Table 3.6 Assessment and management of potential postoperative problems in AVSDs (for detailed management of individual problems, see Chapters 10 and 11)

Left atrioventricular valve incompetence predisposing to congestive heart failure and low cardiac output:
- Assess for increasing left and right atrial pressures which may indicate left atrioventricular valve incompetence
- 15% will require left atrioventricular valve replacement in the future

Heart block and junctional arrhythmias due to the septal surgery

Pulmonary hypertension and hyper-reactive pulmonary vasculature

Chest infection

Problems associated with Down's syndrome:
- Earlier development of pulmonary hypertension perhaps due to the child having upper airway obstruction[47, 48] due to enlarged adenoids, tonsils, laryngomalacia and sleep apnoea
- Increasing respiratory requirements causing prolonged ventilation due to reduced numbers of alveoli with a subsequent reduction in alveolar surface area[3]. Additionally decreased muscle tone compromises respiratory expansion[11]

(contd)

Table 3.6 (contd)

- Once extubated, children with Down's syndrome appear to be more prone to episodes of stridor and may require intravenous dexamethasone, epinephrine nebulisers and humidified oxygen
- Due to the depressed nasal bridge in children with Down's syndrome, there is a reduction in the ability of the nose to drain mucus. This predisposes to a stuffy nose, causing the child to mouth breathe, thus reducing the amount of natural humidity, making secretions much more thick, and drying out the mouth and tongue. Mouth care is important. Synthetic saliva is available on prescription
- Dry, cracked skin is a problem for children with Down's syndrome. This requires the use of emollients. Furthermore, the skin is prone to cutis marmorata (mottling) which may not necessarily be due to low cardiac output

---

The key postoperative management issues are shown in Table 3.6. The postoperative course is determined to a degree, by the preoperative condition of the patient.

Long-term follow-up

- Subsequent problems will depend on any residual defect. The occurrence of pulmonary vascular obstructive disease is not usually totally prevented by surgical repair.
- Life-long follow-up is necessary.
- Life-long antibiotic prophylaxis for bacterial endocarditis is required.

Patent (persistent) ductus arteriosus (PDA)

Aetiology

Patent (persistent) ductus arteriosus (PDA) accounts for 5–12% of congenital heart disease[4, 10]. It is more prevalent in premature babies, being related to gestational age — the more premature, the higher the incidence. In term babies, a PDA is more common in females than males.

Definition

The ductus arteriosus is a normal structure connecting the systemic and pulmonary circulations in utero. Once closed it is termed the ligamentum arteriosum. Closure normally starts within hours of birth, being sealed completely at 2–3 weeks of age. Thus a PDA can be defined as delayed closure of the ductus arteriosus postnatally. See Figure 3.4.

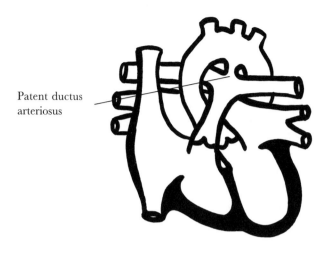

Patent ductus
arteriosus

Figure 3.4 Patent ductus arteriosus (PDA)

Occurrence

A PDA is present in several circumstances:

- As an isolated defect in the otherwise normal term baby.
- As an isolated defect in the premature baby.
- In association with other congenital heart defects.
- As a life-saving conduit in ductus dependent congenital heart defects, providing perfusion of the systemic and pulmonary circulations[9].

Anatomy and pathophysiology

Embryonic and fetal

The ductus arteriosus develops between the fifth and seventh weeks of gestation, from the sixth paired aortic arch branch[11]. It is a wide tube, varying in size and length, depending on the existence of other lesions and is comprised of specialised tissue[9]. The ductus arteriosus connects systemic and pulmonary circulations in utero.

In the normal fetal heart, approximately 60% of the normal right heart's cardiac output is directed to the duct and into the aorta[9]. The duct at this time is as large as the descending aorta.

Neonatal

Initially at birth, the lungs expand. This fall in the pulmonary vascular resistance changes the pressures and flow, now passing from the left (aorta) to the right (pulmonary artery).

Right to left shunting will remain should the pulmonary vascular resistance not fall. This is termed persistent fetal circulation.

The size of the shunt is dependent on two factors:

- The size — width and length — of the duct.
- The pulmonary and systemic vascular resistances. A low pulmonary vascular resistance, with a wide, short ductus will result in a large left to right shunt[10]. This subsequently produces symptoms — see below.

Closure of the duct at birth depends on two factors:

- In the term baby, the first breaths result in a rise in the circulatory oxygen level. This causes constriction of ductal tissue over the subsequent 24–48 hours and permanent closure within 2–3 weeks as the tissues obliterate and fibrose.
- There is a reduction in the naturally occurring circulating prostaglandins precipitating contraction of the muscular ductal tissue.

Reasons for non-closure of the PDA

The reasons for non-closure of the PDA are shown in Table 3.7.

Table 3.7 Reasons for non-closure of PDA

The premature baby
- The ductus is significantly less sensitive to the increase in the partial pressure of oxygen resulting in a persistent ductus arteriosus[9]
- If the premature baby requires mechanical ventilation and administration of diuretics, this triggers an increase in the circulating prostaglandins, relaxing the muscle wall of the ductus[49]
- Development of the contractile tissue in the ductus arteriosus occurs only after 30 weeks gestation[3]

Reduced partial pressure of oxygen due to:
- A cyanotic heart defect
- Living at high altitude
- Respiratory distress syndrome[50]

The normal newborn
- Indicative of an intrinsic abnormality of the ductal response[9]

Maternal infection
- For example rubella syndrome[10]

Signs and symptoms

In the term baby and older patient, symptoms are dependent on the magnitude of duct flow.

The small PDA

The infant and child are asymptomatic, that is, of normal skin colouration with no respiratory distress. It is usually diagnosed by routine examination upon which a continuous murmur is heard[3]. An echocardiogram will confirm the patency of the duct. The patient is at risk of bacterial endocarditis.

A medium-sized PDA

This presents from 8–20 weeks of age.

Cardiovascular signs and symptoms

- Congestive cardiac failure.
- Low diastolic blood pressure causing large volume peripheral pulses.

Respiratory signs and symptoms

- History of chest infections.
- Shortness of breath on exertion.
- Increased respiratory rate at rest.

Other signs and symptoms

- Slow to feed.
- Slightly below normal weight.

Sepsis

- Potential bacterial endocarditis

A large PDA

Symptoms occur early in infancy.

Cardiovascular signs and symptoms

- Congestive cardiac failure.

- Low diastolic blood pressure causing bounding pulses.
- Active precordium.
- Initially left to right shunting, however, if the pulmonary vascular resistance increases, the shunt will reverse resulting in right heart failure.

Respiratory signs and symptoms

- Pulmonary congestion.
- Very breathless at rest and feeding.
- Chest infections.
- Severe pulmonary hypertension, the pulmonary artery pressure equal to or higher than the systemic pressure. If untreated it can lead to pulmonary vascular disease.
- Cyanosis if right to left shunt.

Other signs and symptoms

- Failure to thrive.
- Poor feeding.

Sepsis

- Risk of bacterial endocarditis.

Diagnosis

- Chest x-ray: Cardiomegaly.
- Echocardiography: Left atrial and biventricular enlargement, the presence of the duct. Doppler studies indicate the magnitude of the shunt.
- Cardiac catheterisation: Not normally indicated in the presence of an isolated PDA.

Differential diagnosis

Other conditions which present with a continuous murmur include coarctation of the aorta with collateral circulation, pulmonary atresia with VSD and MAPCAs, pulmonary, systemic and coronary arteriovenous fistula, aortopulmonary window, venous hum and VSD with aortic regurgitation[4].

PDA in the premature baby

Symptoms usually occur within the first week of life and are similar to those of a large PDA with the following features:

Cardiovascular signs and symptoms

- Congestive cardiac failure with hepatomegaly and oedema, active precordium.

Respiratory signs and symptoms

- Respiratory distress is worsened by the presence of a PDA. There is an increased need for ventilatory support.

Gastrointestinal signs and symptoms

- The run-off perfusion from the aorta into the pulmonary artery may result in hypoperfusion of the gut predisposing the patient to necrotising enterocolitis.

Medical management

Closure of the PDA can sometimes be achieved non-surgically by one of two methods:

- Administration of either oral or intravenous prostaglandin synthetase inhibitor indomethacin: This is the first treatment in the premature neonate if the duct is large. It is not effective in term babies. Once diagnosed, the indomethacin must be promptly administered. The doses are given 12–24 hours apart, on two or three occasions, depending on the response. There are several contraindications to its use including low urine output, hyperbilirubinaemia, sepsis, gut ischaemia and clotting dysfunction[3,9] Should the ductus arteriosus fail to close on administration of indomethacin, early surgical intervention should be undertaken to reduce not only mortality but also significant morbidity[3] and overall length of hospital stay.
- Catheter closure of a PDA is possible in the term baby and older child, using one of a variety of devices. It is not a consideration in the premature baby as the procedure is thought to be too risky and impractical, as the catheter device has too large a sheath for a small baby to accommodate.

Key preoperative management issues

The key preoperative management issues are shown in Table 3.8.

Table 3.8 Assessment and management of potential preoperative problems in PDA (for detailed management of individual problems, see Chapters 10, 11 and 13)

Congestive heart failure

Respiratory distress

Pulmonary hypertension

Failure to thrive

Surgical management

In the patient with symptoms, surgery should be undertaken as soon as possible. In the asymptomatic patient, surgery should be taken on diagnosis. Outside the neonatal period, PDA is nearly always managed by cardiac catheterisation. During the neonatal period cardiac catheterisation carries too many risks.

The surgical procedure entails:

- Ligation of the patent ductus arteriosus by performing a left thoracotomy.
- Collapsing of the left lung to reach the PDA.
- The ductus arteriosus can be ligated or clipped, thus reducing the risk of haemorrhage which is greater should the surgeon decide to divide and oversew the lesion. However, if the duct is large, division is necessary.

Key postoperative management issues

The key postoperative management issues are shown in Table 3.9.

Table 3.9 Assessment and management of potential postoperative problems in PDA (for detailed management of individual problems see Chapters 10–12)

Pain from the thoracotomy:
- Use of a paravertebral block in babies over 2 kg
- Intravenous infusion of morphine is given, continually assessing the baby for pain

Respiratory distress due to:
- Collapsing of the left lung during surgery with subsequent atelectasis
- The premature neonate with pre-existing respiratory distress syndrome
- Chest infection related to pre-existing congestive heart failure

Pulmonary hypertension due to delayed closure of the ductus or the patient with a large PDA

(contd)

Table 3.9 (contd)

Haemorrhage due to:
- Surgical ligation of the PDA
- Tearing of the ductus if the tissue is friable (rare)

Residual PDA

Ligation of the wrong structure — this is possible especially in the very small premature baby resulting in poor systemic perfusion to the lower half of the body. Monitor for:
- Absence of leg pulses
- Increase in core:peripheral temperature gradient
- Reduction in urine output
- Gut ischaemia

Long-term follow up

- Prophylaxis for bacterial endocarditis is necessary for six months postoperatively or after cardiac catheterisation closure if the duct is completely closed.
- The parents should be reassured that a normal life can be enjoyed with no restriction on physical activity.

Management of the neonate with a duct dependent circulation

Neonates with life-threatening congenital heart lesions may rely on a patent ductus arteriosus for survival. Examples of such lesions include severe coarctation of the aorta, transposition of the great arteries, hypoplastic left heart syndrome and pulmonary atresia. If the duct starts to close with a defect reliant upon a patent ductus arteriosus, the infant will deteriorate within a few hours.

Signs and symptoms

Cardiovascular signs and symptoms:

- Low cardiac output.
- Reducing to absent peripheral pulses.
- Increased ventricular afterload.
- Cardiovascular collapse.

Respiratory signs and symptoms:

- Falling oxygen saturations.
- Hypoxia.

- Severe cyanosis in pulmonary atresia.
- Respiratory distress.
- Respiratory arrest.

Renal signs and symptoms:

- Oliguria to anuria.
- Metabolic acidosis.

Skin:

- Poor peripheral perfusion.
- Prolonged capillary refill.
- Mottled, grey, cold skin.

A neonate dependent on a PDA for survival, can often be mistaken for a baby in septic shock when presenting in an accident and emergency department.

Key management issues

The key management issues in a neonate with duct dependent circulation are shown in Table 3.10.

Since the 1970s, prostaglandin E_1 has been shown to have the most effect on dilation of the pulmonary vascular bed and ductus arteriosus[51, 52]. This finding revolutionised the management of duct dependent lesions, increasing initial survival.

Aortopulmonary window (AP window)

Aetiology

Aortopulmonary window (AP window) comprises less than 1% of congenital heart disease[10] and is usually associated with defects such as coarctation of the aorta, interrupted aortic arch, atrial and ventricular septal defects and patent ductus arteriosus[9, 20].

Definition

There is a communication between the ascending aorta and usually the main pulmonary artery resulting in a left to right shunt. It is due to incomplete septation of the aorta and pulmonary artery[10] and is thought to be related to truncus arteriosus[9]. See Figure 3.5.

Table 3.10 Assessment and management of potential problems for the neonate with duct dependent circulation (for detailed management of individual problems see Chapters 10–13)

Establishment and maintenance of a patent ductus arteriosus:
- Commence prostaglandin E_1 infusion intravenously at 5–100 ng/kg/min
- Use either a central or peripheral line. However, if a peripheral line is used, it must be continually observed for infiltration as the half-life of prostaglandin is very short. If a baby has to remain on the drug for several weeks (after ballooning of the pulmonary valve in critical pulmonary stenosis), hourly oral administration is possible should venous access become a problem
- Observe the baby for signs that the duct is closing — cooling peripheries, prolonged capillary refill, mottled, grey appearance, dropping oxygen saturations, acidosis, reduced urine output, poor/absent peripheral pulses, arrhythmias and hypotension

Metabolic acidosis and hypoxia:
- Administer intravenous sodium bicarbonate to correct the acid-base balance
- Ventilate to correct the pH and probable hypercapnia
- Use as little oxygen as possible as it is potentially associated with ductus arteriosus closure although this is debatable. Have an air/oxygen mixer attachment by the bedside for hand ventilation
- Administer prescribed plasma
- Repeat blood gases at frequent intervals

Management and the side-effects associated with the infusion of prostaglandin E_1:
- Respiratory effects include apnoea if the infusion is above 20 ng/kg/min, hand ventilate or assist in intubation if the neonate is very sick
- Cardiovascular effects include bradycardia, arrhythmias, hypotension, peripheral vasodilation
- Neurological effects include hyperthermia — do not rule out the possibility of infection if the baby has had episodes of hypoperfusion, twitching limbs, etc.
- Skin effects include flushing due to peripheral vasodilatation

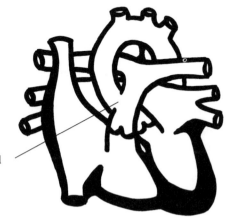

Communication between aorta and pulmonary artery

Figure 3.5 Aortopulmonary window

Anatomy and pathophysiology

The size of an AP window can vary. An isolated lesion has haemodynamic properties similar to a large patent ductus arteriosus; namely a large left to right shunt. Due to the position of the window, the pulmonary artery receives high pressure, high flow blood from the aorta. This predisposes to the early development of congestive heart failure and pulmonary hypertension, especially after the first month of life. If the lesion is small, the left to right shunt is reduced accordingly, resulting in milder symptoms.

Signs and symptoms

Cardiovascular signs and symptoms

- Congestive cardiac failure.
- Bounding pulses.

Respiratory signs and symptoms

- Respiratory distress.
- Chest infections.
- Pulmonary hypertension.
- Pulmonary vascular obstructive disease leading to irreversible Eisenmenger's syndrome if left untreated.

Other signs and symptoms

- Failure to thrive.

Diagnosis

- Auscultation: Continuous murmur[20].
- ECG: Biventricular hypertrophy.
- Chest x-ray: Enlarged left atrium and ventricle, ascending aorta and pulmonary artery.
- Echocardiography: Position of the window. Doppler studies show the magnitude of the shunt.
- Cardiac catheterisation: Calculates the pulmonary vascular resistance and the use of contrast shows the left to right shunt.

Differential diagnosis

Large patent ductus arteriosus, large ventricular septal defect, truncus arteriosus[9, 20].

Key preoperative management issues

The key preoperative management issues are shown in Table 3.11.

Table 3.11 Assessment and management of potential preoperative problems in AP window (for detailed management of individual problems, see Chapters 10 and 11)

Congestive heart failure
Chest infections
Pulmonary hypertension and pulmonary vascular obstructive disease

Surgical management

This defect is potentially fatal if left untreated, with death occurring within the first year of life if the defect is large[9]. Early intervention is therefore necessary to prevent complications associated with the large AP window and should be undertaken on the neonate or infant.

- Median sternotomy.
- Cardiopulmonary bypass: In neonates or small infants, deep hypothermic circulatory arrest is undertaken. In older infants, hypothermic low flow is performed.
- The window is closed with a patch.

Key postoperative management issues

The key postoperative management issues are shown in Table 3.12.

Table 3.12 Assessment and management of potential postoperative problems in AP window (for detailed management of individual problems, see Chapters 10–12)

Haemorrhage due to surgery on the aorta
Low cardiac output
Congestive heart failure
Pulmonary hypertension
Residual shunting if the patch or suture leaks

Long-term follow-up

- Long-term follow-up is required to monitor for pulmonary artery distortion[9].

- Antibiotic prophylaxis.
- The prognosis is good if the baby is operated on before the development of pulmonary vascular obstructive disease.

Partial anomalous pulmonary venous drainage (PAPVD)

Aetiology

This lesion accounts for less than 1% of all congenital heart disease. It is often associated with the sinus venosus type of ASD.

Definition

Between one and three of the pulmonary veins drain into the right atrium, coronary sinus or venae cavae. There may be an associated ASD.

Anatomy and pathophysiology

The anatomy and pathophysiology are as for the definition above, with haemodynamics similar to that of an ASD.

Signs and symptoms

The clinical features resemble those of an ASD, in that most patients will be asymptomatic. If left untreated, pulmonary vascular obstructive disease may develop from around 30 years of age. Echocardiography will confirm the diagnosis. Details of abnormal drainage may need confirmation by angiography.

Nursing and surgical management

The nursing and surgical management are as for ASD.

Chapter 4
Obstructive defects

Coarctation of the aorta (CoAo)

Aetiology

Coarctation of the aorta accounts for 6–12% of all congenital heart disease[3, 4, 10, 53]. It is more common in boys than girls in the approximate ratio of 2:1. Lesions associated with coarctation of the aorta occur in approximately 50% of patients[54] and include PDA, ASD, VSD[55], hypoplastic left heart syndrome, TGA, mitral valve abnormalities and aortic stenosis[9].

Definition

Coarctation of the aorta (CoAo) is a constriction or narrowing of the aorta which is variable in its severity. It occurs usually in the thoracic and very rarely in the abdominal aorta. It becomes of significance when there is a pressure gradient of more than 20 mmHg across the aortic narrowing[53, 56]. See Figure 4.1.

Classification

Several classifications exist. The most useful is to divide the condition into pre- and postductal, which classifies the blood flow of the anomaly.

- Preductal CoAo: The coarctation is found proximal to the ductus arteriosus. It is frequently associated with major abnormalities[57, 58].
- Postductal CoAo: The coarctation is found distal to the ductus arteriosus. This is the more common form[57, 58].

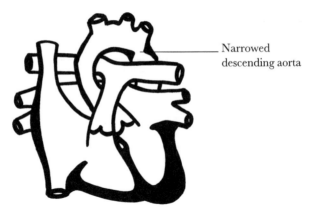

Narrowed
descending aorta

Figure 4.1 Coarctation of the aorta (CoAo)

Anatomy and pathophysiology

CoAo is thought to be caused by specialised ductal tissue migrating to the aorta which constricts after birth causing various degrees of obstruction[59]. Alternative causes may be attributed to hypoplasia of the aortic arch or isthmus distal to the left subclavian artery[20, 60]. The obstruction results in an increased resistance to flow from the ascending aorta to the descending aorta with a subsequent drop in systemic blood pressure. The kidneys respond to the hypoperfusion by secreting renin which vasoconstricts the arteries in an attempt to raise the distal pressure but may result in hypertension in the proximal (upper) segment. Perfusion of the lower limbs will depend on collateral circulation.

Preductal CoAo

In the preductal form, fetal blood flow is unchanged in the presence of a PDA; blood from the right ventricle enters the ductus arteriosus discharging its contents into the descending aorta. The left ventricular blood flows into the ascending aorta to supply the upper body. Once the ductus arteriosus starts to close and pulmonary vascular resistance falls, the baby will show signs of heart failure and if untreated, circulatory collapse will result as little blood can flow from the ascending to the descending aorta in the presence of a severe coarctation.

Postductal CoAo

In a postductal coarctation, the obstruction has implications for the fetus as the constriction reduces blood flow from the ductus arteriosus. Therefore, the contents of the right ventricle, which normally flow through the ductus arteriosus, are impeded. The left ventricle still perfuses the upper body and head via the ascending aorta. As this obstruction affects the fetus, a variable collateral circulation develops, from the proximal to the distal aorta[10].

Signs and symptoms

The signs and symptoms are different depending on whether the lesion is pre- or postductal.

Preductal CoAo

If the lesion is severe, it normally presents within the first few of days of life as the ductus arteriosus closes. Neonatal presentation can be mistaken for septic shock.

Cardiovascular signs and symptoms

- Congestive heart failure (particularly if a VSD is present).
- Femoral pulses weak or absent.
- Right brachial pulses full and bounding.
- If the CoAo is proximal to the left subclavian artery, the left arm pulse will be poor and the blood pressure the same as in the legs. The right radial pulse will be strong with an increase in blood pressure in that arm. Conversely, if the CoAo is distal to the left subclavian artery, hypertension in both arms with hypotension in both lower limbs will be present.

Respiratory signs and symptoms

- Tachypnoea.
- Dyspnoea.
- Shortness of breath on feeding.
- Hypoxia when ductus arteriosus closing.
- Cyanosis in lower limbs as perfusion is dependent from the right ventricle via the PDA.

Gastrointestinal signs and symptoms

- Liver enlargement.
- Risk of necrotising enterocolitis if the duct closes[61].

Renal signs and symptoms

- Oliguria to anuria if the duct closes.
- Metabolic acidosis when PDA closing.

Other signs and symptoms

- Grey and mottled appearance.

Diagnosis

- Auscultation: No murmur unless VSD present.
- ECG: Right ventricular hypertrophy.
- Chest x-ray: Enlarged heart with pulmonary venous congestion.
- Echocardiography: Doppler studies will show the reduced blood flow post coarctation.
- Cardiac catheterisation: This identifies the location of the narrowing with angiography, but is not indicated in the critically ill patient with isolated CoAo.

Postductal CoAo

Postductal CoAo usually presents in the older child. The child is commonly asymptomatic and the lesion is found on medical examination.

Cardiovascular signs and symptoms

- Absent pulses in the legs and hypertension in the arms with strong brachial pulses.
- Rarely, congestive heart failure if left untreated.
- Development of collateral vessels.

Neurological signs and symptoms

- Intracranial bleed if the blood pressure is high.
- Headaches.

Renal signs and symptoms

- Renal failure if left untreated.

Other signs and symptoms

- Leg pain (claudication).
- Nosebleeds.
- Fatigue.

Diagnosis

- Auscultation: Systolic murmur or continuous murmur in the back.
- ECG: Left ventricular hypertrophy.
- Chest x-ray: Slightly enlarged heart, rib notching in an older child.
- Echocardiography: Diagnostic. Doppler examination shows narrowing of the aorta in the region of the coarctation with increased Doppler velocity and diastolic "tail".

Key preoperative management issues

The key preoperative management issues are shown in Table 4.1.

Table 4.1 Assessment and management of potential preoperative problems in CoAo (for detailed management of individual problems, see Chapters 10–12)

Immediate establishment and maintenance of a PDA to temporarily secure systemic blood flow

Treatment of metabolic acidosis, hypoxia and multi-organ failure should the PDA have closed

Management of neonatal coagulopathy

Assessment of limb pressures:
- Record four limb blood pressure and report differences promptly, noting whether differences in both arms or if the right arm is higher than the left

Congestive heart failure

Medical management

Medical management is usually reserved for recoarctation after surgical intervention. However, many centres are now using it as a primary method of correction outside the neonatal period, in which a balloon coronary angioplasty catheter is placed across the coarctation via the femoral artery[62].

Surgical management

The aim of surgery is to relieve the constriction before the hypertension causes complications or becomes irreversible[20]. If the baby arrives collapsed due to ductal closure, the duct needs to be re-established, and stabilisation after resuscitation is required for at least 24 hours. Should the duct have closed but the baby is stable, initial treatment is for the hypertension. The choice of operation is depends on the surgeon's preference, each operation having its pros and cons.

Subclavian flap repair

This operation theoretically has the most potential for aortic growth.

- Left thoracotomy.
- The left subclavian artery is ligated and divided.
- The aorta is cross clamped.
- An aortic incision is made and extended up to the left subclavian artery.
- The descending aorta excision is extended to below the level of the PDA and reconstructed.
- The divided end or subclavian flap is brought down as a patch and sewn to the aorta.

End-to-end anastomosis

This operation has the advantage of being able to remove completely any ductal tissue which is associated with recoarctation[58, 63].

- Left thoracotomy.
- The narrowed segment of the aorta is excised.
- The aorta is then rejoined end to end.

Coarctation with VSD

If the VSD is large, a pulmonary artery band may be considered at the time of CoAo repair. This remains a topic of debate as a pulmonary artery band may heighten risks[64]. The VSD can be closed at the time of surgery or at a later date once the baby has recovered from the aortic cross clamping performed during the coarctation repair. A sternotomy is performed for coarctation with hypoplastic aortic arch.

Key postoperative management issues

The key postoperative management issues are shown in Table 4.2.

Long-term follow-up

- Patients are usually followed up for 6–12 months where four limb blood pressures are recorded to detect the formation of a recoarctation and residual hypertension. A significant gradient is

Table 4.2 Assessment and management of potential postoperative problems in CoAo (for detailed management of individual problems, see Chapters 11–13)

Complications associated with cross clamping the aorta:
- Rarely, 1% of patients will suffer spinal cord ischaemia resulting in paraplegia or parasthesia[65, 66]. The patient should be observed for lack of lower limb movement, absent or weak reflexes and a reduction in perfusion and circulation
- Renal failure may occur if the spinal cord is damaged. The patient should be observed for difficulty in passing urine and subsequent development of an enlarged bladder

Reactive hypertension resulting in the development of postcoarctectomy syndrome:
- This is due to the release of catecholamines and renin when the aorta is cross clamped[38]
- The patient must be observed for signs of left ventricular failure
- Haemorrhage
- Mesenteric arteritis — abdominal pain, distension, vomiting, gastrointestinal bleeding, bowel ischaemia. Enteral feeds must be introduced slowly
- Hypertension is treated aggressively

Hypoperfusion of major organs due to poor condition preoperatively

Reduction in perfusion to the left hand following subclavian flap repair for CoAo[67, 68]:
- Circulatory check monitoring skin colour, temperature and perfusion should be performed hourly for the first 24 hours. Collateral circulation will develop in the first few days but the arm may be slightly growth retarded long-term
- Avoid taking cuff pressures on the left arm as they will be inaccurate
- Avoid intravenous and arterial line siting on the left arm which may further reduce perfusion

Pain due to the thoracotomy:
- Use of paravertebral blocks and pain assessment tools
- Opiate intravenous infusion can be instituted should the block not be sufficient

Bacterial endocarditis

Recoarctation of the aorta due to stenosis of the aorta:
- Record four limb pressures regularly, reporting gradients promptly
- If a recoarctation occurs, it may be treated in the catheter laboratory by a balloon dilatation[69, 70]

---

present when the leg blood pressure is greater than 20 mmHg lower than the right arm.
- Antibiotic prophylaxis is required for life.
- Postoperative drug therapy may include digoxin, diuretics and an angiotensin converting enzyme (ACE) inhibitor (although this drug is contraindicated if any obstruction or renal impairment is present).

Cor triatriatum

Aetiology

This is a very rare anomaly[71], accounting for less than 0.1% of all congenital heart defects[20].

Definition

Cor triatriatum is a fibromuscular diaphragm which septates the left atrium into two compartments. The pulmonary veins thus become obstructed as blood cannot flow easily through the lower atrial chamber and mitral valve. See Figure 4.2.

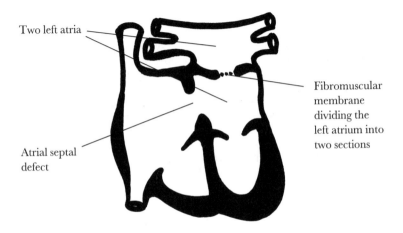

Two left atria

Atrial septal defect

Fibromuscular membrane dividing the left atrium into two sections

Figure 4.2 Cor triatriatum

Anatomy and pathophysiology

The left atrium is composed of two chambers with the pulmonary veins emptying into the top chamber. The bottom chamber resembles the normal atrium in that the mitral valve is present. The lesion is similar to mitral stenosis in that blood leaving the lungs is obstructed resulting in severe pulmonary hypertension. An ASD may be present.

Signs and symptoms

This defect usually presents within the first two years of life although symptoms are often misdiagnosed. However if the obstruction is severe, it can present in the neonate as low cardiac output.

Respiratory signs and symptoms

- Cough.
- Shortness of breath on exertion.
- Pulmonary oedema.
- Pulmonary vascular obstructive disease and pulmonary hypertension.
- Haemoptysis.

Diagnosis

- Auscultation: Soft murmur.
- ECG: Right atrial and ventricular hypertrophy, left atrial hypertrophy.
- Chest x-ray: Pulmonary venous congestion, right-sided enlargement, pulmonary artery enlargement.
- Echocardiography: Diagnostic.
- Cardiac catheterisation: Pulmonary artery hypertension.

Key preoperative management issues

The key preoperative management issues are shown in Table 4.3.

Table 4.3 Assessment and management of potential preoperative problems in Cor triatriatum (for detailed management of individual problems see Chapters 10 and 11)

Low cardiac output in the severely obstructed patient

Pulmonary hypertension

Pulmonary oedema

Surgical management

The only treatment for this condition is excision of the fibromuscular diaphragm.

- Median sternotomy.
- Cardiopulmonary bypass using low flow or deep hypothermic circulatory arrest is performed as there is a high pulmonary venous return.

- Excision of the fibromuscular membrane.
- Closure of the ASD if present.

Key postoperative management issues

The care of the patient should be routine. However, approximately 5% of patients will have developed pulmonary vascular obstructive disease[20]. This group of patients may require a heart-lung transplantation in later life.

Long-term follow-up

- A normal life should be enjoyed unless pulmonary hypertension has developed.

Aortic stenosis (AS)

Aetiology

Aortic stenosis (AS) is responsible for 5–8% of all congenial heart disease[3, 4, 10] and occurs more frequently in males than females in a ratio of approximately 4:1[4]. Valvular aortic stenosis may be associated with hypoplastic left ventricle, coarctation of the aorta, PDA and mitral regurgitation and is the most common type of obstruction of the left ventricular outflow tract[72]. Subvalvular aortic stenosis may be linked with VSD, PDA, AVSD and pulmonary stenosis. Supra-aortic stenosis occurs with William's syndrome, VSD, coarctation of the aorta and pulmonary stenosis[9].

Definition

AS may be defined as left ventricular outflow tract obstruction. The stenosis can occur at a valvular, subvalvular and supravalvular level. See Figure 4.3. Critical aortic stenosis is a term used to describe valvular aortic stenosis presenting in the neonatal period with associated heart failure.

Classification

- Valvular aortic stenosis: The stenosis occurs at the level of the aortic valve. It is the most common type.
- Subvalvular aortic stenosis: The stenosis occurs below the level of the valve and is the second most common type.

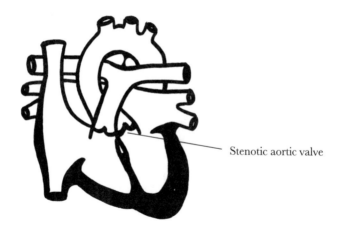

Figure 4.3 Aortic valve stenosis

- Supravalvular aortic stenosis: The stenosis occurs above the level of the valve and is the least common.

Anatomy and pathophysiology

Valvular AS

The aortic valve is thickened with fused cusps. It is usually bicuspid, instead of the normal three cusps. However, a unicusp can occur in the severely stenotic valve. This is normally found in the neonate and is termed critical aortic stenosis (CAS).

Subvalvular AS

The stenosis is normally attributed to a fibrous membrane beneath the aortic valve being attached to the mitral valve and intraventricular septum[3]. Occasionally subvalvular AS may be caused by a hypertrophied muscle (hypertrophic subaortic stenosis) which is progressive in nature.

Supravalvular AS

This stenosis is related to either a fibrous constriction above the aortic valve or to a diffuse or discrete narrowing/hypoplasia in the ascending aorta. The left ventricle is often hypertrophied with reduced coronary blood flow in diastole and especially during exercise-induced tachycardia[73]. The coronary arteries may be thickened and distended.

Haemodynamics

Haemodynamic effects are related to the degree of obstruction. That is, the pressure gradient between the left ventricle and aorta in systole. Thus, in mild stenosis the gradient is less than 30 mmHg, moderate stenosis, less than 50 mmHg and severe stenosis, greater than 80 mmHg up to a maximum of 200 mmHg. Obstruction to the flow of blood out of the left ventricle will increase left ventricular pressure resulting in left ventricular hypertrophy. Hypertrophy will worsen symptoms especially in subvalvular stenosis and there may be increased coronary artery oxygenation demands which cannot be met. This may result in myocardial ischaemia and ultimately, angina.

Severe valvular AS

Signs and symptoms

Most patients present with an asymptomatic murmur. The severity of the stenosis dictates the severity of the symptoms. Severe valvular AS presents in the neonatal period as critical AS. It is responsible for approximately 10% of all AS presentations[9].

Cardiovascular signs and symptoms:
- Low cardiac output.
- Collapse as PDA closes.
- Mitral regurgitation.
- Intractable heart failure.
- Small pulse volume progressing to absent pulses when PDA closes.
- Pressure gradient up to a maximum of 200 mmHg.

Respiratory signs and symptoms:
- Hypoxia when PDA closes.
- Respiratory distress.

Renal signs and symptoms:

- Oliguria to anuria as PDA closes.
- Metabolic acidosis as PDA closes.

Gastrointestinal signs and symptoms:

- Hepatomegaly.

Other signs and symptoms:

- History of poor feeding.

Diagnosis

- Auscultation: Soft murmur.
- ECG: Left ventricular hypertrophy.
- Chest x-ray: Cardiomegaly due to left ventricular dilatation with heart failure.
- Echocardiography: Shows the thickened valve, left ventricular hypertrophy or dilatation. Doppler studies will assess the gradient but can be low if the left ventricle is failing.
- Cardiac catheterisation: Balloon dilatation can be considered.

Mild to moderate AS

Mild to moderate AS presents in childhood.

Signs and symptoms

Cardiovascular signs and symptoms:

- Mitral regurgitation.
- Pressure gradient 20–50 mmHg.
- Angina.
- Syncope due to a reduction in cardiac output on exertion.

Other signs and symptoms:

- Dizziness.
- Fatigue.
- Risk of endocarditis.

Diagnosis

- Auscultation: Systemic murmur and ejection click.
- ECG: Left ventricular hypertrophy.
- Chest x-ray: Normal heart size with calcification of the cusps in the older child.
- Echocardiogram: Diagnostic. Doppler assessment will assess the gradient.

Key preoperative management issues

The key preoperative management issues are shown in Table 4.5.

Table 4.5 Assessment and management of potential preoperative/preprocedural problems in AS (for detailed management of individual problems, see Chapters 10–13)

Immediate establishment and maintenance of a PDA to temporarily secure systemic blood flow
Low cardiac output
Metabolic acidosis, hypoxia and multi-organ failure
Management of neonatal coagulopathy
Bacterial endocarditis

Medical management

A percutaneous balloon valvuloplasty which tears and separates the valve leaflets can be performed in the neonatal period or in the older child with AS[10]. The pressure gradient should reduce immediately. This procedure is the one of choice for the sick neonate. Surgical valvotomy has risks of up to 20%.

Surgical management

The various surgical approaches depend on the degree of left ventricular outflow tract obstruction with the principal aim of relieving the obstruction. However, surgical approaches have their disadvantages in paediatrics as any replacement valve will not grow with the child, making regular replacements necessary. Additionally, anticoagulants for prosthetic valves will be required, with their associated problems. Thus, only severe stenosis is treated surgically when no other form of treatment is available. The Ross procedure[75] is an alternative form of surgical management (see p. 76).

In both valvotomy and ballooning of the valve, 75% of patients will require further intervention in the future.

Valvular AS

Should repeated valvotomies be required for significant aortic stenosis and regurgitation, an aortic valve replacement may be necessary. Alternatively a Ross procedure may be performed whereby replacement of the aortic valve with the patient's own pulmonary valve can be used.

Subvalvular AS

Indications for surgery with this type of AS are worsening symptoms.

- Median sternotomy.
- Cardiopulmonary bypass.
- If a fibrous membrane is present, the membrane is excised through the aortic valve.
- Alternatively, if there is severe tunnelling or narrowing, the aortic root and outflow tract are enlarged, and the aortic valve replaced (Konno procedure). This is a much riskier procedure. The Ross procedure is an alternative option in such cases.

Supravalvular AS

Again, the indications for surgery are worsening symptoms.

- Median sternotomy.
- Cardiopulmonary bypass.
- The wall of the ascending aorta being thickened and narrowed, is repaired with a patch.
- If there is a large stenotic area it is enlarged with a pericardial patch.

Key postoperative management issues

Valvular AS repair

The key postoperative management issues are shown in Table 4.6.

Table 4.6 Assessment and management of potential postoperative problems in valvular AS (for detailed management of individual problems, see Chapters 11 and 12)

Poor ventricular function or less commonly aortic valve regurgitation resulting in low cardiac output and congestive heart failure

Haemorrhage from multiple suture lines

Residual stenosis

Subvalvular AS

The key postoperative management issues are shown in Table 4.7.

Table 4.7 Assessment and management of potential postoperative problems in subvalvular AS (for detailed management of individual problems, see Chapter 11)

Complete heart block following the Konno procedure due to tissue resection near the bundle of His

Supravalvular AS

The key postoperative management issues are the same as for valvular AS.

Long-term follow-up

- Very close follow-up is required by the cardiologist to detect any deterioration promptly.
- Regular exercise is encouraged but restriction from competitive sports is advised if the AS is moderate.
- Stringent antibiotic prophylaxis is required to prevent bacterial endocarditis.
- Anticoagulation is required if prosthetic valve present.

The Ross procedure

Definition

The Ross procedure is a pulmonary autograft in which the aortic valve is replaced with the patient's own pulmonary valve. The coronary arteries are reattached and the right pulmonary valve is replaced with an allograft (donor valve).

Applications

This procedure is of particular use in the infant or child requiring aortic valve replacement normally due to aortic valve disease, critical aortic stenosis, endocarditis affecting the aortic valve or a left ventricular outflow tract obstruction[74, 75]. Normal sized ventricles are required.

Advantages of the Ross procedure

There are advantages to this procedure over mechanical valve replacement:

- An autograft is the only surgical option that has some growth potential[76], without the disadvantage of valvular insufficiency.
- The growth potential of the autograft is supposedly good thereby avoiding the need for regular mechanical valve replacements and the risks associated with re-operation.
- Anticoagulation therapy is unnecessary, unlike the situation in mechanical valve replacement, as there is potentially a very low risk of thromboembolic development.
- There are fewer valve-related complications with the Ross procedure[76].
- Haemodynamics are improved with the Ross procedure.
- There is a significant improvement in left ventricular wall thickness which is not apparent in patients who have undergone allograft valve replacements[77].
- There are few limitations on patient activity.

Disadvantages of the Ross procedure

- The pulmonary allograft may require repeated replacements.
- The Ross procedure is a technically challenging operation.

Postoperative complications following the Ross procedure

- Post-pericardiotomy syndrome.
- Supraventricular tachycardia and ventricular tachycardia in approximately 29% of patients[78].
- There is a risk of transient heart block due to the preoperative volume overload and associated hypertrophied ventricle.
- Aortic regurgitation in children who have had aortic root replacement. This is probably attributed to excessive tissue growth[74, 79].

Long-term follow-up

- The mid-term results look very encouraging as morbidity and mortality are significantly less than with repeated mechanical valve replacements[76].
- The child will be followed up indefinitely.

Pulmonary stenosis (PS)

Aetiology

Isolated pulmonary stenosis accounts for 5–10% of all congenital heart disease[3, 4, 20]. It can be associated with other congenital lesions including VSD, Noonan's syndrome and is an integral clinical aspect of tetralogy of Fallot (TOF).

Definition

PS is a partial obstruction of varying degree, occurring either from below the level of the pulmonary valve, at the level of the valve or above the level of the valve.

Classification

Valvular PS

Valvular PS is at the level of the pulmonary valve and is the most common, accounting for approximately 90% of PS (see Figure 4.4).

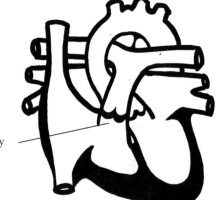

Stenotic pulmonary valve

Figure 4.4 Pulmonary valve stenosis

Subvalvular PS

Subvalvular PS is below the level of the valve, in the infundibular region of the right ventricle and is associated with TOF. It is discussed further in the section on TOF in Chapter 5.

Supravalvular PS

Supravalvular PS is above the level of the valve, that is, in the main pulmonary artery itself.

Anatomy and pathophysiology

The right ventricle has to pump against an obstruction resulting in an increase in right ventricular pressure. This predisposes to the development of right ventricular hypertrophy and possible tricuspid regurgitation. The right atrial pressure subsequently rises and may result in a right to left shunt across the patent foramen ovale in a neonate. A gradient thus develops between the right ventricle and pulmonary artery and is measured in mmHg. In mild stenosis, the gradient will be less than 30 mmHg, in moderate stenosis, less than 50 mmHg, and in severe stenosis, the gradient can be as high as 200 mmHg. This gradient increases when cardiac output increases, for example in pyrexia or with exercise.

Severe PS

Signs and symptoms

Symptoms depend on the severity of the valvular stenosis. Severe PS normally presents as a neonate and is termed critical PS. However, it can develop progressively throughout childhood.

Cardiovascular signs and symptoms:

- Low cardiac output to collapse when PDA closes.
- Congestive heart failure.
- Pressure gradient up to 200 mmHg.

Respiratory signs and symptoms:

- Respiratory distress.
- Hypoxia as PDA closes.
- Cyanosis if pulmonary blood flow inadequate.

Gastrointestinal signs and symptoms:

- Hepatomegaly.

Renal signs and symptoms:

- Metabolic acidosis.

Diagnosis

- Auscultation: Systolic murmur.
- ECG: Right ventricular hypertrophy.
- Chest x-ray: Right ventricular dilatation and enlargement of main pulmonary artery.
- Echocardiography: Thickened valve, post stenotic dilation of the pulmonary artery, right ventricular hypertrophy. Doppler studies will assess the pressure gradient.
- Cardiac catheterisation: Interventional.

Mild PS

Children are usually asymptomatic in mild cases.

Signs and symptoms

Cardiovascular signs and symptoms:

- Pressure gradient below 20 mmHg.

Other signs and symptoms:

- Increased risk of bacterial endocarditis.

Diagnosis

- Auscultation: Systolic murmur with an ejection click.
- ECG: Usually normal but mild right ventricular hypertrophy can occur.
- Chest x-ray: Pulmonary artery enlargement.
- Echocardiography: Diagnostic and Doppler studies will assess the pressure gradient, the thickened pulmonary valve and the post-stenotic dilatation.

Key preintervention management issues

The key preintervention management issues are shown in Table 4.8.

Medical management

Severe PS

A percutaneous pulmonary balloon valvuloplasty is performed which

Table 4.8 Assessment and management of potential preinterventional problems in PS (for detailed management of individual problems, see Chapters 10–13)

Immediate establishment and maintenance of a PDA to temporarily secure pulmonary blood flow

Low cardiac output

Metabolic acidosis, hypoxia and multi-organ failure

Management of neonatal coagulopathy

Congestive heart failure

Bacterial endocarditis

Preparation of the patient for interventional cardiac catheterisation

tears the valve. Prostaglandin E_1 infusion is maintained until the hypoplastic right ventricle is able to cope with the new volume. It is slowly weaned observing for signs of low cardiac output. If the percutaneous valvuloplasty fails, a surgical approach will be required.

Moderate PS

In the child with symptoms, a percutaneous valvuloplasty is performed sooner rather than later and in the asymptomatic child, a routine percutaneous valvuloplasty is performed when the gradient reaches 40 mmHg.

Mild PS

The cardiologist should examine the child regularly, monitoring the gradient on echocardiogram.

Key postprocedural management issues

The key postprocedural management issues are shown in Table 4.9.

Table 4.9 Assessment and management of potential postprocedural problems in PS (for detailed management of individual problems see Chapter 11)

Pulmonary valve regurgitation develops after percutaneous valvuloplasty. It manifests as right sided heart failure or low cardiac output

Right ventricular failure due to hypoplastic right ventricle

Arrhythmias

Complications from the cardiac catheterisation

Surgical management

Should percutaneous valvuloplasty fail then a surgical approach will be required. Surgical management for severe pulmonary stenosis is most likely to be a modified Blalock–Taussig shunt (see Chapter 6 for details of palliative procedures) as an open pulmonary valvotomy is very dangerous in this age of patient.

- Median sternotomy.
- Cardiopulmonary bypass.
- A blade incision to the stenotic valve is made which will decompress the right ventricle.
- The patent foramen ovale is closed if patent.

Key postoperative management issues

The key postoperative management issues are shown in Table 4.10.

Table 4.10 Assessment and management of potential postoperative problems in PS (for detailed management of individual problems, see Chapter 11)

Pulmonary valve regurgitation always occurs but there is no treatment
Congestive heart failure
Low cardiac output

Long-term follow-up

- The cardiologist will see the child at regular intervals monitoring for re-stenosis.
- Antibiotic prophylaxis is required for bacterial endocarditis.

Interrupted aortic arch (IAA)

Aetiology

This is a very rare anomaly accounting for approximately 1% of critically ill neonates with congenital heart disease[4]. This defect is associated with a VSD, normally perimembranous, and the maintenance of a patent ductus arteriosus (PDA). This ensures a right to left shunt thus enabling survival of the neonate. The baby will die if the PDA closes. Associated problems include the chromosomal abnormality Di George syndrome, a bicuspid aortic valve, mitral valve deformity, truncus arteriosus and/or sub-aortic stenosis[80].

Definition

IAA is the complete separation of two segments of the aortic arch[20].

Classification

IAA is an acyanotic, obstructive defect that relies on a right to left shunt through the PDA. The classification of IAA depends on which segment of aortic arch is interrupted. The arch is composed of three segments.

Type C

Type C is between the innominate artery to the left common carotid artery. It accounts for approximately 4% of IAA. The left ventricle ejects blood into the ascending aorta to supply the right common carotid and right subclavian arteries. The right ventricle supplies blood via the PDA to the left common carotid and left subclavian arteries[10] (see Figure 4.5).

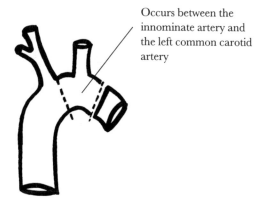

Occurs between the innominate artery and the left common carotid artery

Figure 4.5 Interrupted aortic arch — Type C

Type B

Type B is from the left common carotid artery to the left subclavian artery. It accounts for 55–69% of IAA (see Figure 4.6).

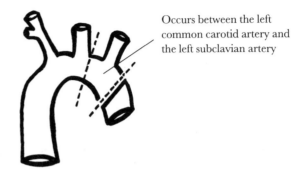

Occurs between the left common carotid artery and the left subclavian artery

Figure 4.6 Interrupted aortic arch — Type B

Type A

Type A occurs after the left subclavian artery, in the direction of the descending aorta. It accounts for 26–41% of IAA[4] (see Figure 4.7).

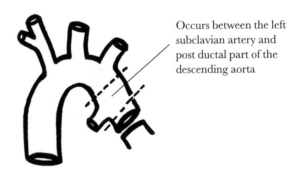

Occurs between the left subclavian artery and post ductal part of the descending aorta

Figure 4.7 Interrupted aortic arch — Type A

Anatomy and pathophysiology

There are several considerations regarding the pathophysiology and haemodynamics:

- The right ventricular pressure rises to supply the distal circulation[20]. This has potential implications for the neonate as the right ventricle delivers blood to the descending aorta via the PDA, predisposing the child to low cardiac output when the PDA closes.
- Perfusion of the lower half of the body is from the right ventricle into the descending aorta via the PDA. Right ventricular and pulmonary artery flow also goes to the lungs. Pulmonary resistance will rise. If the PDA closes, there will be no lower body blood flow.
- As approximately 20% of patients have sub-aortic stenosis, the left ventricular outflow tract may be too severe to undergo the usual surgery for repair of IAA.

Signs and symptoms

The baby usually presents when the PDA is closing or has closed in which case circulatory collapse prevails. This often results in a multi-organ insult as organs become hypoperfused and ischaemic. It must, however, be differentiated from hypoplastic left heart syndrome, aortic atresia and severe coarctation of the aorta.

Cardiac signs and symptoms

- There are poor or absent peripheral pulses:
  Type A may have a pulse in the right arm.
  Type B may have a pulse in the arm but leg pulses are weak or absent.
  Type C may have pulses only felt in the neck[3].
- No murmur until the PDA has opened.
- Severe congestive cardiac failure resistant to medical treatment.
- Profound low cardiac output.

Respiratory signs and symptoms

- Respiratory distress despite pulmonary blood flow being adequate.
- Cyanosis, although classified as an acyanotic defect due to the right to left shunt across the PDA.
- Oxygen saturations in the right arm will be 100% but only about 70% in the feet.

Renal signs and symptoms

- Severe metabolic acidosis.

Other signs and symptoms

- The kidneys, brain, liver and intestines may all be hypoperfused due to the duct dependent circulation thus predisposing to multi-organ failure.

Diagnosis

- ECG: Biventricular hypertrophy.
- Chest x-ray: Enlarged heart with pulmonary congestion[3].
- Echocardiography: Preferred investigation for this critically ill neonate, who will tolerate little handling, as it is non-invasive. The echo will show the level of interruption. Doppler studies will show the interrupted blood supply.
- Cardiac catheterisation: This procedure is too invasive for such a sick baby.

Key preoperative management issues

The baby normally presents in a critical, even moribund condition as the PDA is closing or has closed. Resuscitation and stabilisation are the main aims. Surgical reconstruction is delayed until stability with good/improving renal function has been achieved. This may take several days. A multidisciplinary approach is used to assess, plan, implement and evaluate the care for a neonate with such a life-threatening condition (see Table 4.11).

Surgical management

Uncorrected IAA is incompatible with life unless the ductus arteriosus is patent. Surgery is postponed until resuscitation and stabilisation are achieved[82]. Surgery is the only definitive treatment for survival[83]. During transportation of the baby to theatre, the same care must be taken that has been employed on the intensive care unit.

IAA with VSD repair

There are several possible surgical approaches but the commonly preferred one is by median sternotomy, a one-stage repair directly anastomosing the interrupted segments of aortic arch and closure of the VSD[84-87].

- If not already *in situ*, the anaesthetist may place two arterial lines to measure the blood pressure before and after the subsequent

Table 4.11 Assessment and management of potential preoperative problems in IAA (for detailed management of individual problems, see Chapter 11)

Immediate establishment and maintenance of a PDA to temporarily secure systemic blood flow

Low cardiac output

Metabolic acidosis, hypoxia and multi-organ failure

Management of neonatal coagulopathy

Avoidance of hyperventilation in too high a concentration of oxygen, when hand-ventilating or mechanically ventilating the baby. This would predispose to respiratory alkalosis and lowering of the pulmonary vascular resistance

Management of Di George syndrome[81]:
- Blood must be taken for T cell subset and chromosomal analysis to establish whether the baby has the syndrome. The sample must be taken before any blood products are administered as they could affect the results of the chromosomal analysis
- The baby must be monitored for hypocalcaemia and the associated effects. This is a feature of Di George syndrome as there is absence of the parathyroid glands. Administration of prescribed calcium should preferably be via a central venous line as extravasation of calcium into a peripheral line will cause a significant burn to the tissues
- There is a risk of infection in children with Di George syndrome due to the congenital absence of a thymus with the subsequent reduction in immunocompetence. Irradiated, cytomegalovirus negative blood must be ordered from the transfusion department. Non-irradiated blood products must not be given to the patient due to the reduction in immunocompetence

anastomosis. The right radial and femoral artery or umbilical artery are usually chosen. This then allows any pressure gradient to be assessed across the repair and evaluation of the perfusion of the separate upper and lower body circulation during cardiopulmonary bypass[9].
- Median sternotomy.
- Two arterial cannula are placed. Deep hypothermic circulatory arrest, cooling the baby to 18°C is undertaken. The flow through the distal body is maintained by the PDA until this time.
- The PDA is ligated, the interrupted segments anastomosed and the VSD closed. A pulmonary artery band may be considered if VSD closure is not possible at this time.

Key postoperative management issues

The postoperative management of the baby is critical and is influenced by the baby's condition preoperatively (see Table 4.12). This once lethal condition has dramatically improved chances of survival due to the advent of prostaglandin E_1[80]. In 1974 there was an approximately 70% chance of death up to two weeks postoperatively and just 13 years later, only an approximately 10% risk[9]. This remarkable change around may be attributed to two main areas:

- The importance of preoperative resuscitation[9].
- The management of neonates.

Table 4.12 Assessment and management of potential postoperative problems in IAA (for detailed management of individual problems, see Chapters 10–13)

Haemorrhage due to the numerous suture lines, preoperative neonatal coagulopathy, friability of tissue due to the severity of preoperative acidosis

Multi-organ failure after bypass if the preoperative condition has been critical

Residual VSD

Phrenic nerve damage

Late complications

- Potential pressure gradient across the arch — this is significantly reduced in patients who have had a direct anastomosis[9]. A balloon dilatation in the cardiac catheter laboratory can relieve most gradients[84, 88]. However, some require re-operation.
- Potential left ventricular outflow tract obstruction — this is not uncommon in patients with an associated perimembranous VSD[9, 80]. It usually requires surgical relief of the obstruction several years after initial repair.
- Potential left bronchial obstruction — the left main bronchus passes under the aortic arch. If the anastomosis was tight it can result in air being trapped in the left lung, shown on chest x-ray. This rare complication can be prevented by adequate mobilisation of the ascending and descending aorta[9]. Should it occur, an ascending to descending aortic conduit may be necessary.

Long-term follow-up

- Life-long antibiotic prophylaxis is necessary for dental extractions and other surgical procedures.
- Life-long regular follow-up in the outpatient department.

Vascular ring and sling

Aetiology

This lesion accounts for approximately 1% of all congenital heart disease[4]. It is associated with other defects, namely TOF, VSD, ASD[89] and is an important consideration in patients with upper airway obstruction[90].

Definition

The term vascular ring encompasses several anomalies in which abnormal branches of the aortic arch surround and compress the trachea and oesophagus. If the encircling is complete, it is known as a vascular ring, if incomplete, a sling. See Figures 4.8–4.11.

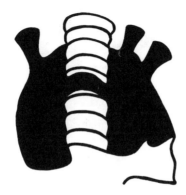

Figure 4.8 Vascular ring — double aortic arch

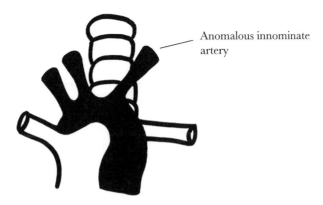

Anomalous innominate artery

Figure 4.9 Vascular sling — anomalous innominate artery

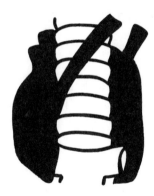

Figure 4.10 Vascular ring — right aortic arch and ligamentum

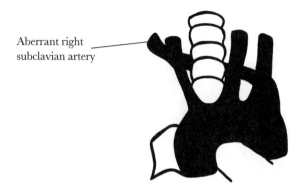

Aberrant right
subclavian artery

Figure 4.11 Aberrant right subclavian artery

Embryology

In the developing embryo, there are six pairs of aortic arches which develop into facial arteries, pulmonary arteries, the carotid artery and aortic arch branches. Should these structures fail to fuse and reabsorb, a vascular ring or sling will occur[9].

Anatomy and pathophysiology

Several abnormal structures can arise:
- Double aortic arch (left and right arches): This forms the ascending aorta where both left and right arches join to meet the ascending

aorta. The right arch is normally the dominant one. This is known as a vascular ring (Figure 4.8).
- Anomalies in the innominate artery — a vascular sling (Figure 4.9).
- Right aortic arch and left ligamentum — a vascular ring (Figure 4.10).
- Aberrant right subclavian artery — a vascular ring (Figure 4.11).

Whatever the presentation, the ring causes obstruction of the airways by encircling both the trachea and oesophagus.

Signs and symptoms

Symptoms present in early infancy if significant.

Cardiovascular signs and symptoms

- Normal findings.

Respiratory signs and symptoms

- Respiratory distress.
- Stridor and wheeze which reduce when the patient is sitting up.
- History of chest infections from aspiration of feeds flowing into the lungs (not reflux).
- Cyanosis indicates severe obstruction leading to respiratory arrest, bronchomalacia, tracheomalacia.

Other signs and symptoms

- Dysphagia especially when solids are introduced.
- Failure to thrive.

Diagnosis

- Chest x-ray: Pneumonia — consolidation and atelectasis. The x-ray is always abnormal[91].
- Angiography: Gives the most accurate diagnosis.
- MRI: is very informative.
- Bronchoscopy: Diagnostic.
- Barium swallow: Diagnostic.
- Oesophagoscopy: Diagnostic.

Key preoperative management issues

The key preoperative management issues are shown in Table 4.13.

Table 4.13 Assessment and management of potential preoperative problems in a child with a vascular ring (for detailed management of individual problems, see Chapters 10 and 13)

Respiratory distress. Place the child in an upright position to minimise tracheal compression and subsequent dyspnoea

Failure to thrive

Surgical management

The indications for surgery are the presence of symptoms. The procedure is normally by a left thoracotomy whereby the vascular ring is divided. Mobilising the tissue surrounding the trachea and oesophagus is required[20]. Aortoplexy may be considered if tracheomalacia and compression of the trachea are present.

Key postoperative management issues

The key postoperative management issues are shown in Table 4.14.

Table 4.14 Assessment and management of potential postoperative problems in a child with a vascular ring (for detailed management of individual problems, see Chapter 10)

Increased secretions released by surgical intervention. Pulmonary toileting is very important

Localised oedema at the site of operation, causing the same symptoms as preoperatively, can take days to settle so the child may not appear to have improved postoperatively

Persistent respiratory distress if the obstruction was severe. This may be present for several months after surgery

Long-term follow-up

- If the obstruction was severe, the baby will still need to be placed in an upright position to relieve the tracheal compression and prevent aspiration of feeds from oesophagus. Thirty per cent of patients can have upper and lower airway symptoms on late follow-up[92].

- Otherwise, the baby should be able to enjoy a normal life.

Chapter 5
Cyanotic defects

Tetralogy of Fallot (TOF)

Aetiology

This is the most common lesion of the cyanotic group accounting for approximately 5–10% of congenital heart disease[3, 4, 10, 20]. It may present in conjunction with other congenital heart diseases: aortopulmonary window, atrioventricular septal defect, vascular ring[93] and with non-cardiac anomalies such as: Di George syndrome, tracheo-oesophageal fistula and imperforate anus. Without treatment, approximately 50% of children die before the age of three[3].

Definition

Tetralogy of Fallot (TOF) was first described in detail by Fallot in 1888[10]. It is a cyanotic lesion with right to left shunting, characterised by four main anomalies (see Figure 5.1):

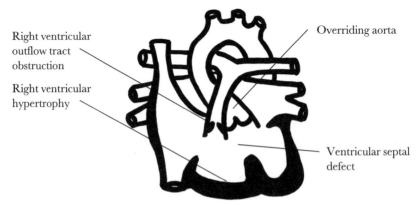

Right ventricular outflow tract obstruction

Right ventricular hypertrophy

Overriding aorta

Ventricular septal defect

Figure 5.1 Tetralogy of Fallot (TOF)

- Ventricular septal defect (VSD).
- Right ventricular outflow tract obstruction (RVOTO).
- Overriding aorta.
- Right ventricular hypertrophy.

However, the VSD and RVOTO are essentially the two main components of TOF, the severity of which is solely based upon the degree of the infundibular and pulmonary valve abnormalities.

Anatomy and pathophysiology

In relation to the formation of the embryonic heart, tetralogy is the abnormal development of the infundibulum causing varying degrees of RVOTO. The most common form of obstruction is a hypoplastic infundibulum with mild stenosis of the pulmonary valve[9]. This abnormal development, or hypoplasia, results in a hypoplastic, displaced, short, thin and shallow infundibulum[9]. Consequently, these features cause malalignment of the infundibular septum producing a large unrestricted outlet VSD and overriding of the aorta in varying degrees; the severe form being double outlet right ventricle, discussed in Chapter 6.

The right ventricular hypertrophy is attributed to the degree of right ventricular outflow tract obstruction and the presence of an unrestricted VSD.

Haemodynamics

The haemodynamic features in response to TOF are related to the degree of RVOTO. Pressures in both ventricles are normally equal. In mild pulmonary and infundibular stenosis, there is little shunting across the VSD as pulmonary blood flow resistance is similar to systemic resistance[10]. If however, pulmonary and infundibular stenosis is significant, the resistance to flow causes a right to left shunt through the VSD[11]. This produces varying degrees of cyanosis as the greater the resistance to pulmonary blood flow, the larger the right to left shunt[10]. Additionally, as the baby becomes older, the degree of infundibular obstruction, due to muscle hypertrophy, increases resulting in a greater degree of cyanosis[20]. Furthermore, crying and exercising may predispose to episodes of cyanosis. The stenosis does have the advantage of protecting the lungs from high pressure/high flow systemic blood as would happen in the presence of a VSD without pulmonary stenosis. Pulmonary hypertension, however, can occur as a result of an elevated packed cell volume with reduced pulmonary blood flow[94]. The low pulmonary blood flow is the cause of the raised blood viscosity[10].

To summarise, the venous blood enters the right ventricle via the right atrium. Most blood flows into the area of least resistance, that is, the left ventricle and on into the aorta. Subsequently, there is little flow of deoxygenated blood into the lungs and reduced flow from the lungs, potentially giving rise to a hypoplastic left ventricle[20].

Signs and symptoms

Cardiovascular signs and symptoms

At birth there is usually a left to right shunt. As the degree of infundibular obstruction increases, a right to left shunt develops. Congestive heart failure can occur from three months if there is mild pulmonary stenosis. The pulses are full and bounding.

Respiratory signs and symptoms

At birth there is likely to be minimal cyanosis due to the lungs receiving an adequate flow from the patent ductus arteriosus. Once the duct closes, the degree of cyanosis is dependent on the level of RVOTO but by 4–6 months this will be progressive due to increasing infundibular obstruction. Furthermore, cyanosis will be exacerbated by crying and exercising. Respiratory distress, hypoxaemia, acidosis, and "spelling" develop (see below).

Neurological signs and symptoms

Cerebral abscess and cerebral vascular accident can occur if the cyanosis is severe and untreated.

Haematological signs and symptoms

Polycythaemia develops as a compensatory mechanism to hypoxaemia, increasing the risk of cerebral vascular accident. Hypervolaemia and an increased red cell count with a packed cell volume of approximately 0.55% occurs. The patient is prone to bleeding as thrombocytopenia is present.

Gastrointestinal signs and symptoms

Poor feeding as the baby is too tired to feed due to the hypoxaemia. The older child can be poorly nourished if untreated.

Sepsis

Increased risk of bacterial endocarditis due to cyanosis.

Other signs and symptoms

If the child has presented late or has not been operated on at an early age, squatting (see below) and clubbing of the fingers and toes due to the effects of chronic cyanosis will develop. This is rarely seen in developed countries.

Diagnosis

- Auscultation: Systolic murmur.
- ECG: Right ventricular hypertrophy.
- Chest x-ray: Classic boot-shaped heart due to the small pulmonary artery. In approximately 25% of patients the aortic arch is on the right.
- Echocardiography: Diagnostic. Doppler studies show the ventricular pressures.
- Cardiac catheterisation: Measures the left and right ventricular pressures and saturation of oxygen. Angiography shows the degree of RVOTO and pulmonary artery anatomy.

Cyanotic "spelling"

This is representative of a sudden severe reduction in pulmonary blood flow and is a unique feature of TOF. It can occur from infancy, in mild or severe tetralogy and usually as a result of crying and feeding during the morning[10], although it can occur after a period of rest and factors causing vasodilation, e.g., warm bath, warm bed. The parents are usually the first to report the episodes which must be taken seriously. See Figure 5.2.

Signs and symptoms of a spell

A spell can occur at any age producing hypercyanosis, accompanied by crying as if in pain or irritability. The baby becomes pale, breathless, sweaty, limp and unconscious with hypoxia, acidosis, hypercapnia, myocardial hypoperfusion (low cardiac output) and cerebral hypoperfusion (potential brain damage). Once the cycle is broken, the infundibulum relaxes and the infant regains consciousness.

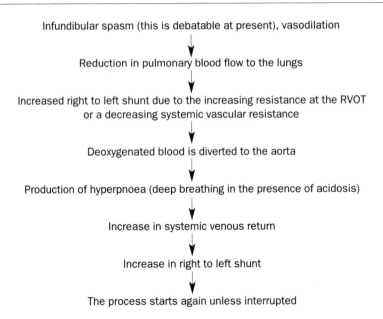

Infundibular spasm (this is debatable at present), vasodilation

Reduction in pulmonary blood flow to the lungs

Increased right to left shunt due to the increasing resistance at the RVOT or a decreasing systemic vascular resistance

Deoxygenated blood is diverted to the aorta

Production of hyperpnoea (deep breathing in the presence of acidosis)

Increase in systemic venous return

Increase in right to left shunt

The process starts again unless interrupted

Figure 5.2 Mechanism of a cyanotic spell[4]

Treatment of a cyanotic spell

This is discussed in detail below. However, a baby can die during a cyanotic spell so surgery should be planned as a matter of urgency, once a history of spelling has been established.

Squatting

This phenomenon is also attributed to TOF and although a classic sign of a child with tetralogy, squatting is rarely seen in developed countries due to early surgical intervention. It usually occurs when the toddler has exercised, resulting in the child bringing his knees up to his chest, and is thought to:

- Decrease venous return from the lower limbs by flexing the legs. This allows the arterial oxygen to increase gradually[3].
- Reduce the right to left shunt by increasing systemic arterial blood flow. This subsequently increases pulmonary blood flow[10].

Key preoperative management issues

The key preoperative management issues are shown in Table 5.1.

Table 5.1 Assessment and management of potential preoperative problems in TOF (for detailed management of individual problems, see Chapters 10 and 12)

Cyanosis

Bacterial endocarditis

Haemorrhage due to the thrombocytopenia associated with polycythaemia

Increased risk of cerebral abscess due to hypoxaemia

Cyanotic spelling — prevention is the aim. As most spells will occur at home and be quite mild in nature, advising the parents what to do in the event of a cyanotic spell is important — see below. If the spell is severe all steps must be followed as the child will be hospitalised
- During the spell, hold the child over an adult's shoulder or in the knee–chest position
- Administer oxygen
- Administer prescribed propranolol — if the patient is on the maximum oral dose, the intravenous dose cannot be given. The patient can stay on the beta blocker until surgery is performed. It is thought to reduce the infundibular spasm
- Administer prescribed IV morphine at 0.1 mg/kg. Morphine, being a respiratory depressant will correct hyperpnoea[4]
- Administer prescribed phenylephrine which increases the systemic vascular resistance and encourages blood flow to the lungs[4]
- Acidosis must be treated aggressively with intravenous sodium bicarbonate and blood gases checked accordingly
- If this occurs in the toddler, exercise does not have to be restricted as the toddler will self-restrict

Medical management

Most children will undergo cardiac catheterisation and pulmonary valvuloplasty although this will depend on the cardiologist's preferred method of treatment.

Surgical management

Surgery for TOF can be staged. However, this choice remains controversial.

Palliative surgery

The aim of palliative surgery is to increase pulmonary blood flow in the severely cyanotic infant. It usually consists of a modified Blalock–Taussig shunt[95] (see Chapter 6). In some centres it is required in approximately 50% of patients should a total correction be postponed past early infancy[96]. However, it is associated with risks, the main one being pulmonary artery hypoplasia[97].

Corrective surgery

This carries an approximate 5% risk of mortality[10, 20]. It is usually performed from four months of age. However, in some centres, surgeons prefer to do a total correction in the newborn period[96, 98–101]. Both approaches have pros and cons — if the surgery is performed in the newborn it will prevent the baby from developing the complications associated with cyanosis and spelling. Additionally, primary repair within the first year of life is shown to have a faster regression of right ventricular hypertrophy thus reducing the risk of impaired myocardial function and the potential for arrhythmias[102]. However, surgery in the younger patient can be associated with a greater degree of mortality and morbidity.

The main indications for surgery are increasing and/or uncontrollable hypoxaemia, the oxygen saturations generally being below 80% and the packed cell volume, being approximately 60%. It has the aim to relieve the RVOTO and close the VSD. Risks are increased when the baby has underdeveloped pulmonary arteries and left ventricle[20].

Surgical procedure

- Median sternotomy.
- Cardiopulmonary bypass.
- Taking down any palliative shunts if present.
- A transatrial approach is preferred to avoid a ventriculotomy.
- The VSD is closed.
- The RVOTO is resected/reconstructed/widened as required. Widening of the outflow tract is accomplished with a transannular patch if the tract is hypoplastic or small. There are associated complications with using a transannular patch — pulmonary valve incompetence and potential right ventricular failure, which may not be a problem unless there is a residual pulmonary stenosis. An alternative to the transannular patch is a pulmonary homograft.

Key postoperative management issues

The key postoperative mangement issues are shown in Table 5.2.

Late complications

- Ventricular arrhythmias resulting in sudden death which is related to a late repair of the condition[103].
- There is a small risk of severe pulmonary valve insufficiency (although in the majority of patients it is quite mild) with the use of a transannular

Table 5.2 Assessment and management of potential postoperative problems in TOF (for detailed management of individual problems, see Chapters 11 and 12)

Heart block due to the patch repair of the septum

Bleeding due to the chronic thrombocytopenia

Congestive heart failure due to residual VSD

Right ventricular failure — this can occur if a ventriculotomy is performed resulting in low cardiac output. Additionally, right ventricular failure may occur due to a residual RVOTO or VSD:
- Right ventricular failure requires a central venous pressure of 16–18mm Hg to increase contractility and overcome right sided heart obstruction[38]. This can be achieved by infusing plasma
- Capillary leak may subsequently occur with fluid overload so diuretics must be administered
- Pleural effusions and ascites may develop requiring chest drains and a peritoneal catheter to drain the fluid
- After the patient has been fluid loaded, inotropes must be considered to support the left side of the heart
- Digitalisation is normally required

---

patch. This may result in a pulmonary valve homograft replacement.
- Residual RVOTO and VSD require re-operation.

Long-term follow-up

- Electrophysiological studies and haemodynamic evaluation are required due to potential ventricular arrhythmias.
- Exercise may have to be limited due to reduced exercise tolerance especially in the patient with a transannular patch[104].
- Antibiotic prophylaxis is required for life.

Pulmonary atresia with VSD (PA VSD)

Aetiology

This defect accounts for approximately 1% of congenital heart disease[3]. It is more frequent in males than females and is linked with the incidence of Di George syndrome.

Definition

Pulmonary atresia with ventricular septal defect (PA VSD) can be thought of as the extreme form of tetralogy of Fallot, with severe pulmonary stenosis and no communication between the right ventricle and pulmonary artery. It is a cyanotic lesion with right to left shunting across the VSD. The positioning of the atresia may vary. In two-thirds of cases pulmonary blood flow is dependent upon the presence of a PDA and in one third of cases, major aortopulmonary collateral arteries (MAPCAs) will develop[4].

Classification

The classification is dependent on the size and origin of the pulmonary blood supply[9]:

- Type 1 has well-developed pulmonary arteries. The pulmonary blood supply is reliant upon the presence of a PDA (see Figure 5.3).

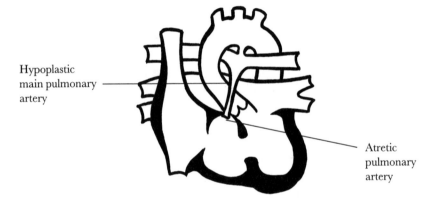

Hypoplastic
main pulmonary
artery

Atretic
pulmonary
artery

Figure 5.3 Pulmonary atresia with VSD — Type I

- Type ll has well-developed pulmonary arteries but the main pulmonary artery can be absent. The pulmonary blood supply is reliant on the presence of a PDA (see Figure 5.4).
- Type lll has hypoplastic pulmonary arteries which can be disconnected from each other. The main pulmonary artery is absent. The pulmonary blood supply is via the MAPCAs. There is a small PDA (see Figure 5.5).
- Type lV has no pulmonary arteries, main pulmonary artery, or PDA so totally relies upon the presence of MAPCAs for pulmonary blood supply (see Figure 5.6).

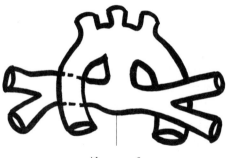

Absence of
main pulmonary artery

Figure 5.4 Pulmonary atresia with VSD — Type II

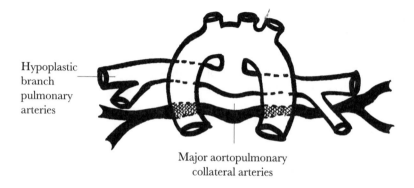

Hypoplastic
branch
pulmonary
arteries

Major aortopulmonary
collateral arteries

Figure 5.5 Pulmonary atresia with VSD — Type III

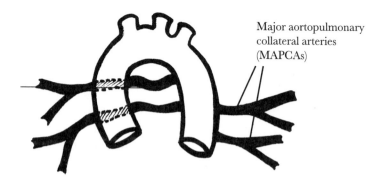

Major aortopulmonary
collateral arteries
(MAPCAs)

Figure 5.6 Pulmonary atresia with VSD — Type IV

Anatomy and pathophysiology

Blood empties from the venae cavae into the right atrium, through the tricuspid valve and into the right ventricle. Blood shunts from the right ventricle across the VSD into the aorta, mixing deoxygenated blood with oxygenated blood, giving rise to cyanosis.

Pulmonary blood flow is reliant on a PDA and the MAPCAs, if present, as the central source of pulmonary blood is usually poor. The collateral blood supply normally develops off the aortic arch from branches of brachial arteries, which join pulmonary arteries before entering the lungs. The vessels are large until reaching the lungs where stenosis may occur[3], minimising the risk of pulmonary vascular obstructive disease. However, if there is no collateral circulation and the PDA closes, the baby will collapse due to profound cyanosis and hypoxia. The lungs receive blood from the collateral arteries and/or PDA. Blood re-enters the heart via the pulmonary veins but as there is reduced pulmonary blood flow, the left ventricle can be small. The atresia may occur in either the infundibular, valve or pulmonary artery areas or in a combination of each. The other anatomical and physiological aspects of this lesion are similar to those of tetralogy of Fallot.

Signs and symptoms

The signs and symptoms are present at birth or shortly afterwards.

Cardiovascular signs and symptoms

- If no collateral circulation, collapse will occur once the PDA closes.
- Increased pulse volume.
- Rarely, congestive heart failure if there is increased pulmonary blood flow.

Respiratory signs and symptoms

- Severe cyanosis at birth, its degree depends on flow through the PDA and the collateral circulation.
- Hypoxia when the PDA closes as there is no collateral circulation.
- Pulmonary vascular obstructive disease in the presence of a collateral circulation.

Gastrointestinal signs and symptoms

- Failure to thrive in the presence of MAPCAs or a severe reduction in pulmonary blood flow.

Renal signs and symptoms

- Metabolic acidosis when the PDA closes.

Diagnosis

- Auscultation: No murmur.
- ECG: Right ventricular hypertrophy.
- Chest x-ray: Normal heart size but boot-shaped appearance of heart. Decreased pulmonary vascular markings unless MAPCAs large and absent pulmonary artery.
- Echocardiography: Diagnostic.
- Cardiac catheterisation with angiography: For assessment of collateral circulation and size of pulmonary arteries.

Key preoperative management issues

The key preoperative management issues are shown in Table 5.3.

Table 5.3 Assessment and management of potential preoperative problems in PA VSD (for detailed management of individual problems, see Chapters 6 and 10–12)

Immediate establishment and maintenance of a PDA to temporarily secure pulmonary blood flow

Treatment of metabolic acidosis, hypoxia and multi-organ failure should the PDA have closed

Management of neonatal coagulopathy

Establishment of a more secure pulmonary blood flow

Later, management of congestive cardiac failure if collateral blood supply large

Medical and surgical management

Staged intervention is usually necessary with the ultimate aim of establishing a right ventricular dependent pulmonary circulation[9]. The plan of treatment can be difficult and vary enormously for each patient with risks from 5–50%.

Initial medical management includes:

- Maintenance of the PDA.
- Pulmonary valvotomy by ablation of the atretic valve in the catheter laboratory. Additionally, cardiac catheterisation may dilate stenotic pulmonary arteries and occlude MAPCAs once detailed angiograms have identified their individual blood supply.

Surgical management

Surgical management is tailored to the individual patient as there are many anatomical variables to take into account.

- Good sized central pulmonary artery: A primary repair can be undertaken when the central pulmonary artery is of good size. This involves placing a conduit between the right ventricle and the central pulmonary artery. The VSD is closed.
- Small pulmonary arteries: Should the branch pulmonary arteries be small, a central shunt is performed on the main pulmonary artery to stimulate growth of the branch pulmonary arteries. This will make unifocalisation easier.
- Presence of MAPCAs: In the majority of cases, MAPCAs are stenotic. If the child is well oxygenated, surgical correction can be elective. If the stenosis is severe with hypoxia, a shunt should be performed early. Rarely there is no stenosis with systemic pressures in the MAPCAs.

The aim of the surgery is to recruit blood vessels for each segment of the lung then reconnect them to the heart. This unifocalisation of the pulmonary blood flow (MAPCAs) or anastomosis of the vessels to a branch pulmonary artery will promote growth of the branch pulmonary arteries. Single stage unifocalisation is now being performed with excellent results[105]. At the same time as the unifocalisation, a right ventricle conduit to the pulmonary artery can be created[106]. Should the pulmonary arteries not be of adequate size, a modified central shunt can be performed and the VSD left open. This will further enhance growth of the pulmonary arteries with the increased intracardiac shunt becoming left to right and congestive heart failure developing. This is the indication for closure of the VSD. Should the pulmonary arteries not grow, only palliative surgery can be undertaken with a view to heart–lung transplantation at a later date.

Key postoperative management issues

The key postoperative management issues are shown in Table 5.4.

Table 5.4 Assessment and management of potential postoperative problems in PA VSD (for detailed management of individual problems, see Chapters 10–12)

Congestive heart failure related to a large modified BT shunt, remaining collateral circulation or pulmonary insufficiency from regurgitation of blood from the pulmonary artery to the right ventricle

Pulmonary vascular obstructive disease related to a large modified BT shunt or large left to right shunt

Residual hypoxia and cyanosis related to the modified BT shunt being too small

Low cardiac output related to compression of the right ventricle to pulmonary artery conduit if the chest is closed

Right ventricular dysfunction due to stenosis of the conduit, resulting in an increase in right ventricular pressure. If the VSD was closed in the presence of small pulmonary arteries, this may also cause right ventricular dysfunction

Haemorrhage may occur due to the multiple suture lines when unifocalisation is performed

Complications pertaining to the VSD surgery — see section on VSD, Chapter 3

Long-term follow-up

- Indefinite antibiotic prophylaxis.
- Exercise restriction in most patients will be required.
- Follow-up for life.

Pulmonary atresia with intact ventricular septum (PA IVS)

Aetiology

This defect accounts for 1–3% of congenital heart disease[3, 4, 20, 55].

Definition

Pulmonary atresia with intact ventricular septum (PA IVS) can be described as hypoplastic right heart syndrome in which the pulmonary valve is atretic with varying degrees of right ventricle and tricuspid valve hypoplasia. The pulmonary arteries are usually of normal size[107] due to having a blood supply from the patent ductus arteriosus (PDA). The baby is dependent on a PDA and intra-atrial communication[44]. This lesion represents a wide spectrum of anomalies which determine the patient's management. It is a cyanotic defect with right to left shunting at atrial level (see Figure 5.7).

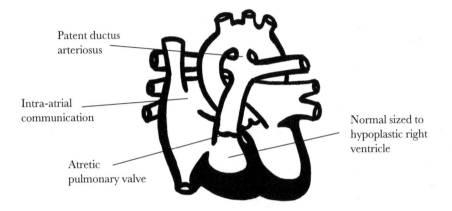

Patent ductus arteriosus

Intra-atrial communication

Normal sized to hypoplastic right ventricle

Atretic pulmonary valve

Figure 5.7 Pulmonary atresia with intact ventricular septum

Anatomy and pathophysiology

Anatomy

The right ventricle is small and hypoplastic in the majority of cases. In the normal right ventricle, there are three compartments — inlet, trabecular and outlet[108]. In PA IVS, only two compartments are commonly found. However, if the right ventricle is severely hypoplastic, there may only be one compartment[3]. Alternatively, all three compartments may be present but each is hypoplastic.

The pulmonary valve is atretic and the tricuspid valve is affected by either becoming thickened, having fused cusps, or resembling the tricuspid valve found in Ebstein's anomaly[20, 109]. The coronary arteries may be dilated due to the retrograde blood flow from the presence of sinusoids which are irregular channels in which blood vessels anastomose. This may result in ischaemic ventricles[110] and suprasystemic right ventricular pressures.

Pathophysiology

Blood enters the right atrium from the venae cavae and either flows through the tricuspid valve into the hypoplastic right ventricle or passes directly across the intra-atrial communication. If the blood passes into the right ventricle, it will not be able to enter the main pulmonary artery due to the atretic valve, so flows back into the right atrium — tricuspid regurgitation. This causes hypertrophy of the right atrium with a concomitant increase in right atrial pressure, causing the reopening of the foramen ovale. Blood therefore flows into the left atrium across this communication allowing systemic venous blood to mix with pulmonary venous blood resulting in cyanosis.

Pulmonary blood flow would be absent if it were not for the presence of a ductus arteriosus which enables the flow of systemic blood into the pulmonary arterial circulation. Additionally, sinusoids may be present between the right ventricle and coronary arteries providing an extra communication so as to decompress the elevated suprasystemic right ventricular pressure[111, 112]. There may be coronary artery anomalies such as stenosis or atresia, which can significantly alter the prognosis[113, 114].

Signs and symptoms

This defect presents at birth with increasing cyanosis as the child develops.

Cardiovascular signs and symptoms

- Collapse as the PDA closes.
- Congestive heart failure with systemic venous obstruction, elevated right atrial pressure and suprasystemic right ventricular pressures.
- Tricuspid valve regurgitation.
- Sinusoids cause low cardiac output. This is due to ischaemic left and right ventricles from the dilated coronary arteries. Ventricular arrythmias may occur due to the associated myocardial ischaemia.

Respiratory signs and symptoms

- Increasingly severe hypoxia and cyanosis as the PDA closes.
- Tachypnoea.

Gastrointestinal signs and symptoms

- Enlarged liver due to systemic venous congestion.

Renal signs and symptoms

- Increasing metabolic acidosis.

Other signs and symptoms

- Periorbital oedema due to systemic venous obstruction.

Diagnosis

- Auscultation: Murmur from the PDA.
- ECG: Right atrial hypertrophy, left ventricular hypertrophy.
- Chest x-ray: Normal sized heart with reduced pulmonary blood flow.
- Echocardiography: Diagnostic. Doppler shows absent blood flow through the pulmonary valve.
- Cardiac catheterisation: Angiograms are required to examine the coronary blood flow. Right ventricular pressures measured.

Key preoperative management issues

The key preoperative management issues are shown in Table 5.5.

Table 5.5 Assessment and management of potential preoperative problems in PA IVS (for detailed management of individual problems, see Chapters 10–12)

Immediate establishment and maintenance of a PDA to temporarily secure pulmonary blood flow

Treatment of metabolic acidosis, hypoxia and multi-organ failure should the PDA have closed

Management of neonatal coagulopathy

Preparation of the baby for cardiac catheter

Low cardiac output due to the presence of sinusoids

Congestive heart failure due to the presence of sinusoids

Detection and management of ventricular arrhythmias due to myocardial ischaemia caused by the presence of sinusoids

Medical and surgical management

The aims of treatment are to establish a pulmonary blood flow, decompress the right ventricle and create a systemic and pulmonary circulation. Risk of mortality can be as high as 15–20%[20] and will depend on the size of the right ventricle and the presence of sinusoids, which are associated with a poorer prognosis.

Right ventricle of adequate size

A transannular patch or closed transcatheter pulmonary valvotomy is performed to connect the right ventricle and main pulmonary artery. This decompresses the right ventricle and allows for its growth along with the tricuspid valve. A transcatheter is becoming the procedure of choice as it is both safe and effective. A two ventricle circulation can be achieved in the majority of patients despite subnormal right ventricular growth[115, 116]. A modified Blalock–Taussig shunt will be required if the prostaglandin E_1 infusion cannot be weaned after valvotomy so as to maintain the pulmonary blood flow and increase the saturations of oxygen until the right ventricle has grown sufficiently. The shunt can be closed in the catheter laboratory at a later date[3, 4, 117]. If the right ventricle does not grow, a Fontan procedure will be required (see Chapter 6).

Hypoplastic right ventricle with sinusoids

A modified BT shunt is performed to increase the pulmonary blood supply. As perfusion of the coronary arteries is retrograde through to the right ventricle, systemic pressure may need to be maintained in the right ventricle. Thus decompression of the right ventricle may predispose to ischaemia of the myocardium. A Fontan procedure will be required at a later date[118, 119] (see Chapter 6).

Long-term follow-up

- Antibiotic prophylaxis will be required for life.
- Long-term survival rates are variable for patients who have undergone a Fontan procedure.
- Exercise tolerance will depend on any residual problems.

Transposition of the great arteries (TGA)

Aetiology

Transposition of the great arteries (TGA) is the second most common cyanotic heart lesion accounting for 4–5% of all congenital heart disease[3, 4]. It is frequently associated with other anomalies — ASD, VSD, DORV[9], pulmonary stenosis and VSD[4]. TGA is found to be more prevalent in boys than girls in a ratio of 3:1. If left untreated approximately 90% will die during the first year of life[9].

Definition

The aorta arises from the right ventricle anteriorly and the pulmonary artery from the left ventricle posteriorly. This can further be described as atrioventricular concordance with ventriculoarterial discordance. If no other cardiac defect is present, it is termed simple transposition, whereas the presence of other defects reclassifies it as complex transposition, see Figures 5.8 and 5.9.

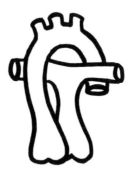

Figure 5.8 Transposition of the great arteries

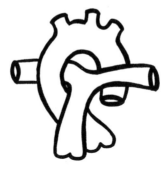

Figure 5.9 Normal position of the aorta and pulmonary artery

Anatomy and pathophysiology

TGA has wide variations in its anatomical presentation[120]. It was initially thought to occur as a result of inappropriate septation and spiralling of the truncus arteriosus during embryonic development[10]. However, the cause of TGA is now thought to be attributable to the abnormal growth of the subpulmonary and subaortic infundibular muscle areas[121].

With the aorta being dextrotransposed (D-transposition), that is, lying anteriorly to the pulmonary artery, two separate circulations occur. Venous blood enters the right atrium from the venae cavae, passing through the tricuspid valve into the right ventricle. From here, deoxygenated blood enters the aorta into the systemic circulation. Oxygenated blood from the lungs enters the left atrium, passes to the left ventricle and into the pulmonary artery, thus re-entering the lungs. This is only compatible with life in the presence of a structure allowing the mixing of oxygenated and deoxygenated blood. Therefore, once the patent ductus arteriosus starts to close, a neonate will become profoundly cyanotic, acidotic and will collapse without the aid of an ASD or VSD. Additionally, the number of communications and degree of shunting that occurs through the communication depict the neonate's level of oxygenation (see Table 5.6). However, the increased pulmonary blood flow in patients with or without VSDs predisposes the infant to an increase in pulmonary artery pressure with subsequent development of pulmonary vascular obstructive disease making early surgical intervention a necessity. In infants with severe pulmonary hypertension, the outcome is not necessarily fatal and can be reversed by surgery[122].

Table 5.6 The haemodynamic effects of various defects

Defect	Effect of communication on haemodynamics
TGA and PDA	Bidirectional shunting occurs until the pulmonary vascular resistance falls upon which blood shunts from the aorta into the pulmonary artery[3, 10]. A more permanent source of shunt will then be required until definitive surgery is performed
TGA and PFO	A neonate with a restrictive PFO will present with severe cyanosis and hypoxia. However, if the PFO is large, bidirectional shunting will occur minimising the cyanosis and hypoxia[4, 10]
TGA and VSD	Again, depending on the size of VSD, bidirectional shunting can occur, that is, during ventricular diastole, a left to right shunt occurs and a right to left shunt in ventricular systole[9, 10]. This provides oxygenation of the systemic circulation until pulmonary vascular resistance falls. The shunt then becomes right to left with blood flowing into the pulmonary artery, under high pressure, predisposing to congestive heart failure and pulmonary vascular obstructive disease. Nonetheless, a higher degree of saturated oxygen will be observed than in simple transposition. Pulmonary venous return will therefore be increased resulting in a left to right shunt at atrial level, across the foramen ovale[10] again providing a means of oxygenating the severely hypoxic systemic circulation
TGA and VSD with pulmonary stenosis	In the neonate with moderate pulmonary stenosis, the lungs will be protected from high pressure, high blood flow, thus making the development of pulmonary vascular obstructive disease and congestive heart failure less likely[3, 4, 10]. In contrast, severe pulmonary stenosis will significantly reduce pulmonary blood flow predisposing the baby to severe hypoxia and acidosis. Additionally, an elevation in left ventricular pressure results in left to right shunting

Signs and symptoms

Simple transposition: Despite the classification, infants with simple transposition are often initially the most sick as they are solely reliant upon a PDA. Presentation usually occurs during the first day of life. Sudden death may occur if the PDA and/or the PFO close[123].

Cardiovascular signs and symptoms

- Precordium is quiet.
- Pulses normal.
- Cardiovascular collapse when PDA closes.

Respiratory signs and symptoms

- Increasingly severe cyanosis as the duct closes.
- Developing hypoxia.
- Risk of pulmonary vascular obstructive disease later, if untreated.
- Dyspnoea.
- Tachypnoea.
- Hyperpnoea (deep breathing with use of abdominal muscles. Acidosis is usually present).

Renal signs and symptoms

- Increased metabolic acidosis when PDA closes

Complex transposition: If there is an ASD, VSD or PDA, the baby may not present for several weeks.

Cardiovascular signs and symptoms

- If a large VSD without pulmonary stenosis, congestive heart failure develops when the pulmonary vascular resistance falls at 2–6 weeks.

Respiratory signs and symptoms

- Varying levels of cyanosis depending on the degree of shunting.
- Increased pulmonary blood flow due to falling pulmonary vascular resistance resulting in an increase in pulmonary artery pressure and pulmonary vascular obstructive disease.

- Dyspnoea.
- Tachypnoea.

Gastrointestinal signs and symptoms

- History of poor feeding.
- Necrotising enterocolitis if hypoperfusion has occurred.

Diagnosis

- Auscultation: No murmur at birth.
- ECG: Persistent right ventricular hypertrophy due to right ventricular hypertension.
- Chest x-ray: Heart is of normal size. Due to the position of the aorta and pulmonary artery, the x-ray image resembles an egg on its side. Normal pulmonary vasculature.
- Echocardiography: Diagnostic, showing the abnormal positioning of the great vessels.

Key preoperative management issues

The key preoperative management issues are shown in Table 5.7.

Table 5.7 Assessment and management of potential preoperative problems in TGA (for detailed management of individual problems, see Chapters 10–12)

Simple TGA:
- Immediate establishment and maintenance of a PDA to temporarily secure systemic blood flow
- Treatment of metabolic acidosis, hypoxia and multi-organ failure should the PDA have closed
- Management of neonatal coagulopathy
- Urgent preparation of the neonate for an atrial septostomy should there be inadequate mixing of blood with just the PDA or if the PDA fails to open with prostaglandin E_1
- Low cardiac output

Complex TGA:
- Congestive heart failure if VSD present
- Pulmonary hypertension

Simple and complex TGA:
- Complications of chronic hypoxaemia

Medical management

Should severe hypoxia persist despite a PDA, an urgent balloon atrial septostomy will be performed to increase interatrial mixing of oxygenated and deoxygenated blood. This is referred to as the Rashkind procedure[124]. This is performed in the catheter laboratory or in emergency situations, on the intensive care unit under echocardiography control. If the neonate fails to increase arterial saturations after septostomy, the pulmonary vascular resistance is probably still too high and surgical intervention will be required. Neonates with TGA and a large VSD do not normally require such a procedure as adequate mixing of circulations usually occurs.

Surgical management

In the patient with simple transposition, an arterial switch procedure is performed electively within the first few weeks of life. Should the patient with a complex transposition present later, a switch procedure can be performed up to three months of age. After this there is the risk of the patient developing pulmonary vascular obstructive disease.

Palliative surgery

Pulmonary artery banding is considered for TGA with a large VSD. This will help in the prevention of pulmonary vascular obstructive disease and also train the left ventricle for a systemic circulation prior to definitive surgery. Occasionally, a modified BT shunt for TGA with pulmonary stenosis and VSD is performed.

Corrective surgery

Arterial switch (referred to as the Jatene procedure) is now the preferred method of correction for simple transposition, TGA with VSD, or Taussig–Bing anomaly[120, 125–127]. It is performed in patients with a left ventricle that can support the systemic circulation, and who have a normal pulmonary valve and a normal left ventricular outflow tract[20]. It is usually performed within the first few weeks of life, but is not attempted when pulmonary vascular resistance is too high, or when the pulmonary vascular resistance has fallen to such an extent that the musculature of the left ventricle has wasted[20].

The procedure for the switch operation is as follows:

- Median sternotomy.
- Cardiopulmonary bypass.
- Intracardiac defects repaired.
- Transection of both great vessels.

- Reimplantation of the coronary arteries to the old pulmonary artery, that is, the new aorta.
- Reconnection of the blood vessels to the anatomically correct position.
- Intracardiac shunts are closed.

Intra-atrial repair or venous switch procedures: the Mustard or Senning procedures are more or less obsolete but are described here as older patients may still present with associated problems.

Mustard procedure

- Atrial septum removed.
- A baffle is sutured into the atria to direct blood from the venae cavae through the baffle, to the mitral valve, left ventricle and into the pulmonary artery.
- Blood from the pulmonary veins enters the atria and is directed into the baffle, through the tricuspid valve, into the right ventricle and into the aorta.

Senning procedure

This is similar to the Mustard procedure but uses the patient's own tissue instead of prosthetic material.

Rastelli procedure

- This procedure is for the patient with TGA, VSD or severe pulmonary stenosis[120, 128]. The timing of surgery depends on the clinical condition and the desire to do the operation when the child is older so that the conduit can be of adult size. See Figure 5.10.

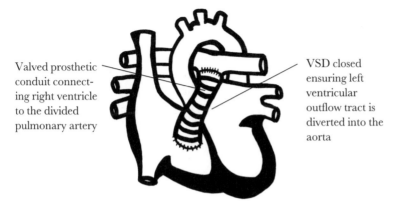

Valved prosthetic conduit connecting right ventricle to the divided pulmonary artery

VSD closed ensuring left ventricular outflow tract is diverted into the aorta

Figure 5.10 Rastelli procedure

- The pulmonary artery is divided from the left ventricle.
- An intracardiac patch is placed across the VSD incorporating the aorta into the left ventricle.
- The right ventricle is connected to the pulmonary artery by aortic homograft or valved conduit.

Key postoperative management issues

The key postoperative management issues are shown in Table 5.8.

Table 5.8 Assessment and management of potential postoperative problems in TGA (for detailed management of individual problems, see Chapters 10–12)

Arterial switch procedure:
- Myocardial ischaemia resulting in low cardiac output due to
  1. Poor left ventricular performance found initially in most infants following arterial switch[129]
  2. Obstruction to the coronary arteries due to reimplantation and kinking
  3. Debris in the coronary arteries following reimplantation
  4. Preoperative low cardiac output
- Haemorrhage due to the multiple suture lines and complications of polycythaemia
- Right ventricular dysfunction due to increased pulmonary vascular resistance preoperatively resulting in pulmonary hypertension

Intra-atrial procedures:
- Atrial and junctional arrhythmias
- Systemic venous return obstruction resulting in high superior vena cava pressures causing facial oedema or with high inferior vena cava pressures, ascites and liver obstruction. Balloon expandable stents for the obstruction have been shown to be effective and safe in the short term, and years after the initial surgery[130]
- Pulmonary venous obstruction resulting in pulmonary hypertension and pulmonary oedema
- Late myocardial failure as the anatomic right ventricle is still the systemic pump

Long-term complications

- After the arterial switch repair, aortic regurgitation, supravalvular pulmonary stenosis and coronary artery occlusion are associated long-term complications[131]. Late coronary artery complications are at present low, although results from long-term follow-up studies have yet to be established[132].
- After the intra-atrial repair, sudden death can occur, usually due to cardiac arrhythmias.
- Right ventricular failure may also occur.

Long-term follow-up

- Life-long follow-up will be required.
- Exercise limitation will be required should there be any residual complications.
- Antibiotic prophylaxis will be required for life.

Total anomalous pulmonary venous drainage (TAPVD)

Aetiology

Total anomalous pulmonary venous drainage (TAPVD) is responsible for approximately 1% of congenital heart disease[3, 4, 10]. The infracardiac type of disorder is the more common in boys[4]. Other defects linked with TAPVD include dextracardia and lung hypoplasia[133], tetralogy of Fallot and double outlet right ventricle[134], ventricular septal defect[3] and right atrial isomerism.

Definition

TAPVD is manifested as failure of the four pulmonary veins to drain into the left atrium. Instead, they connect directly or indirectly to the right atrium by way of the systemic veins. The correct nomenclature thus being total anomalous pulmonary venous connection.

Classification

The classifications of TAPVD are related to where the pulmonary veins connect to the systemic venous circulation. There are four types: supracardiac, cardiac, infracardiac and mixed. Additionally, each type may be obstructed or unobstructed, the management changing drastically if of the obstructed type.

Supracardiac

This accounts for approximately 45–50% of all cases[4, 9, 10]. The pulmonary veins connect to the systemic veins by a vertical vein which then joins the superior vena cava and empties into the right atrium. The unobstructed form is more common with this type and also with the cardiac type (see Figure 5.11).

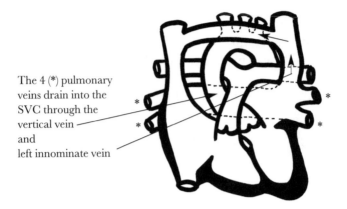

The 4 (*) pulmonary
veins drain into the
SVC through the
vertical vein
and
left innominate vein

Figure 5.11 Total anomalous pulmonary venous drainage — supracardiac

Cardiac

This is responsible for 20–25%[4, 9] of cases. The pulmonary veins connect directly to the coronary sinus or the right atrium (see Figures 5.12 and 5.13).

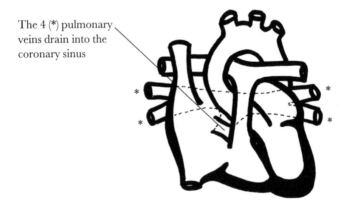

The 4 (*) pulmonary
veins drain into the
coronary sinus

Figure 5.12 Total anomalous pulmonary venous drainage — cardiac, draining into the coronary sinus

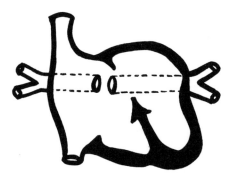

Figure 5.13 Total anomalous pulmonary venous drainage — cardiac, draining into the right atrium

Infracardiac

This is responsible for approximately 20%[4, 135] of cases. The pulmonary veins join to form a vertical vein which empties into the ductus venosus, portal vein, hepatic vein or inferior vena cava, then emptying into the right atrium. Obstruction occurs more frequently with this type (see Figure 5.14).

The 4 (*) common pulmonary veins drain into portal vein, hepatic vein or IVC

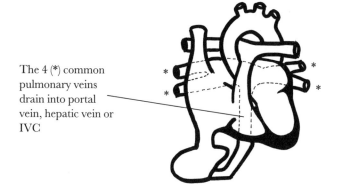

Figure 5.14 Total anomalous pulmonary venous drainage — infracardiac

Mixed

This is the least common accounting for approximately 10% of all cases[4, 10]. At least one pulmonary vein is connected to a different systemic vein from all other remaining anomalous veins.

Anatomy and pathophysiology

With any type of TAPVD, pulmonary venous return ultimately empties into the right atrium where it meets and mixes with systemic venous return.

Unobstructed types

If the defect is unobstructed, a large volume of mixed blood, including all the oxygenated blood, fills the right atrium. Some of this mixed blood is shunted across a life-saving intra-atrial connection, right to left, whether it be a true atrial septal defect or patent foramen ovale. This results in a varying degree of cyanosis depending on the amount of shunted blood, but is usually mild. The remainder empties into the right ventricle which becomes dilated, and then up into the pulmonary artery. Once pulmonary vascular resistance falls, the majority of blood will invariably empty into the right ventricle predisposing the infant to congestive cardiac failure and pulmonary vascular obstructive disease.

Obstructed types

Obstructed TAPVD is present in approximately 30% of patients, being most prevalent as the infracardiac type. If obstruction to the pulmonary veins is present, pulmonary venous return is reduced resulting in minimal shunting across the intra-atrial communication. Cyanosis is therefore severe. Additionally, pulmonary venous obstruction results in frank pulmonary oedema due to interstitial oedema[9] and secondary pulmonary arterial hypertension occurs from an early age.

Signs and symptoms

Clinical features depend on the degree of pulmonary venous obstruction.

Obstructed types

Obstructed types present within hours of birth.

Cardiovascular signs and symptoms

- Low cardiac output resulting in cardiovascular collapse.
- Poor pulses, tachycardia.

Respiratory signs and symptoms

- Respiratory distress.
- Profound cyanosis.
- Hypoxia, no response to oxygen therapy.
- Frank pulmonary oedema.
- Pulmonary hypertension.
- Increased pulmonary vascular resistance.

Renal signs and symptoms

- Profound metabolic acidosis.

Diagnosis of obstructed types

- Auscultation: No murmur.
- ECG: Right atrial and ventricular hypertrophy.
- Chest x-ray: Ground glass appearance, pulmonary congestion, right ventricular enlargement once pulmonary vascular resistance high.
- Echocardiography: Diagnostic and presence of intra-atrial communication shown.
- Cardiac catheterisation: This is not indicated in such a sick neonate as it has a high risk of mortality.

Unobstructed types

Unobstructed types present from three months of life.

Cardiovascular signs and symptoms

- Features are similar to a large atrial septal defect.
- Congestive heart failure.

Respiratory signs and symptoms

- Minimal cyanosis that increases on crying.
- Progressive pulmonary hypertension.
- History of chest infections.

Gastrointestinal signs and symptoms

- Failure to thrive.

Diagnosis of unobstructed types

- Auscultation: Murmur due to increased pulmonary blood flow through tricuspid and pulmonary valves.
- ECG: Right atrial and ventricular hypertrophy.
- Chest x-ray: Cardiomegaly, "sugar loaf" appearance of heart, increased pulmonary vascular markings.
- Echocardiography: Diagnostic, ASD or PFO.

Key preoperative management issues

The key preoperative management issues are shown in Table 5.9.

Table 5.9. Assessment and management of potential preoperative problems in TAPVD (for detailed management of individual problems, see Chapters 10–13)

Obstructed types:
- Immediate establishment and maintenance of a PDA to temporarily secure systemic blood flow
- Treatment of metabolic acidosis, hypoxia and multi-organ failure
- Management of neonatal coagulopathy
- Minimise pulmonary vascular resistance
- Preparation for urgent surgery — this is the only defect that requires definitive surgery within hours of birth

Unobstructed types:
- Congestive heart failure
- Pulmonary hypertension
- Failure to thrive

Surgical management

The main aim of surgery is to establish a connection between the pulmonary veins and left atrium[82]. Risk of mortality for the obstructed type is 15–50%, with the risks being at the higher end of this range for the infracardiac or mixed types. The risks also increase in the neonate who was critically ill preoperatively[20, 133].

Obstructed types

The critically ill neonate requires surgery urgently to relieve the obstructed pulmonary veins. The surgery consists of:

- Median sternotomy.
- Deep hypothermic circulatory arrest.

- Ligation of the PDA.
- The pulmonary veins are reconnected to the left atrium and ligation of the venous connection (vertical vein) is normally performed. Some centres leave the vertical vein open in the obstructed form.
- Closure of the ASD.

Unobstructed types

Once diagnosed, surgery should be performed without undue delay after diagnosis to prevent the development of pulmonary hypertension. It should not be left too long as the secondary complication of cyanosis may occur. The procedure is similar to that for obstructed types but, once the infant weighs over 8 kg, deep hypothermic circulatory arrest cannot be used.

Key postoperative management issues

The key postoperative management issues are shown in Table 5.10.

Table 5.10 Assessment and management of potential postoperative problems in TAPVD (for detailed management of individual problems, see Chapters 10–13)

Obstructed types:
- Management of low cardiac output and multi-organ failure which will persist if present preoperatively
- A slightly hypoplastic left ventricle will require higher left atrial pressures
- Management of pulmonary hypertension
- Detection and management of atrial arrhythmias
- Management of congestive heart failure

Unobstructed types:
- Management is similar to that of a large ASD

Later complications

Approximately 5–10% of infants will present with re-obstruction of the pulmonary veins within 3–6 months[136, 137].

Long-term follow-up

- Antibiotic prophylaxis is required for all types and should be continued long term if there are any residual cardiac lesions.
- Follow-up depends on the degree of residual problems.
- There is a small risk of the development of arrhythmias in the later postoperative period.

Ebstein's anomaly of the tricuspid valve

Aetiology

This defect accounts for approximately 1% of congenital heart disease[3, 4]. It is associated with other cardiac lesions namely, ASD, VSD, corrected TGA, RVOTO and arrhythmias — SVTs from Wolff–Parkinson–White syndrome[138]. The lesion is linked to a maternal history of taking lithium[3].

Definition

Ebstein's anomaly can be defined as a malformed and displaced tricuspid valve[20] see Figure 5.15.

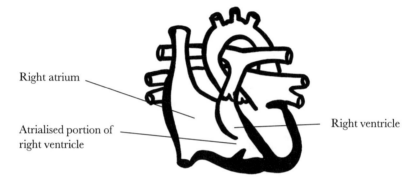

Right atrium

Atrialised portion of
right ventricle

Right ventricle

Figure 5.15 Ebstein's anomaly of the tricupsid valve

Anatomy and pathophysiology

The posterior and septal leaflets of the tricuspid valve are displaced downwards and into the right ventricle. This creates an atrialised right ventricle whereby part of the right ventricle is integrated into the right atrium[4]. This results in a small hypoplastic right ventricle which cannot eject its contents efficiently, causing a reduction in pulmonary blood flow and varying degrees of cyanosis. Blood thus passes back into the atrialised right ventricle through to the right atrium and shunts right to left across the ASD or PFO. A neonate with associated high pulmonary vascular resistance and pulmonary artery pressure will further compound the problem, as right to left shunting at atrial level will be greater, resulting in an increase in tricuspid regurgitation. Other physiological aspects include atrial arrhythmias developing from the increased right atrial pressure and supraventricular tachycardias occurring from accessory pathways[44]. An increased right atrial pressure and tricuspid regurgitation may predispose to systemic venous obstruction[10].

Signs and symptoms

This lesion can be detected *in utero*, but may present with profound cyanosis in the neonate when pulmonary vascular resistance (PVR) is high. If the tricuspid valve anomaly is mild, the defect may not present until childhood.

Cardiovascular signs and symptoms

- Congestive cardiac failure until PVR falls.
- Right to left shunt.
- Low cardiac output due to systemic venous obstruction.
- Pulses of small volume.

Respiratory signs and symptoms

- Severe cyanosis until PVR falls. After the neonatal period, cyanosis may only occur with exercise.
- Tachypnoea.
- Dyspnoea in the older child.

Haematological signs and symptoms

- Polycythaemia with severe cyanosis.
- Paradoxical emboli.

Other signs and symptoms

- Fatigue in the older child.
- Clubbing of the fingers and toes.

Diagnosis

- Auscultation: Systolic murmur related to tricuspid regurgitation.
- ECG: SVT, first degree heart block, right bundle branch block, right atrial hypertrophy.
- Chest x-ray: Cardiomegaly with decreased pulmonary vascular markings.
- Echocardiography: Diagnostic. Doppler studies assess the degree of tricuspid regurgitation and the morphology of the tricuspid valve.

- Cardiac catheterisation: High risk as it can predispose to the development of arrhythmias.

Key preoperative management issues

The key preoperative management issues are shown in Table 5.11.

Table 5.11 Assessment and management of potential preoperative problems in Ebstein's anomaly (for detailed management of individual problems see Chapters 10–12)

The neonate with a high pulmonary vascular resistance:
- Immediate establishment and maintenance of a PDA to temporarily secure pulmonary blood flow
- Treatment of metabolic acidosis, hypoxia and multi-organ failure should the PDA have closed
- Management of neonatal coagulopathy
- Congestive heart failure
- Arrhythmias
- Management of the effects of cyanosis

The older child:
- If the older child is asymptomatic, there is no treatment

Surgical management

The indications for surgery are increasing congestive heart failure, cyanosis, tricuspid regurgitation, arrhythmias and increasing polycythaemia. However, surgery is best avoided in the neonatal period as there is an approximately 20% risk of mortality[44].

The aims of surgery are to restore the competency of the tricuspid valve[20].

The surgical approaches include the following:

- Tricuspid valve repair: This is the procedure of choice with additional VSD closure if technically possible. If the anterior leaflet of the tricuspid valve is normal, a tricuspid valve annuloplasty and plication of the atrialised portion of the right ventricle can be achieved[44, 118, 139, 140].
- Tricuspid valve replacement and VSD closure: This is the procedure of second choice and is associated with higher mortality rates[141].
- A modified cavopulmonary anastomosis will be required if there is severe hypoplasia of the right ventricle[141–143].
- A modified Fontan procedure is required should the right ventricle be very small with associated pulmonary stenosis or atresia.
- Cardiac transplantation is considered in centres outside the UK.

Key postoperative management issues

Postoperative management depends on the procedure undertaken (Table 5.12). See Chapter 6 for the management of a Fontan operation.

Table 5.12 Assessment and management of potential postoperative problems in Ebstein's anomaly (for detailed management of individual problems, see Chapters 10 and 11)

Arrhythmias
Low cardiac output
Right ventricular failure
Residual cyanosis if the intra-atrial communication is not closed in surgery

Long-term follow-up

- Exercise restriction may be necessary but tolerance should improve after surgery.
- Antibiotic prophylaxis for life.
- Arrhythmia follow-up in approximately 10–20% of patients[4].

Hypoplastic left heart syndrome (HLHS)

Aetiology

This accounts for approximately 1–2% of congenital heart defects[4, 10, 144] and is responsible for the highest cause of death (approximately 95%) attributed to heart failure in the first four weeks of life[144–147]. However, a defect once described as fatal now has an improved chance of survival due to refinements in the preoperative, surgical and postoperative management. It is associated with DORV, complete AVSD[147] and approximately 50% of patients have been found to have coarctation of the aorta[146].

Definition

Hypoplastic left heart syndrome (HLHS) is a collective name for a wide spectrum of abnormalities related to the left side of the heart. Structures involved include a hypoplastic left ventricle, mitral valve stenosis or atresia and aortic valve stenosis or atresia, all of which predispose to a hypoplastic ascending aorta and arch. A PDA is required for survival in the neonatal period.

Anatomy and pathophysiology

Castañeda et al.[9] classify HLHS into four subgroups depending on the characteristics of the left heart valve:

- Type 1: Aortic valve stenosis and mitral stenosis.
- Type 2: Aortic valve atresia and mitral atresia.
- Type 3: Aortic valve atresia and mitral stenosis.
- Type 4: Aortic valve stenosis and mitral atresia.

In the types with aortic valve atresia, there is often associated ascending aorta and aortic arch hypoplasia with the ascending aorta being reduced in size to approximately 2.5 mm in diameter. Conversely with aortic valve stenosis, the aorta may be doubled in size at 4–5 mm in diameter[9]. The left ventricle is hypoplastic and the left atrium small. Related mitral valve stenosis or atresia is usually present.

Blood flow is essentially provided from the right ventricle through the PDA. It varies depending on the degree of resistance to flow from any associated stenosis or atresia. Pulmonary venous blood enters the left atrium and if mitral stenosis is present, a small amount enters the left ventricle and aorta, the majority shunting left to right across the foramen ovale. This increases left atrial pressure and pulmonary blood flow resulting in pulmonary oedema and pulmonary venous congestion. If, however, atresia of the mitral and aortic valves is present, blood flow is accomplished entirely from the pulmonary artery through the PDA which thus supplies the aortic arch, coronary arteries and descending aorta[10].

Survival therefore depends on a PDA and equally, the fine balance between the pulmonary and systemic vascular resistances. Once born, the neonate will undergo several physiological changes which disturb this balance. The increased fetal pulmonary vascular resistance will start to fall causing a reduction in blood flow from the right side of the heart and through the PDA thereby affecting systemic blood supply. This fall in pulmonary vascular resistance, accompanied by closure of the ductus arteriosus results in reduced systemic perfusion, low cardiac output with a subsequent reduction in perfusion of the coronary arteries, metabolic acidosis, congestive heart failure, absent peripheral pulses, shock, cardiovascular collapse and eventually death.

Signs and symptoms

The lesion presents within days of life due to alterations in the pulmonary and systemic vascular resistances and closure of the PDA.

Cardiovascular signs and symptoms

- Progressive congestive heart failure.
- Tachycardia.
- Poor peripheral pulses, which become absent when the PDA closes.
- Low cardiac output.
- Cardiovascular collapse when the PDA closes.

Respiratory signs and symptoms

- Mild cyanosis.
- Increasing respiratory distress.
- Pulmonary oedema.
- Only a slight reduction in pO_2 until the duct closes then profound hypoxia and eventual cardiovascular collapse.

Renal signs and symptoms

- Severe metabolic acidosis.

Other signs and symptoms

- Multi-organ failure due to cardiovascular collapse and acidosis: renal, hepatic, neurological, gut and liver involvement.

Diagnosis

- Auscultation: Systolic murmur.
- ECG: Right ventricular hypertrophy.
- Chest x-ray: Pulmonary venous congestion, pulmonary oedema.
- Echocardiography: Diagnostic from 16–20 weeks gestation.
- Cardiac catheterisation: There is too high a risk to the neonate to justify a cardiac catheterisation.

Key preperative management issues

The key preoperative management issues are shown in Table 5.13.

Table 5.13 Assessment and management of potential preoperative problems in HLHS (for detailed management of individual problems see Chapters 10–13)

Immediate establishment and maintenance of a PDA to temporarily secure pulmonary and systemic blood flow

Treatment of metabolic acidosis, hypoxia and multi-organ failure

A neonate with HLHS should be continuously monitored and assessed for deterioration in vital signs. Subtle changes in parameters may indicate the start of the neonate's deterioration so the nurse plays a valuable role in detecting, reporting and acting on these changes

Achieving a balance between systemic and pulmonary blood flows by manipulation of systemic and pulmonary vascular resistances. This is essential to prevent shifts in perfusion predisposing to cardiac arrest:

- If possible, allow spontaneous respiration. However, if large doses of prostaglandin E_1 are required to maintain duct patency, prostaglandin-induced apnoeas may occur requiring mechanical ventilation. The aim is to reduce pulmonary blood flow, increase pulmonary vascular resistance and reduce the work of breathing
- Increased pO_2 acts as a potent vasodilator, thereby lowering pulmonary vascular resistance and increasing systemic vascular resistance. This causes excessive pulmonary blood flow, pulmonary oedema, metabolic acidosis, poor systemic perfusion (hypotension), cool peripheries, wide pulse pressures (diastolic 20–30 mmHg) with poor coronary artery perfusion. Intervention to increase pulmonary vascular resistance and lower systemic vascular resistance includes:
  1. Aiming for oxygen saturations of 70–75%, in room air (O_2 levels of 21%) or even adding nitrogen to the ventilator circuit to achieve O_2 levels of 18%
  2. Ensuring the hand ventilation set is attached to an air/oxygen blender to avoid hand ventilation with 100% oxygen
  3. Setting the PEEP between 4–6 slightly vasoconstricts the blood vessels
  4. The minute volume should be adjusted to achieve a pH of 7.34–7.40[145, 148]. pH appears to be the main factor influencing the pulmonary vascular resistance[145]. Some centres will allow the neonate to become mildly acidotic to increase pulmonary vascular resistance, thus increasing the systemic blood flow. This could predispose to a decline in the neonate's condition if there is failure to intervene should the neonate become severely acidotic[9].
- A decreased pO_2 acts as a potent vasoconstrictor, thereby increasing pulmonary vascular resistance and reducing systemic vascular resistance. This causes a reduction in pulmonary blood flow, pulmonary venous hypertension, acidosis, hypoxaemia with oxygen saturations of 55–60%, and congestive heart failure. Intervention to decrease pulmonary vascular resistance and increase systemic vascular resistance includes:
  1. Hyperventilation to achieve a pH of 7.5–7.6, a pCO_2 of 30–35
  2. Increasing the inspired oxygen level
  3. Management of the congestive heart failure
- Barnea et al.[149] devised a mathematical model for both the systemic arterial and venous saturations in HLHS. They found when there is an increased systemic arterial and low venous saturation, pulmonary blood flow is low. Conversely when both systemic arterial and systemic venous saturations are low, flow is directed to the pulmonary circulation
- Frequent assessment of arterial blood gases with small, minute to minute alterations of mechanical ventilation are necessary[9]. Large, infrequent changes may upset the fine balance between the circulations

(contd)

Table 5.13 (contd)

- Avoidance of noxious stimuli is most important — minimal handling must be employed with co-ordination of nursing care. Suctioning may be very precarious so should be undertaken only when indicated. In-line suction catheters may be beneficial but it must be remembered that the catheter will increase the dead space, necessitating initial frequent gases
- Adequate sedation and analgesia can be given in the form of fentanyl. Fentanyl infusion has been shown to relax or blunt the stress response to the pulmonary vasculature[150]. Paralysis is normally required if ventilated to decrease the work of breathing, enable full compliance with the ventilator and manipulation of the pH

Maintenance of cardiac output:
- Contractility of the myocardium can be enhanced with inotropic support. However, it must be remembered that if high dose inotropes are used, it may result in an increased systemic vascular resistance upsetting the fine balance between the systemic and pulmonary vascular resistances. The nurse should observe for hypertension which may increase shunt flow into the pulmonary circulation[144]. Dopamine at 3–5 µg/kg/min should improve cardiac output and renal perfusion by increasing contractility but not systemic vascular resistance. Should the blood pressure fall, avoid bolusing inotropes as again, it could upset the fine balance between the circulations
- Preload can be manipulated by infusing colloid preparations to maintain adequate filling pressures and cardiac output. Care must be taken not to bolus colloids, with the aim of avoiding peaks and troughs in filling pressure and associated cardiac instability
- Afterload reduction must be undertaken with caution as pulmonary blood flow may decrease pulmonary resistance[144]. Colloid infusion may be necessary to support the afterload reduction and the associated vasodilation

Preoperative neurological assessment is required as a significant percentage of neonates with HLHS will have a congenital neurological disorder. It also serves as a baseline with which to assess the baby postoperatively or after episodes of hypotension and hypoperfusion to organs

Management of neonatal coagulopathy

Maintaining the haematocrit to 0.4–0.5 will help the oxygen-carrying capacity if hypoxaemia is present

Parental support:
- Many parents will have been aware from 16–20 weeks gestation that their baby will be born with HLHS. Some will elect to terminate the pregnancy after receiving appropriate counselling, others will be faced with the decision whether to let their baby die peacefully at birth or take the surgical option with all the uncertainty which that brings. Diagnosis antenatally has the advantage that should the parents decide to have treatment for their baby, the mother can be transferred to a specialist neonatal centre, close to a paediatric cardiac centre, for the birth and immediate aftercare
- The surgical options include the Norwood procedure[144] for which the success rate is variable[144] or neonatal heart transplantation which is rarely performed in the UK. The appropriate decision must be made, in conjunction with the parents, who must be fully informed and supported throughout this very difficult time

Surgical management

The management of the baby with HLHS is both complex and controversial. Cardiac transplantation has not been found to be successful in the neonatal period and will not be discussed here[144]. Several stages exist in the surgical management of the neonate with HLHS. It commences with palliation, the first stage of the Norwood procedure[145], followed by a bidirectional Glenn operation and then the modified Fontan operation (both covered later in this chapter) with a possible heart transplant at a later age. Unfortunately, due to the neonate's immature lungs and the increased pulmonary vascular resistance, a Fontan procedure cannot be undertaken in this period[145, 147].

Palliative surgery

Surgical atrial septectomy

Should there be severe hypoxia due to a restrictive foramen ovale, a surgical septectomy may be required[9].

First stage palliation, the Norwood procedure

This procedure is designed to physiologically rather than anatomically correct the neonatal circulation. The aims of the procedure are to establish an unobstructed arterial blood flow, to provide a secure source of pulmonary blood flow and establish unobstructed pulmonary venous return[10]. Ideally it is performed when the baby has recovered from any resuscitation and stabilisation, usually at between 5 and 7 days old. The procedure carries a substantial risk of death and involves the following:

- Median sternotomy is performed.
- Cardiopulmonary bypass is instituted, the baby being cooled to 18°C[144, 147].
- PDA is ligated.
- An atrial septectomy is performed to encourage intra-atrial mixing and prevent pulmonary venous hypertension as blood flow will thus be unrestricted.
- The main pulmonary artery is divided, thus disconnecting the branch pulmonary arteries. The distal end is closed.

- Provision of a systemic to pulmonary shunt with reconstruction of the hypoplastic aortic arch is undertaken. The proximal pulmonary artery is sutured to the hypoplastic ascending aorta and aortic arch. An allograft is used which may improve subsequent growth of the neoaorta[151].
- A central shunt is performed to increase pulmonary blood flow.
- The right ventricle now receives both pulmonary and systemic venous blood, ejecting the mixed blood into the aorta from the right ventricle. This ensures a right ventricle to aorta connection thereby providing an unobstructed blood flow from the right ventricle to the systemic circulation[147]. Pulmonary blood flow is achieved by blood entering the systemic to pulmonary artery shunt which then returns to the common atrium via the pulmonary veins. See Figure 5.16.

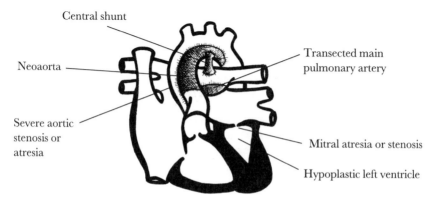

Figure 5.16 Norwood procedure for hypoplastic left heart syndrome

- A bidirectional Glenn procedure is performed at around 6 months of age. This delay allows time for growth of the pulmonary vasculature and a reduction in pulmonary artery pressure (see later in this chapter).
- Completion of modified Fontan operation is performed from age 18 months. See Chapter 6. This step will separate the systemic and pulmonary circulations but with the associated risk that the right ventricle will not function indefinitely as the systemic pump.
- A heart transplantation will probably be needed in future years.

Key postoperative management issues

The key postoperative management issues are shown in Table 5.14.

Table 5.14 Assessment and management of potential postoperative problems in HLHS (for detailed management of individual problems, see Chapters 10–13)

Managing the balance between systemic and pulmonary blood flows:
- This is necessary for the first 48 hours postoperatively after which stability is normally achieved

Management of potential decreased pulmonary blood flow:
- Manipulation of the ventilation to achieve hyperventilation in conjunction with sodium bicarbonate will ensure mild metabolic alkalosis and pulmonary artery dilatation
- Administration of colloids to increase the intravascular volume may lower the pulmonary vascular resistance. Colloids should be infused rather than bolused to prevent a shift in the balance of circulations
- The systemic to pulmonary artery shunt may be too small with severe hypoxia (oxygen saturations of 55–60%) in extreme cases. Inhaled nitric oxide may be delivered in an attempt to dilate the pulmonary vasculature. If this step fails, the shunt will have to be revised as prolonged hypoxia and acidosis will compromise the pulmonary blood flow. The pulmonary vascular resistance will be high therefore predisposing to an inadequate systemic blood flow

Management of potential increased pulmonary blood flow resulting in congestive heart failure:
- Oxygen saturations of 85–90% may result in low cardiac output with hypotension, poor peripheral perfusion and metabolic acidosis therefore reduce the oxygen, and maintain the pCO_2 at 40 mmHg. This will maximise pulmonary vascular resistance and minimise systemic vascular resistance
- Clipping of the shunt may be necessary to reduce pulmonary blood flow
- Aggressive treatment of the congestive heart failure is required
- Revision of the shunt may be necessary

Management of low cardiac output:
- As for preoperatively, these infants need a systolic blood pressure of 65–70 mmHg as the systemic–pulmonary shunt is reactive to the systolic blood pressure. The diastolic pressure also needs to be adequate for coronary perfusion but the shunt may cause the diastolic pressure to be low

Management of an adequate intravascular volume:
- To keep the central venous pressure 9–12 mmHg in the patient with decreased ventricular function

Management of the open chest

Management of potential bleeding

Management of the late development of coarctation of the aorta next to the reconstruction site. See Chapter 4

Management of the late development of right ventricular failure

Management of nutrition is very important in a baby who faces a long-term recovery. A significant percentage of babies with HLHS have proven swallowing co-ordination problems and can aspirate easily. Some centres now perform a gastrostomy following the Norwood procedure which allows for safe weight gain

Long-term follow-up

- Early death appears to be attributed to the surgical technique associated with inadequate perfusion of the lungs, myocardium and systemic organs[152]. Additionally, failure to maintain the balance between the pulmonary and systemic circulations accounts for a significant number of deaths in the early postoperative period.
- Close monitoring for life will be required.
- Cardiac catheterisation by 3 months followed by a bidirectional Glenn procedure — see Chapter 6.
- Completion of modified Fontan at 18 months to 3 years of age —see Chapter 6.
- Support for the parents when the baby is discharged from the ward should be provided as they are often very apprehensive at taking home a potentially unstable baby. Good communication should be maintained between the multidisciplinary team (hospital and community). Both parents and community staff need to be aware of the signs of deterioration and how to perform cardiopulmonary resuscitation.

Chapter 6
Defects that may be acyanotic or cyanotic

Double outlet right ventricle (DORV)

Aetiology

This is a rare anomaly accounting for less than 1% of all congenital heart disease[4, 55]. Additional defects are present in approximately 50% of patients with double outlet right ventricle (DORV)[10]. These include ASD, anomalous coronary arteries, heterotaxia, asplenia and mitral atresia[9, 10, 153].

Definition

DORV is a defect in which the great vessels (aorta and pulmonary artery) originate from the right ventricle. To meet this definition one of the vessels and at least 50% of the other must arise from the right ventricle[9, 20]. See Figure 6.1.

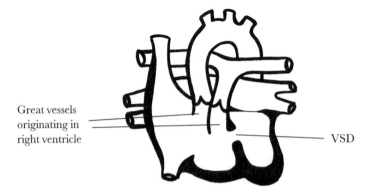

Great vessels
origining in
right ventricle

VSD

Figure 6.1 Double outlet right ventricle (DORV)

Classification

DORV encompasses a wide spectrum of defects from tetralogy of Fallot to transposition of the great arteries. Additionally there may be two functional ventricles or a very underdeveloped left ventricle resulting in a single ventricle scenario. A ventricular septal defect (VSD) is almost always present, the position of which classifies the type of DORV[153, 154].

- Subpulmonary VSD, no pulmonary stenosis (referred to as the Taussig–Bing defect).
- Subaortic VSD, no pulmonary stenosis — 50–70% of cases are this type[4].
- Subaortic VSD and pulmonary stenosis.
- Doubly committed VSD.

Anatomy and pathophysiology related to the classification

DORV results from the abnormal rotation of the truncus arteriosus during embryonic development[10].

DORV with subpulmonary VSD, no pulmonary stenosis

During the first month of life, deoxygenated blood flows from the right ventricle into the aorta resulting in severe cyanosis. The neonate is reliant upon a patent ductus arteriosus. Oxygenated blood flows from the left ventricle into the pulmonary artery predisposing to the early development of pulmonary hypertension. This resembles transposition of the great arteries and is named a Taussig–Bing defect. Once the pulmonary vascular resistance falls, congestive cardiac failure will prevail due to blood from both ventricles entering the area of least resistance, that is, the pulmonary artery[9].

DORV with subaortic VSD, no pulmonary stenosis

With this type, the haemodynamics are relatively normal in that blood enters the aorta from the left ventricle and deoxygenated blood enters the pulmonary artery from the right ventricle. There is little cyanosis but once the pulmonary vascular resistance falls, congestive cardiac failure and pulmonary hypertension can occur due the increase in pulmonary blood flow[4]. This type of DORV is similar to a large VSD.

DORV with subaortic VSD with pulmonary stenosis

This type of DORV is similar to tetralogy of Fallot. Therefore, if the right ventricular outflow tract obstruction is severe, a right to left shunt occurs, resulting in cyanosis.

DORV with doubly committed VSD

This rare type of DORV results in a large VSD situated close to both pulmonary and aortic valves.

Signs and Symptoms

Clinical features are related to the type of DORV:

- DORV with subpulmonary VSD, no pulmonary stenosis: The symptoms are similar to those of an infant with transposition of the great arteries with VSD (see Chapter 5).
- DORV with subaortic VSD, no pulmonary stenosis: The symptoms are similar to those of an infant with a large VSD with pulmonary hypertension and congestive heart failure (see Chapter 3).
- DORV with subaortic VSD and pulmonary stenosis: The symptoms are similar to those of an infant with tetralogy of Fallot (see Chapter 5).
- DORV with doubly committed VSD: The symptoms include increased pulmonary blood flow, congestive heart failure and mild cyanosis.

Key preoperative management issues

See Chapters 3 and 5 for details of preoperative management of a large VSD, transposition of the great arteries and tetralogy of Fallot.

Surgical management

The surgical management, both palliative and corrective, again depends on the anatomical type of DORV:

- DORV with subpulmonary VSD, no pulmonary stenosis: This repair carries a relatively high mortality rate of 15–20%[20, 155]. The VSD is patched then an arterial switch, Senning or Mustard procedure is performed, resulting in normal anatomy and physiology (see Chapter 5). Some children, however, will require a Fontan type repair[155] (see p. 160).
- DORV with subaortic VSD, no pulmonary stenosis: An intracardiac patch is sutured to the septum thus ensuring left ventricular blood empties into the aorta and right ventricular blood empties into the pulmonary artery. The associated risks increase with pre-existing pulmonary hypertension.

- DORV with subaortic VSD and pulmonary stenosis: The repair resembles the surgery for tetralogy of Fallot (see Chapter 5). If there is an anomalous coronary artery close to the right ventricular outflow tract, a conduit from the right ventricle to the pulmonary artery may be required[10] and is best approached via a transverse ventriculotomy. This ensures adequate viewing of the intracardiac defect in the presence of an anomalous coronary artery[156].

Key postoperative management issues

See Chapters 3 and 5 for details of postoperative management of large VSD, transposition of the great arteries and tetralogy of Fallot.

Long-term follow-up

- Follow-up depends on the type of repair and any residual complications.
- Antibiotic prophylaxis again depends on the type of repair.

Truncus arteriosus

Aetiology

Truncus arteriosus is responsible for 0.5–2% of all congenital heart defects[3, 55]. In the majority of cases it is associated with a VSD. Other links with congenital heart disease include interrupted aortic arch and single ventricles. Di George syndrome is present in approximately 30% of cases[4].

Definition

Truncus arteriosus is a defect in which the truncus arteriosus fails to divide in the developing fetus. Therefore, the two great vessels are united to form a common great vessel providing both systemic and pulmonary circulations.

Classification

There are four types of truncus arteriosus:

- Type 1: There is a common trunk with the main pulmonary artery branching off it. There are left and right pulmonary arteries. It is responsible for approximately 80% of cases[3]. See Figure 6.2.

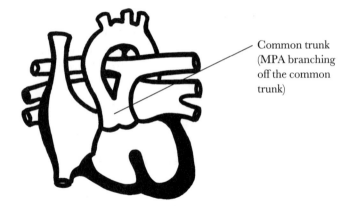

Common trunk
(MPA branching
off the common
trunk)

Figure 6.2 Truncus arteriosus — Type 1

- Type 2: There is a common trunk but no main pulmonary artery. The left and right pulmonary arteries develop from the centre back of the common trunk. See Figure 6.3.

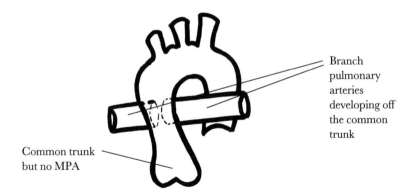

Branch
pulmonary
arteries
developing off
the common
trunk

Common trunk
but no MPA

Figure 6.3 Truncus arteriosus — Type 2

- Type 3: There is a common trunk but no main pulmonary artery. The left and right pulmonary arteries develop from the sides of the common trunk. See Figure 6.4.
- Type 4: There is a common trunk with no main pulmonary artery. Collateral vessels develop from the descending aorta supplying the pulmonary arterial circulation. This is now classified as pulmonary atresia. See Figure 6.5.

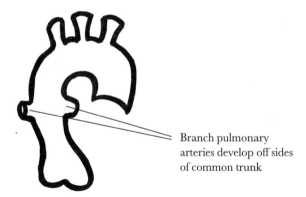

Branch pulmonary
arteries develop off sides
of common trunk

Figure 6.4 Truncus arteriosus — Type 3

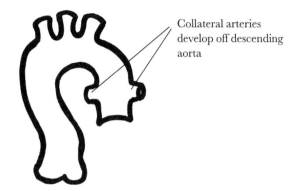

Collateral arteries
develop off descending
aorta

Figure 6.5 Truncus arteriosus — Type 4

Anatomy and pathophysiology

The common trunk overrides both ventricles and in most circumstances a large VSD is present. There is a common valve — the truncal valve — with one to four cusps. It is usually dysplastic and dysfunctional[157]. Oxygenated blood from the left ventricle and deoxygenated blood from the right ventricle empty into the common trunk. Cyanosis is usually minimal due to the VSD being unrestricted which allows equalisation of blood flow from each circulation.

After the first month of life, when pulmonary vascular resistance has fallen, blood flows through to the area of least resistance, that is, from the common trunk into the pulmonary circulation, resulting in congestive cardiac failure and pulmonary vascular obstructive disease.

Conversely, in the presence of pulmonary stenosis or atresia, pulmonary blood flow will be reduced resulting in increased cyanosis. Approximately one third of patients have right aortic arches[10]. Should the common truncal valve be incompetent or stenosed, congestive heart failure will worsen.

Signs and symptoms

This defect usually presents within the first month of life when pulmonary vascular resistance has fallen.

Cardiovascular signs and symptoms

- Bounding pulses.
- Congestive heart failure which presents early, especially if the valve is incompetent.

Respiratory signs and symptoms

- Pulmonary hypertension.
- Mild to moderate cyanosis from birth.
- Breathlessness.
- Tachypnoea.

Gastrointestinal signs and symptoms

- Failure to thrive.

Diagnosis

- Auscultation: Systolic murmur caused by turbulence across the truncal valve.
- ECG: Biventricular hypertrophy.
- Chest x-ray: Cardiomegaly with increased pulmonary vascular markings.
- Echocardiography: Diagnostic.

Key preoperative management issues

The key preoperative management issues are shown in Table 6.1.

Table 6.1 Assessment and management of potential preoperative problems in truncus arteriosus (for detailed management of individual problems see Chapters 10–12)

Aggressive management of congestive cardiac failure

Management of pulmonary vascular obstructive disease

The baby with pulmonary stenosis and truncus arteriosus:
- Immediate establishment and maintenance of a PDA to temporarily secure pulmonary blood flow
- Management of metabolic acidosis, hypoxia and multi-organ failure
- Management of neonatal coagulopathy

Surgical management

Palliative treatment

Very few surgeons perform a palliative procedure, preferring instead to proceed directly to corrective surgery. However, if performed, a pulmonary artery band can be placed in small babies to decrease pulmonary blood flow thus protecting the lungs from pulmonary vascular obstructive disease and congestive cardiac failure. There is a high mortality rate associated with this so the risks must be balanced against the option of corrective surgery.

Corrective surgery

Surgeons now prefer to operate on the baby at 1–2 months of age to lower risks associated with palliative surgery[20, 158]. There is an approximately 20% risk of mortality. Several surgical options are available:

Type 1 truncus arteriosus:
- The pulmonary artery is detached from the truncus (aorta).
- The hole on the truncus is closed.
- The truncal valve is repaired.
- A ventriculotomy is performed and the VSD is closed.
- A Rastelli procedure, joining the right ventricle to the pulmonary artery by means of a conduit, is performed[158, 159].

Types 2 and 3 truncus arteriosus
The pulmonary arteries are disconnected from the common trunk and attached to the valved conduit. Then the steps outlined above are performed.

Key postoperative management issues

The key postoperative management issues are shown in Table 6.2.

Table 6.2 Assessment and management of potential postoperative problems in truncus arteriosus (for detailed management of individual problems see Chapters 10–12)

Truncal valve regurgitation

Low cardiac output

Congestive heart failure

Bleeding

Right ventricular dysfunction in patients who have had a right ventriculotomy for VSD closure

Pulmonary hypertension

Bacterial endocarditis following conduit or valve insertion

Thrombus formation following conduit or valve insertion

Long-term follow-up

- The conduit will have to be replaced as the child grows[160].
- The pulmonary vascular obstructive disease will need to be closely monitored.
- Warfarin is required if the baby has had a valve replacement.
- No contact sports should be allowed.

Corrected transposition of the great arteries (CTGA)

Aetiology

This lesion represents less than 1% of all congenital heart defects[4]. It is more commonly associated with other heart defects, namely, VSD, pulmonary stenosis, tricuspid valve abnormality, heart block and supraventricular tachycardia[3, 4, 9].

Definition

Corrected transposition of the great arteries (CTGA) is a lesion whereby the aorta lies anteriorly and the pulmonary artery posteriorly. This is similar to transposition of the great arteries but the difference lies in the fact that the aorta is on the left of the pulmonary artery instead of the right and the ventricles are transposed[3]. Other definitions include left transposition which is representative of the aorta lying on the left side and atrioventricular discordance with ventriculoarterial discordance. This can be described anatomically as the great vessels are transposed (ventriculoarterial), and physiologically as the right atrium is connected to the left ventricle and the left atrium is connected to the right ventricle (atrioventricular discordance)[20]. See Figures 6.6 and 6.7.

Note position of ascending aorta to main pulmonary artery

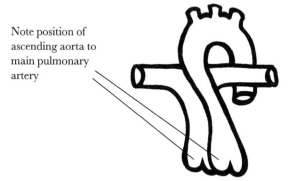

Figure 6.6 Corrected transposition of the great arteries

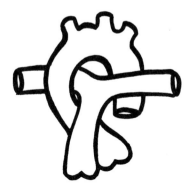

Figure 6.7 Normal position of the aorta and pulmonary artery

Anatomy and pathophysiology

- The great vessels: As mentioned previously, the aorta lies anterior to and to the left of the pulmonary artery. The pulmonary artery lies posterior to and to the right of the aorta. Accordingly the aorta leaves the morphological right ventricle, and the pulmonary artery leaves the morphological left ventricle.

- Chambers: Morphologically and anatomically, the right atrium is connected to the morphological left ventricle, and the morphological and anatomical left atrium is connected to the morphological right ventricle.
- Valves: The morphological right ventricle has a tricuspid valve but anatomically it is the left ventricle, that is, the systemic ventricle. There is a high incidence of tricuspid valve abnormality. The morphological left ventricle has a mitral valve but anatomically is the right ventricle, that is, the pulmonary ventricle.
- Conduction system: There is an elongated pathway with fibrosis between the atrioventricular node and the bundle of His[9, 20].
- Blood flow: The inferior and superior venae cavae empty into the anatomical and morphological right atrium. From here blood passes through a mitral valve into the morphological left ventricle. Deoxygenated blood leaves this systemic ventricle and enters the pulmonary artery before reaching the lungs. Oxygenated blood enters the pulmonary veins and discharges into the anatomical left atrium. From here blood passes through the tricuspid valve and into the morphological right ventricle. Blood subsequently leaves the pulmonary ventricle and enters the aorta supplying the systemic circulation. If a VSD is present, there is left to right shunting. However, if pulmonary stenosis is present, a right to left shunt may occur if the stenosis is moderate to severe.

Signs and symptoms

If other defects are present, symptoms present in infancy. If isolated CTGA occurs, symptoms may not occur until adulthood.

Cardiovascular signs and symptoms

- If there is a large VSD present, congestive heart failure with other symptoms similar to a VSD will occur.
- There may be tricuspid valve regurgitation due to the circulation being served by a right-sided valve and ventricle.

Respiratory signs and symptoms

- If a VSD and pulmonary stenosis are present, varying degrees of cyanosis with other features similar to that of tetralogy of Fallot will occur.

Diagnosis

- Auscultation: A murmur may be present, representing a VSD or tricuspid regurgitation.
- ECG: First to third degree heart block, SVTs.
- Chest x-ray: Increased pulmonary vascular markings unless there is pulmonary stenosis and VSD in which case the pulmonary vascular markings will be reduced. There is cardiomegaly.
- Echocardiography: Diagnostic.

Key preoperative management issues

The key preoperative management issues are shown in Table 6.3.

Table 6.3 Assessment and management of potential preoperative problems in corrected TGA (for detailed management of individual problems, see Chapters 10 and 11)

Congestive heart failure if VSD present
Complications of cyanosis if VSD and pulmonary stenosis present
Arrhythmias

Surgical management

This is dependent on the associated lesions:

- CTGA with VSD and pulmonary stenosis: Initially, surgery is performed to increase pulmonary blood flow, for example, a modified Blalock–Taussig shunt, followed by a patch closure of VSD and a valved cardiac conduit to relieve the pulmonary stenosis[20]. Resection of the pulmonary stenosis is contraindicated due to an increased risk of complete heart block in these patients[9].
- CTGA with VSD: A pulmonary artery band is undertaken in infancy to prevent pulmonary hypertension and to reduce the risk of congestive heart failure. Patch closure of the VSD is performed at the age of 1–2 years. It is delayed until this time as the VSD tends to be malaligned increasing the risk of complete heart block, requiring permanent pacing[161]. However, some centres would opt for earlier closure.

- Tricuspid valve abnormality: An abnormality is frequently present due to the valve being under increased haemodynamic pressure[162]. For the first year of life it is treated medically, followed by a valve replacement at a later date.
- Double switch procedure: This is a relatively new method of intervention addressing the long-term complications of a morphological right ventricle and valve supporting the systemic circulation[163, 164]. It involves an atrial switch (Mustard or Senning procedure; see Chapter 5) and an arterial switch operation thus correcting the atrioventricular and ventriculoarterial discordance (see Chapter 5). Initial results suggest low rates of early mortality and surgical heart block[125, 165].

Key postoperative management issues

The key postoperative management issues are shown in Table 6.4.

Table 6.4 Assessment and management of potential postoperative problems in corrected TGA

CTGA with VSD and pulmonary stenosis, see Chapter 5 on tetralogy of Fallot

CGTA with VSD, see Chapter 3 on VSD

For the double switch procedure, see Chapter 5 on TGA

Long-term follow-up

- Electrophysiological studies are required in the presence of heart block and pacemaker insertion.
- CTGA may not be diagnosed until the fourth or fifth decade, therefore a double switch procedure will not be an option. Subsequently there will be progressive right (systemic) ventricle dysfunction, tricuspid regurgitation and arrhythmias[166].

Single ventricle (univentricular heart)

Aetiology

The single-ventricle disorders are responsible for approximately 1–4% of congenital heart disease[4]. The occurrence is dependent on the presenting defect.

Definition

A variety of heart defects fall into this category, but according to Jordan and Scott[3], the heart must have only one complete ventricle, encompassing an inlet, atrioventricular valve and outlet portion. Thus, mitral atresia, hypoplastic left heart syndrome, tricuspid atresia and extreme forms of double outlet right ventricle may be classed as a single ventricle. However, the most common presentation of single ventricle is double inlet left ventricle (DILV) which will be used here to demonstrate aspects of a univentricular heart. See Figure 6.8.

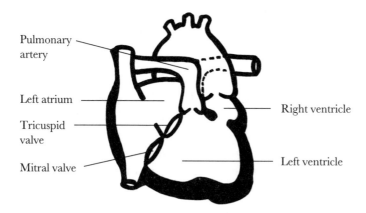

Figure 6.8 The most common form of a single-ventricle heart (double inlet left ventricle with corrected TGA)

Anatomy and pathophysiology

In the most common form of single ventricle, DILV, both atrioventricular valves arise from a single ventricle which is normally a morphological left ventricle. The right ventricle is present in the form of a small chamber, connected to the main ventricle through a restrictive bulboventricular foramen[4]. In the most typical presentation, there are transposed great vessels or congenitally corrected transposed vessels with the aorta arising from the small right chamber. The pulmonary artery leaves the left ventricle. Pulmonary stenosis may be present.

As blood from the left and right atria empty into the common ventricle, mixing will produce varying degrees of cyanosis. Pulmonary blood flow varies according to the presence of pulmonary stenosis[20]. The consequences of pulmonary stenosis being profound cyanosis once the PDA closes. Conversely, congestive heart failure and pulmonary vascular obstructive disease will prevail if pulmonary stenosis is not present.

Signs and symptoms

Features vary enormously depending on the pulmonary blood flow and the mixing of the systemic and pulmonary circulations:

Cardiovascular signs and symptoms

- Cardiovascular collapse when PDA closes if duct dependent defect.
- Severe congestive heart failure in the absence of pulmonary stenosis.

Respiratory signs and symptoms

- If there is decreased pulmonary blood flow with pulmonary stenosis, the features are similar to tetralogy of Fallot with varying degrees of cyanosis, hypoxia and collapse if the neonate is duct dependent.
- The neonate without pulmonary stenosis will present with mild cyanosis whilst the pulmonary vascular resistance is high.
- Pulmonary hypertension.
- Chest infections.

Gastrointestinal signs and symptoms

- Failure to thrive.
- Hepatomegaly.

Renal signs and symptoms

- Metabolic acidosis.

Diagnosis

- ECG: Ventricular hypertrophy.
- Chest x-ray: With increased pulmonary blood flow, there will be increased pulmonary vascular markings. With decreased pulmonary blood flow, there will be decreased pulmonary vascular markings.
- Echocardiography: Diagnostic.

Key preoperative management issues

The key preoperative management issues are shown in Table 6.5.

Table 6.5 Assessment and management of potential preoperative problems in babies with a single ventricle (for detailed management of individual problems see Chapters 6 and 10–13)

Baby with increased pulmonary blood flow:
- Congestive heart failure
- Pulmonary vascular obstructive disease
- Management of the baby needing pulmonary artery banding to reduce pulmonary blood flow

Baby with reduced pulmonary blood flow:
- Immediate establishment and maintenance of a PDA
- Metabolic acidosis, hypoxia and multi-organ failure should the duct close
- Neonatal coagulopathy
- Management of the baby needing a modified Blalock–Taussig shunt to increase pulmonary blood flow

Failure to thrive

Surgical management

Please refer to tricuspid atresia for palliative and corrective options. Risks of mortality are approximately 10–20% depending on the underlying lesion[167–170].

Postoperative nursing management

See the section on Fontan later in this chapter (p. 160).

Long-term follow-up

See the section on Fontan later in this chapter (p. 160).

Palliative operations and the Fontan procedure

Palliative operations were performed in the past because surgical techniques were not advanced enough for adequate correction of severe defects. However, they are still used in the interim until the patient has grown sufficiently to have the corrective surgery or a Fontan procedure[38]. Various procedures are available but as surgery is now audited, procedures such as the Waterston and Pott's shunt are rarely used due to major complications.

The following palliative operations decrease pulmonary blood flow.

Pulmonary artery banding

Aim

Pulmonary artery banding aims to decrease pulmonary blood flow.

Indications

Indications for this operation have changed over the years. Originally, it was routinely performed on patients with large VSDs, rather than considering a definitive operation. Today it is recognised that pulmonary artery banding has inherent complications, so it is usually reserved for the treatment of complex congenital heart disease[170, 171], in which the volume load on the systemic ventricle is too great, to reduce congestive cardiac failure and for the prevention of pulmonary vascular obstructive disease[9]. Should the patient be a candidate for the Fontan procedure in the future, the banding needs to be carried out in the first month of life. See Figure 6.9.

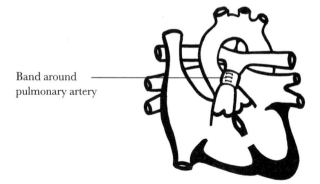

Band around
pulmonary artery

Figure 6.9 Pulmonary artery banding

Procedure

- Median sternotomy is performed.
- Cardiopulmonary bypass is not used.
- A prosthetic band is placed around the main pulmonary artery to restrict pulmonary blood flow to approximately 50% of the right ventricular pressure in patients with a left to right shunt[3, 172]. In right to

left shunts (cyanotic lesions) the aim is to achieve a mean pulmonary artery pressure of 10–15 mmHg. However, the surgeon may have to accept a mean pulmonary artery pressure outside this range so as to balance the oxygen saturations. For example, a mean pulmonary artery pressure of 15 mmHg with oxygen saturations of 60% is not normally acceptable, but equally depends upon the pulmonary vascular resistance and condition of the lungs.

- The chest can be left open to facilitate alteration of the band in the early postoperative period as tightness of the band is difficult to gauge accurately when the patient is anaesthetised. New techniques involve the use of a percutaneous bidirectional adjustable device to compensate for haemodynamic changes postoperatively[170, 171]. However, success with this new technique is still under review.

Key postoperative management issues

The key postoperative management issues are shown in Table 6.6.

Table 6.6 Assessment and management of potential postoperative problems in pulmonary artery banding (for detailed management of individual problems see Chapters 10 and 11)

Congestive cardiac failure, preventing weaning from the ventilator, due to the band being too loose:
- Report oxygen saturations above 90%
- Prepare the patient for tightening of the band

Hypoxia due to the band being too tight:
- Report oxygen saturations below 75%
- Prepare the patient for loosening of the band

Low cardiac output due to increased cardiac afterload after pulmonary artery banding

Pulmonary artery stenosis and deformity:
- This may require reconstruction of the pulmonary artery at the time of corrective surgery

The following systemic artery to pulmonary arterial shunts increase pulmonary artery blood flow.

Blalock–Taussig (BT) shunt

This operation is seldom performed nowadays. The left or right subclavian artery is anastomosed to the same side pulmonary artery. The right sided BT shunt is the procedure of choice as it kinks less readily than a left sided shunt. Blood thus flows from the aorta through the subclavian artery to the pulmonary artery.

Modified Blalock–Taussig shunt

The subclavian artery and pulmonary artery are connected together by means of a Gore-tex™ tube. This allows for an optimal sized shunt[3] especially in a neonate whose own anatomy may be too small. Blood flows from the aorta, through the subclavian artery, down the prosthetic shunt and into the pulmonary artery. See Figure 6.10.

Right subclavian to right pulmonary artery connection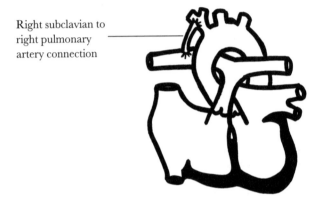

Figure 6.10 Modified right Blalock–Taussig shunt

The advantage of a systemic to pulmonary artery shunt is that the increased blood flow is normally tolerated well by the lungs, thus preventing hypoxia and vascular changes. It is easily taken down at the time of corrective surgery or at a later date in the catheter laboratory using a detachable coil device[173].

Key postoperative management issues

The key postoperative management issues are shown in Table 6.7.

Damas–Kaye–Stansel procedure

This procedure is performed for complex heart disease such as TGA with VSD and subaortic stenosis or single ventricle disorders where the bulboventricular foramen is too small predisposing to haemodynamic and surgical complications[4]. To perform a Damas–Kaye–Stansel procedure, the aortic arch has to have developed, unlike in hypoplastic

Table 6.7 Assessment and management of potential postoperative problems in a baby with a modified BT shunt (for detailed management of individual problems see Chapters 10 and 11)

Management of a potential shunt thrombosis particularly in the cyanotic, polycythaemic baby:
- Report hypoxic episodes manifested by low oxygen saturations or pO_2 — this may indicate shunt blockage
- Assist medical staff in the examination of the baby for a shunt murmur
- Ensure adequate cardiac output to maintain shunt patency, reporting signs of low cardiac output promptly. Consider use of inotropes to manipulate cardiac output
- Observe for signs of dehydration which may contribute to clot formation
- Administer prescribed anticoagulants — initially heparin until the patient is absorbing oral fluids. Aspirin may then be commenced
- Wean ventilation as the effects of positive pressure may exacerbate the problem

Reduction in arterial blood flow to the arm (the side upon which the subclavian artery has been utilised):
- Monitor pulses, colour, perfusion, capillary refill in the affected arm
- Avoid taking cuff blood pressures on the affected arm
- Avoid siting arterial lines on the affected arm

Modified BT shunt too small:
- Monitor for signs of hypoxia that may indicate insufficient pulmonary blood flow caused by a shunt that is too small

Modified BT shunt too large:
- Monitor for a marked increase in oxygen saturations and the development of congestive heart failure, both indicative of the shunt being too large thus providing excessive pulmonary blood flow

Distortion of the pulmonary tree preventing any further surgical intervention[97, 174]

---

left heart syndrome, in which a Norwood procedure is performed to correct the underdeveloped aortic arch. See Figures 6.11, 6.12 and 6.13.

The procedure

- The main pulmonary artery is transected (Figure 6.11).
- An incision is made into the aorta.
- The proximal pulmonary artery is anastomosed end to side to the ascending aorta using Gore-tex™ (Figure 6.12). Blood is then channelled into the aorta.
- In non-single ventricle disorders, the VSD is closed.
- A valved conduit is placed between the distal pulmonary artery and the right ventricle, directing blood from the right ventricle to the branch pulmonary arteries (Figure 6.13)[4].

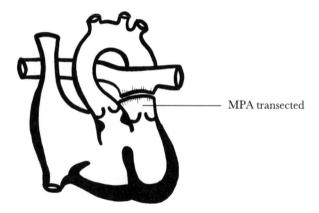

Figure 6.11 Damas–Kaye–Stansel procedure — Part 1

MPA transected

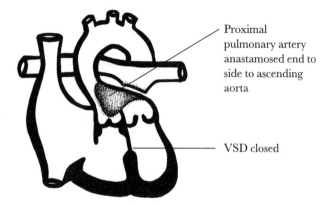

Figure 6.12 Damas–Kaye–Stansel procedure — Part 2

Proximal pulmonary artery anastamosed end to side to ascending aorta

VSD closed

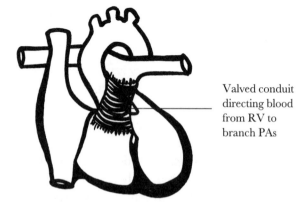

Figure 6.13 Damas–Kaye–Stansel procedure — Part 3

Valved conduit directing blood from RV to branch PAs

Systemic venous to pulmonary artery shunt (cavopulmonary anastomosis)

Glenn procedure

This operation was used for patient palliation in the tricuspid atresia and complex heart patient. The superior vena cava (SVC) is anastomosed end to end with the distal right pulmonary artery. The SVC–right atrial junction and proximal right pulmonary artery are ligated. This procedure has its disadvantages, including arteriovenous fistulae in the right lung and veno-venous collaterals in the left lung[20]. Consequently, it is rarely performed today.

Bidirectional Glenn procedure

This procedure is the one of choice today, being used for patients with tricuspid atresia or complex hearts in preparation for a subsequent Fontan procedure. One major advantage of the bidirectional Glenn procedure over the modified BT shunt is that it preserves left ventricular function, lowers the stroke volume[175], and lowers preload and afterload in single ventricle disorders[176]. The risk factors will be discussed under the Fontan procedure but in addition to these, performing the Fontan operation in infancy can increase mortality significantly[9, 177, 178]. See Figure 6.14.

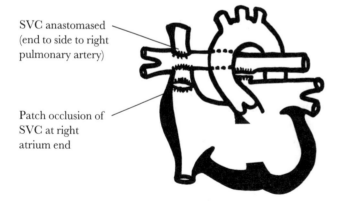

SVC anastomased (end to side to right pulmonary artery)

Patch occlusion of SVC at right atrium end

Figure 6.14 Cavopulmonary anastomosis (bidirectional Glenn)

The procedure:

- Median sternotomy with cardiopulmonary bypass.
- Previous systemic shunts taken down.
- The SVC is divided at the right atrium.

- It is then anastomosed end to side to the right pulmonary artery.
- The main pulmonary artery may be left or oversewn at the bifurcation.
- To prepare the patient further for completion of Fontan, the surgeon may place a patch over the transected right atrium at the junction of the SVC.
- The presence of a restrictive ASD may require an atriotomy[9].

Advantages of the procedure:

The main advantage is in the avoidance of pulmonary vascular obstructive disease by the use of an SVC to pulmonary artery shunt instead of an aortic to pulmonary artery connection. Blood flow is therefore under low pressure as opposed to high pressure from the aortic to pulmonary artery connection via a modified BT shunt. A bidirectional Glenn procedure therefore reduces the volume overload of the ventricle and prepares the ventricle for a subsequent Fontan procedure.

For assessment and management see the section on the Fontan procedure below.

Fontan procedure

The Fontan procedure was initially developed in the late 1960s to bypass the right ventricle in cases of tricuspid atresia. In addition to tricuspid atresia it has now been adopted for complex heart disorders including single ventricles (e.g., double inlet left ventricle, hypoplastic left heart syndrome) and unbalanced AVSDs.

Aim

The Fontan procedure has the ultimate aim of creating two circulations: systemic and pulmonary. It is achieved by anastomosing systemic venous drainage to the pulmonary arteries relying on systemic venous pressures for pulmonary blood flow.

Selection criteria

Choussat[179] stipulated several criteria for successful surgical outcome following the Fontan procedure. See Table 6.8.

Key preoperature management issues

The key preoperative management issues are shown in Table 6.9.

Table 6.8 Criteria for successful surgical outcome

- No haemodynamic complications from previous shunts
- Normal mitral valve function, that is, no left sided obstruction
- Normal systemic venous drainage
- Mean pulmonary artery pressure below 20 mmHg
- Pulmonary vascular resistance below 4 Wood units/m^2
- Pulmonary arteries to be of a good size
- Sinus rhythm
- Left ventricular ejection fraction above 60%
- Ages 4–15 years — now tolerated at earlier ages[180]

Table 6.9 Assessment and management of potential preoperative problems with Fontan procedure (for detailed management of individual problems, see Chapters 10–13)

Problems of chronic cyanosis

Congestive heart failure

Failure to thrive

Management of other problems specific to underlying defect

The procedure

The classic Fontan procedure involves joining the right atrium to the right pulmonary artery with a valveless conduit. Currently, various modified Fontan operations are normally undertaken depending on the patient's underlying condition. They have the advantage over the classic Fontan procedure that they only utilise a small part of the right atrium due to the presence of an extra cardiac conduit, thereby reducing the incidence of right atrial hypertension, atrial arrhythmias and atrial thrombi[10]. The associated risk of mortality is 5–20% depending on the underlying condition[118, 167, 181]. The modified Fontan procedure involves:

- Median sternotomy.
- Cardiopulmonary bypass.
- Taking down any previous systemic to pulmonary shunt.
- If a previous cavopulmonary anastomosis has been performed, completion of the Fontan procedure is the aim (see bidirectional Glenn procedure for the first part of this procedure).
- Completion of the Fontan procedure may include an atrial septostomy if not already performed, although the ASD is closed in tricuspid atresia.

- The patch is removed from the top of the right atrium and SVC junction.
- An intra-atrial baffle is inserted directing the IVC blood flow from the bottom of the right atrium to the SVC.
- Blood then flows from the SVC to the right pulmonary artery and on to the lungs.
- A 4 mm fenestration can be used to decompress the systemic venous flow.
- Two separate circulations are now present (Figure 6.15).

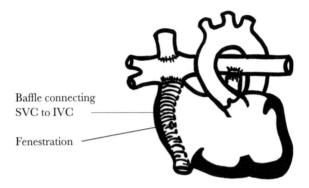

Baffle connecting
SVC to IVC

Fenestration

Figure 6.15 Modified Fontan procedure

Alternatively, an extra cardiac conduit can be used which has two main advantages:

- The procedure can be performed without cross clamping the aorta thus preserving the myocardium.
- There is no suturing of the atrium which reduces the risk of atrial arrhythmias.

The main disadvantage of this method is that the conduit does not grow, making it essential to delay the surgery until the patient's weight is around 15 kg (that is 3–4 years of age). The conduit should then last until adulthood.

Key postoperative management issues

The key postoperative management issues are shown in Table 6.10.

Long-term follow-up

Long-term prognosis is uncertain at present, but right-sided defects with hypoplastic ventricles will presumably tolerate the Fontan procedure

Table 6.10 Assessment and management of potential postoperative problems with Fontan procedure (for detailed management of individual problems see Chapters 10–13)

Minimise elevated SVC pressures to augment pulmonary blood flow by:
- Monitoring for elevated SVC pressures which may compromise
  1. cardiac output
  2. cerebral perfusion pressure especially if low cardiac output is present
- Manipulate ventilation to achieve a low PEEP[2], low peak inspiratory pressures and large tidal volumes of 10–15 ml/kg. This will encourage forward flow of venous blood back to the pulmonary bed
- Avoidance of a high pCO_2 and hypoxia will lower pulmonary artery pressure and increase perfusion pressures[38]. Conversely, a high pCO_2 and hypoxia will increase pulmonary vascular resistance, lower venous return and promote pulmonary constriction
- Allowing the patient to return to spontaneous breathing as soon as possible will enable a negative intrathoracic pressure to be achieved
- Sitting the child up will reduce the SVC pressure, gravity allowing blood to return to the pulmonary bed
- Additionally, venous return and pulmonary blood flow can be maximised by optimising filling pressures — CVP 15–18 mmHg, LAP 12–15 mmHg
- Ensure sinus rhythm is present. Consider pacing if arrhythmias develop
- Use inotropes to dilate the pulmonary vascular bed, to lower the pulmonary vascular resistance and avoid ventricular failure
- Use vasodilators to minimise afterload

Complications associated with an elevated SVC:
- Monitor for the development of pleural effusions, ascites, cerebral oedema and hepatomegaly — the hepatic capillary bed is particularly prone to leaking[9]. Water retention can be dealt with by administering diuretics

Low cardiac output due to preoperative myocardial dysfunction and cardiopulmonary bypass

Atrial arrhythmias

Observation of the child unable to tolerate a Fontan procedure. Monitor for:
- Increasing SVC pressure above 20 mmHg
- Low cardiac output requiring increasing inotropic support
- An increasing left atrial pressure above 15 mmHg
- Oxygen saturations below 90% (if fenestrated Fontan, lower)

Should the above features present, the cardiac surgeon and cardiologist need to consider reversing the Fontan to a cavopulmonary anastomosis to prevent early death

Protein-losing enteropathy is present in approximately 10% of Fontan patients[182] resulting in loss of large proteins responsible for the production of coagulation factors. Other problems related to low protein levels include systemic oedema and low serum albumen[10]. Treatment is the ingestion of enteral proteins so encouragement of a high protein diet is vital. Steroids have been tried with varying degrees of success[182]

Intra-atrial thrombus formation is a potential risk due to right atrial distortion and low flow in the Fontan circulation. Prevention of thrombi is achievable by administering anticoagulants. However, bleeding can be a problem due to the chronic effects of cyanosis and the protein losing enteropathy longer than the hypoplastic left ventricle which will rely on the morphological right ventricle as the pumping chamber. Long-term results are still being assessed and include:

- Exercise tolerance is improved but not normal[3]. Competitive sports should be avoided.
- Tachyarrhythmias may occur resulting in sudden death[20]. Studies suggest the older the child having the procedure, the higher the incidence of atrial and ventricular arrhythmias, whereas in the younger patient, junctional ectopics may occur[183].
- Bacterial endocarditis prophylaxis and anticoagulation are required for life.
- Excessive salt in the diet must be avoided.
- If a fenestrated Fontan has been performed, it can be closed in the catheter laboratory at a later date[184].

Chapter 7
Acquired heart disease

Infective endocarditis

Aetiology

This acquired disease can present at any age in a patient who is predisposed to certain events: e.g., congenital heart lesion, recent heart surgery, recent dental treatment, recent throat/mouth/urine infection, and the presence of central lines or rheumatic fever[185, 186]. Despite the advances in medical science, it still remains problematic for the patient and staff involved[187] and is associated with a poor prognosis, with the overall mortality being approximately 30% and higher (50–100%) in high risk patients[188].

The main cause (80–90%) of the infections predisposing to endocarditis is bacterial (*Streptococcus viridans*, *Streptococcus faecalis*, *Staphylococcus aureus*, *Staphylococcus epidermis*[4, 10, 20]). In children with an *Staphylococcus aureus* infection, morbidity appears more severe than in an infection with *Streptococcus viridans*[189]. Other causes are fungal (e.g. *Candida albicans*), especially in the neonatal or immunocompromised patient. Parasitic and viral infections are also possible[190, 191].

Definition

Infective endocarditis is an infection of the lining of the heart, endocardium and valves.

Anatomy and pathophysiology

Endocarditis occurs frequently in patients with congenital heart disease and bacteraemia. The endocarditis is predisposed to by pressure gradients and turbulent blood flow, the most common defects being VSD,

PDA,coarctation of the aorta and mitral and aortic valve abnormalities[3]. However, any defect is a potential risk, the exception ordinarily being secundum ASDs[4].

Platelets and fibrin adhere to the endocardium resulting in thrombosis formation, termed vegetations, which can damage surrounding tissues and/or embolise to the lungs or systemic circulation[20]. The combative effects of antimicrobial therapy and phagocytosis are reduced due to the fibrin surrounding these vegetations[10]; hence the need for a minimum of four to six weeks of antimicrobial therapy.

Signs and symptoms

Endocarditis may present suddenly or subacutely and may have the following features:

- Septicaemia: Fever, lethargy, headache, loss of weight, arthralgia, pallor, anaemia, backache.
- Changed heart murmur.
- Enlarged spleen.
- Features of embolisation: Localised pain, organ dysfunction: brain (fits, hemiplegia, meningitis), kidneys (haematuria, proteinuria), lungs (chest pain, respiratory distress), skin (Osler nodes — red, tender nodes at end of fingers).

Diagnosis

- Echocardiography: Vegetations seen on scan. This is a very important diagnostic tool and early diagnosis is vital[188].
- Blood tests: Positive blood cultures, raised ESR, CRP, increased white cell count, low haemoglobin.
- Other: Investigations for haematuria.

Key management issues

The key mangement issues are shown in Table 7.1.

Preventative measures

Patient and parental education

- Education of the patient and parent for antibacterial prophylaxis prior to procedures will help in the prevention of endocarditis in high risk

Table 7.1 Assessment and management of potential problems in infective endocarditis (for management of individual problems, see Chapters 10–13 and 15)

Management of infection:
- Initial blood cultures to establish the cause, followed by cultures at regular intervals to assess the effectiveness of therapy
- Administration of high dose antimicrobial therapy for 4–6 weeks, immediately after the initial blood cultures have been taken. The choice of antimicrobial may initially be "blind therapy" but can be tailored to the organism, once known

Management of the pyrexia

Detection and management of emboli and any damage sustained to organs

Management of pain and discomfort (arthralgia and headache)

Management of anaemia

Management of weight loss

Management of the child requiring surgery — this carries a very high risk, approximately 50% risk of mortality[20] — so the initial therapy should be conservative, however if this fails, surgery may be needed:
- To remove vegetations
- To replace damaged heart valves

Psychological preparation of the child is vital for:
- Long-term intravenous antimicrobial therapy and blood cultures
- Understanding the need for bedrest although a stimulating environment needs to be provided whilst on bedrest, for example, encouraging visitors, computer games, videos, school work, board games, music and painting

---

groups (see aetiology). Procedures such as dental work, ear piercing, urinary catheterisation, gastrointestinal, genitourinary, tonsil and adenoid surgery will require prophylaxis.
- Presentation of fever should alert the patient and parents to seek medical help urgently. Self-diagnosis should not be considered.

Antimicrobial prophylaxis

Antimicrobial prophylaxis will be required.

Oral hygiene

Scrupulous oral hygiene is required to prevent mouth infections predisposing to bacteraemia. Encouraging regular visits to the dentist, regular brushing and flossing of teeth, use of fluoride supplements and a low sugar diet will help in the prevention of dental caries and other mouth infections[11].

Patient information card

A card with details of the child's heart lesion and the need for antibiotic prophylaxis should be carried at all times. The child and parents should be encouraged to inform medical and dental practitioners of the underlying problem so prophylaxis can be implemented appropriately.

Long-term care and follow-up

- Upon completion of treatment, the child can be discharged home with the emphasis placed on watching for further episodes of endocarditis. The parents should therefore take the child's temperature regularly, observing for signs of infection and employ the above preventative measures.
- Regular outpatient appointments to assess for damage sustained during the acute phase of the illness and to detect for reoccurrence. Echocardiograms and blood cultures should be performed.

Myocarditis

Aetiology

Myocarditis in an inflammatory process caused by[192, 193]:

- Bacteria.
- Fungi.
- Protozoa.
- Parasites.
- Viruses (responsible for approximately 69% of myocarditis[193]).
- Diseases, e.g., Kawasaki, rheumatic fever, systemic lupus erythematosus.

Definition

Myocarditis is inflammation of the myocardium, the heart muscle.

Anatomy and pathophysiology

The organism damages the heart muscle causing necrosis of the myocardium. As the tissue dies, scar tissue forms in the muscle fibres.

Signs and symptoms

There is commonly a history of respiratory tract infection. The myocardial cell loss can cause the following complications:

Cardiovascular signs and symptoms

- Congestive heart failure.
- Pulmonary oedema.
- Cardiogenic shock.
- Arrhythmias.
- Dilated cardiomyopathy.
- Chest pain.

Other signs and symptoms

- Anorexia.
- Vomiting.
- Diarrhoea.
- Lethargy.

Diagnosis

- Auscultation: Systolic murmur, gallop rhythm.
- ECG: ST changes. Arrhythmias (ectopics, supraventricular or ventricular tachycardias).
- Chest x-ray: Cardiomegaly, pulmonary venous congestion.
- Echocardiography: Left ventricular enlargement and impaired contractility.
- Blood tests: Raised ESR, cardiac enzymes, blood cultures often negative, viral titres.

Key management issues

The key management issues are shown in Table 7.2.

Long-term care and follow-up

- Approximately 30% of patients will die in the acute stages of the disease and approximately 15% will have chronic left ventricular impairment[3].
- Heart transplantation will be required in some cases.

Table 7.2 Assessment and management of potential problems in myocarditis (for management of individual problems see Chapters 10 and 11)

Cardiogenic shock

Congestive heart failure:
- Avoidance of drugs which compound the myocardium, reducing myocardial function is necessary — diuretics, digoxin, ACE inhibitors[194]

Arrhythmias

Pulmonary oedema

Management of the infective process if present

Management of the inflammatory process in patients with a positive biopsy:
- Use of immunosuppressive therapy unresponsive to other treatment[194–196]

Psychological care:
- The child and parents should be kept informed of the condition as sudden death may occur. Reassurance and much support will be required at this distressing time

Pericarditis

Aetiology

Pericarditis is usually due to a viral infection, commonly the coxsackievirus[3] or less commonly, a bacterial source — *Staphylococcus aureus, Haemophilus influenzae, Streptococcus pneumoniae*, tuberculosis or, rarely, meningococcus[197]. Collagen diseases such as rheumatoid arthritis may be a causative factor. Pericarditis with effusion can present postoperatively in approximately 10% of ASDs, VSDs and tetralogy of Fallot.

Definition

Pericarditis is an inflammation or infection of the pericardium.

Pathophysiology

The organisms or disease process inflame and infect the pericardium resulting in the development of a pericardial effusion. Should the fluid accumulation be rapid, a cardiac tamponade may occur[4].

Signs and symptoms

Signs and symptoms include pyrexia, chest pain, pericardial rub, pericardial effusion, cardiac tamponade and ventricular tachycardia.

Diagnosis

- ECG: Small voltage complexes, ST elevation, ventricular tachycardia.
- Chest x-ray: Cardiomegaly.
- Echocardiogram: Pericardial effusion, cardiac tamponade.

Key management issues

The key management issues are shown in Table 7.3.

Table 7.3 Assessment and management of potential problems in pericarditis (for detailed management of individual problems see Chapters 10 and 11)

Pericardial effusion:
- Drain the effusion to relieve cardiac embarrassment
- Send the aspiration fluid for analysis to establish the causative organism

Cardiac tamponade

Pyrexia

Inflammatory/infective process:
- Administration of aspirin and steroids
- Administration of intravenous antimicrobials
- Administration of colchicine if viral cause[198]

Arrhythmias

Long-term care and follow-up

- There is an approximate 15–30% risk of morbidity associated with pericarditis.
- Immunosuppressive therapy is suggested to prevent relapse[199].

Cardiomyopathy

Aetiology

Cardiomyopathy is responsible for approximately 1% of paediatric heart disease[11].

Definition

A cardiomyopathy is a disease of the heart muscle, the myocardium.

Classification

Several classifications exist for cardiomyopathies and are related to the presenting anatomy and physiology[4, 20].

Dilated cardiomyopathy (congestive cardiomyopathy)

In dilated cardiomyopathy, there is gross cardiomegaly resulting in poor ventricular contraction due to dilatation of the chambers[4]. The myocardium is also hypertrophied or thin and stretched. It is associated with a past history of viral, immunological or toxic illness[4, 20, 200]. It is found in all ages of patient and can be familial[201].

Signs and symptoms

Cardiovascular signs and symptoms:

- Congestive heart failure.
- Poor left ventricular contractility.
- Reduced ejection fraction which predisposes to the formation of ventricular thrombi. This is due to the stasis of blood[202].
- Left ventricular enlargement and dysfunction.
- Ventricular arrhythmias[203].

Respiratory signs and symptoms:

- Chest infections.
- Dyspnoea.
- Orthopnoea.
- Respiratory distress.

Other signs and symptoms:

- Fatigue.
- Weakness.
- Reduced exercise tolerance.

Diagnosis

The differential diagnosis is myocarditis.

- Auscultation: Systolic murmur, gallop rhythm.

- ECG: Sinus tachycardia, left ventricular hypertrophy, evidence of ischaemia.
- Chest x-ray: Cardiomegaly.
- Echocardiography: Dilated chambers, left ventricular function reduced.
- Bloods: FBC, ESR, CRP, urea and electrolytes, LFT, thyroid function tests, white blood cell enzymes, carnitine levels, organic acids, viral titres (adenovirus, coxsackievirus, Epstein–Barr virus), TORCH screen in infants.
- Urine: Virology (e.g. CMV), organic acids.
- Stool: Virology.

Key management issues

The key management issues are shown in Table 7.4.

Table 7.4 Assessment and management of potential problems in dilated cardiomyopathy (for detailed management of individual problems see Chapters 11 and 15)

Congestive heart failure:
- Consider the use of vasodilator therapy to reduce heart failure

Arrhythmias to prevent sudden death

Anticoagulation to prevent sudden death from CVA

Poor ventricular contractility:
- Beta blocking therapy[4, 204]
- Inotropes
- Transplantation

Psychological adjustment to the disease:
- To develop such a disease is catastrophic for the child and parents. Their once healthy child now has a condition that could cause sudden death, result in a heart transplant or the child could be left with a degree of heart failure. The family must be kept informed at all times and reassurance given when required as this will be a very worrying and uncertain time

Long-term care and follow-up

Death can occur within a few years of being diagnosed and, realistically, heart transplantation is the only long-term solution[205], but equally this procedure is fraught with problems in the younger child.

Endocardial fibroelastosis

This is a disease related to dilated cardiomyopathy in that both have similar features of dilated heart chambers and poor ventricular function.

However, it differs from true dilated cardiomyopathy in that the endocardial structure consists of a fibrous patchy white lining[3].

The causes of endocardial fibroelastosis are usually viral[206], immunological or toxic. It affects the younger child and infant presenting with similar features to that of dilated cardiomyopathy. According to Park[4], approximately 33% respond to treatment, approximately 33% maintain the status quo, and approximately 33% eventually die.

Hypertrophic cardiomyopathy (hypertrophic obstructive cardiomyopathy — HOCM)

HOCM causes hypertrophy of the myocardium and septum resulting in an obstruction to the left and possibly the right ventricle with a reduction in ventricular compliance[20, 207]. Contractility is enhanced. However, ventricular filling is poor due to left ventricular stiffness[4].

The genetic causes are usually autosomal dominant[207], affecting adolescents and adults between 20–30 years[4].

Signs and symptoms

Cardiovascular signs and symptoms:

- Progressive thickening of the myocardium and septum causing the size of the ventricular cavity to reduce.
- Left ventricular outflow tract obstruction.
- Reduced ventricular compliance.
- Angina pain.
- Syncope.
- Arrhythmias.
- Congestive heart failure.

Respiratory signs and symptoms:

- Dyspnoea.
- Tachypnoea.

Other signs and symptoms:

- Fatigue.

Diagnosis

- Auscultation: Systolic murmur.
- ECG: Left ventricular hypertrophy.
- Chest x-ray: Left ventricular enlargement.
- Echocardiography: Left ventricular hypertrophy.
- Bloods, urine and stool analysis as before.

Key management issues

The key management issues are shown in Table 7.5.

Table 7.5 Assessment and management of potential problems in hypertrophic cardiomyopathy (for detailed management of individual problems, see Chapter 11)

Left ventricular outflow tract obstruction:
- Administration of a beta blocker will help the obstruction and any associated angina pain[4]

Arrhythmias

Prevention of bacterial endocarditis

Congestive heart failure — late onset

Low cardiac output — late onset

Physical exertion:
- The child should be advised against exercise as sudden death can occur

Long-term care and follow-up

Sudden death can occur, probably as a result of increasing left ventricular outflow tract obstruction and arrhythmias[207, 208]. It is documented as a frequent cause of sudden death in young athletes[209].

Preventative measures to avoid sudden death include avoidance of moderate to heavy activity and management of the arrhythmias[210].

Restrictive cardiomyopathy (obliterative)

This variation produces stiff ventricular walls causing abnormal ventricular filling. The atria are enlarged with normal sized ventricles and contraction[4] and there is associated fibrosis of the myocardium[20]. It is a rare cause of cardiomyopathy in childhood[211] and is thought to be caused by repeated exposure to tropical diseases[10].

Signs and symptoms

Cardiovascular signs and symptoms:
- Chest pain.
- Atrial thrombus formation.
- Mitral regurgitation.
- Arrhythmias.

Respiratory signs and symptoms:

- Pleural effusion.
- Pulmonary congestion.

Diagnosis

- Auscultation: Systolic murmur due to mitral regurgitation.
- ECG: Atrial fibrillation.
- Chest x-ray: Cardiomegaly.
- Echocardiography: Diagnostic.
- Blood, urine and stool analysis as before.

Key management issues

The key management issues are shown in Table 7.6.

Table 7.6 Assessment and management of potential problems in restrictive cardiomyopathy (for detailed management of individual problems, see Chapters 10 and 11)

Pulmonary congestion

Arrhythmias

Atrial thrombus

Chest pain

Mitral regurgitation
- Beta blockers will improve diastolic filling[212]

Pleural effusions — rare

Long-term care and follow-up

Heart transplantation may be required as patients may develop a marked pulmonary vascular resistance index[211]. The prognosis is poor except in patients without pulmonary venous congestion where survival rates improve[213].

Kawasaki disease

Aetiology

Kawasaki disease is an acute, febrile vasculitis affecting young children, commonly under 4 years of age[4, 214]. It is associated with infectious diseases resulting in an abnormal response of the immune system[4, 215]. The cause is not known but has been linked to streptococcal infections and certain cleaning products[216]. It is usually unresponsive to antibiotics.

Signs and symptoms

There are three stages to the disease:

- Stage I: Over 3–4 days the child is pyrexial with inflamed mucus membranes and eyes. A skin rash develops.
- Stage II: By days 7–10 the patient's temperature is dropping, but the lymph nodes are enlarged. Skin peels, arthritis develops, diarrhoea presents and cardiovascular features occur.
- Stage III: This period occurs several weeks after the onset of symptoms. It is the recovery phase during which the symptoms gradually disappear.

Cardiovascular signs and symptoms

- Pericardial effusion.
- Arrhythmias.
- Arteritis causing coronary artery aneurysms which, if large, can result in low cardiac output.
- Ischaemic heart disease and calcification of the coronary arteries. Approximately 15–20% of patients develop aneurysms[4] and those at greatest risk are patients under six months of age[217].
- Mitral regurgitation.
- Myocarditis.

Haematological signs and symptoms

- High white cell count.
- High ESR.
- High CRP.
- Low haemoglobin.
- Thrombocytosis (high platelet count).

Immunological signs and symptoms

- Prolonged, unexplained fever.
- Enlarged lymph nodes.

Other signs and symptoms

- Skin rash.
- Hands, feet and mucus membranes are painful, arthritic, oedematous and red with peeling skin (especially in the groin area).
- Diarrhoea.

Table 7.7 Assessment and management of potential problems in Kawasaki disease (for management of individual problems see Chapters 10–13 and 15)

Inflammatory process:
- Aspirin 30–100 mg/kg/day for the first 2 weeks, then 3–5 mg/kg/day if coronary artery abnormalities present
- IV gamma globulin 2 mg/kg/day administered before day 10 significantly reduces the risk of developing coronary artery aneurysms[4, 217]

Thrombosis

Pleural effusion if present, although very rare

Arrhythmias

Coronary artery aneurysms:
- Coronary artery bypass grafting to bypass the obstruction may be necessary in the future

Myocarditis

Low haemoglobin

Pyrexia

Pain (joint, chest)

Conjunctivitis:
- Bathing the eyes with distilled water and administering artificial tears may soothe the eyes if very sore

Dehydration

- Abdominal pain.
- Conjunctivitis.
- Aseptic meningitis.
- Irritability.

Key management issues

Management is largely supportive depending on the presenting features. See Table 7.7.

Long-term care and follow-up

Regular assessment of the aneurysms and coronary arteries will be required. As this disease was first identified in 1967, comprehensive long-term results are not known. However, intermediate follow-ups show ischaemic heart disease occurs in approximately 5%, myocardial infarction in approximately 1.9%, and death in up to 5%[4, 218].

Chapter 8
Cardiopulmonary bypass

Principles of cardiopulmonary bypass

Cardiopulmonary bypass (CPB) is instituted during open heart surgery to allow the surgeon to operate in a bloodless field by stopping either the heart, lungs and heart, or lungs thus maintaining perfusion to vital organs. For example, when performing a Fontan procedure, bidirectional Glenn or reconstruction of the pulmonary artery, the heart will be kept beating but cardiopulmonary bypass will replace lung function.

There are three goals of CPB.

Circulatory aims

- To provide adequate cardiac output to perfuse organs and tissue.
- To control the central venous pressure.

Respiratory aims

- To maintain oxygenation.
- To eliminate carbon dioxide.

Metabolic aims

- A successful combination of the previous aims will usually ensure that metabolic demands are met.

Components of cardiopulmonary bypass

Cannulation

Both arterial and venous access are required to achieve cross circulation between the heart–lung machine and the patient. Ideally, cannulation should allow adequate unobstructed drainage and flow, and perfusion and drainage of all organs[219].

Arterial cannulation

This is normally instituted via the ascending aorta. However, should several previous sternotomies have been performed, bypass can be achieved by cannulating the femoral artery and femoral vein but free flow is hard to achieve. If an interrupted aortic arch is present two arterial cannulae are placed in the ascending and descending aorta respectively[220].

Venous cannulation

This is usually instituted via the two great veins or via the right atrium. Exceptions to this include adults, where use of a single cannula in the atrium is acceptable, as opposed to patients with congenital heart disease in whom the right side of the heart is usually open in some form[220]. Additionally, one cannula is used when the heart is small (e.g., in a baby under 5 kg), during deep hypothermic circulatory arrest[219] or when performing a cavopulmonary anastomosis. During a cavopulmonary anastamosis the heart is still beating and only lung function or right heart function needs to be replaced by cardiopulmonary bypass.

Intracardiac suction

Commonly, several suction lines are used, the most common sites being:

Left atrium or ventricle

To decompress the heart following the initiation of bypass.

Aortic needle

A line is connected to the aortic needle which is then used to infuse the cardioplegic solution and allow suction around the aortic root during bypass. However, its main use is at the end of a period of aortic cross clamping to remove air from the ascending aorta.

Hand held suction

To clear the blood from the site of the operation.

Heat exchange

Heating and cooling of the blood occurs out of the venous reservoir, around the arterial pump, into the heat exchanger and then through the oxygenator.

Oxygenator

There are two types of oxygenators or artificial lungs responsible for ventilation, that is, oxygenation and carbon dioxide elimination.

Bubble oxygenator

Oxygen bubbles through the venous blood in a reservoir. Small bubbles are used, increasing the surface area allowing more oxygenation of blood to take place and effective carbon dioxide removal. The bubbles produce a froth which is then exposed to an antifoaming agent that eliminates the bubbles before the blood is recirculated to the patient[20]. The disadvantages of bubble oxygenators include large prime volumes, injury to the red cells causing haemolysis, thrombocytopaenia, inefficient gaseous exchange at high flow rates and the risk of increasing the development of air emboli[38, 221]. Bubble oxygenators are rarely used in developed countries nowadays[219].

Membrane oxygenator

A semipermeable membrane is present to separate the blood from oxygen and carbon dioxide. Some degree of pressure is required, which has to be applied distally to the pump head, rather than proximally. Membrane oxygenators have the main advantage over bubble oxygenators in that there is less risk of air emboli, and minimal trauma to the red cells resulting in less haemolysis and platelet destruction[222]. They are used more successfully for prolonged periods of bypass greater than two hours.

Arterial filter

After oxygenation, the blood is filtered to remove air and debris before passing back into the patient.

Haemofilter

This filter is responsible for ultrafiltration which removes excess fluid during and after bypass[223].

Pump

There are several types of pumps available for CPB:

Roller pump

A double-armed roller pump, which is non-occlusive, is used to milk the tubing. One of the rollers acts as a valve to reduce the backflow of blood. A constant speed and flow is maintained, regardless of changes in resistance[220].

Centrifugal pump

This is a newer type of pump which gives a continuous flow of blood from its spinning blades. It has the advantage of reducing haemolysis and destruction of platelets[224]. Additionally there is increased perfusion of capillaries resulting in less incidence of acidosis[225]. However, a centrifugal pump has the disadvantage of increased total prime volume[219].

Stages of cardiopulmonary bypass

Whilst the anaesthetist is intubating, inserting central, arterial and other pressure lines, oesophageal and bladder thermometers, the perfusionist sets up and primes the extracorporeal circuit. The patient enters theatre and the surgeon performs a median sternotomy.

Heparinisation is commenced, aiming for an activated clotting time (ACT) of greater than 500 seconds. The venous and arterial cannulae are sited.

The bypass machine is started and the venous cannulae unclamped, venous blood flowing by gravity into the venous reservoir. Over the course of half an hour, the patient's core temperature is cooled to around 18–35°C depending on the procedure to be undertaken. Blood passes from the venous reservoir, around the arterial pump, into the heat exchanger, through the oxygenator and arterial filter into the aorta. Additional blood from the suction tubes passes into the cardiotomy and venous reservoirs, into a filter removing debris before arriving back into the arterial pump, heat exchanger, oxygenator, arterial filter and aorta.

The pump speed starts at the expected normal cardiac output but can be reduced if necessary when the patient is hypothermic and metabolic demands are reduced[38]. Additionally, in paediatric heart surgery, this flow rate needs to be reduced or stopped for intracardiac repairs to take place. Conversely, if most of the surgery is extracardiac, as in adult surgery, a higher flow rate can be maintained[219]. With certain congenital heart lesions (e.g., major aortopulmonary collateral vessels), there will be two circulations to consider: the machine's and the patient's, combining to determine the patient's flow rate[219].

- Neonates start with flow rates of 100 ml/kg/min.
- Infants and children start with flow rates of 2.4 l/m^2/min.

Techniques to protect the myocardium

Several techniques exist to protect the myocardium:

Cardioplegia

Cardioplegia allows the surgeon to cross clamp the aorta with minimal ischaemic damage to the heart in order to perform the specific repair. The technique involves injecting an ice-cold solution (4°C) into the aortic root. A crystalloid or colloid solution containing potassium is used. There are many solutions available, each having its own pros and cons.

Hypothermia

Hypothermia reduces the metabolic rate and oxygen demands of the patient's tissues. When the core temperature drops to 17°C, myocardial oxygen demands are reduced to approximately 12% of that at 37°C[220].

Deep hypothermic circulatory arrest

In neonates with complex heart lesions, it will be necessary to cool the patient using the cardiopulmonary bypass machine. This can achieve temperatures of 18°C whereby the heart can then be stopped, draining the vascular bed into the circuit[20]. This technique enables a shorter bypass time with less insult to the red cells. It also protects the myocardium, allowing the surgeon to perform the operation in the most ideal conditions possible — bloodless field, no cannulae to obscure the view, and shorter ischaemic times[220]. The time period for this procedure varies from 30–60 minutes[226].

Hypothermic low flow bypass

Bypass can continue when complex, prolonged surgery is undertaken with one venous cannula, therefore not obstructing the view. This allows the extra cardiac component of the operation to be repaired, for example, interrupted aortic arch with transposition of the great arteries and VSD[219].

Cross clamping of the aorta

Cross clamping of the aorta is performed in:

- Open heart procedures where the heart has to be arrested by cardioplegia (e.g., ASD, VSD, AVSD, Ross procedures, etc.). Acceptable cross clamp times vary with open heart surgery. However, the myocardium must be protected every 20 minutes with cardioplegia. This can be repeated several times, but the risk of myocardial damage increases the more cardioplegia given.
- Closed heart procedures where the heart is still beating (e.g., coarctation of the aorta when the narrowed sections of the aorta are clamped distally and proximally). Acceptable cross clamp time is 40–60 minutes; the shorter the time, the safer for the patient.

Situations where cross clamping of the aorta is not performed:

- Procedures such as cavopulmonary anastomosis, extra cardiac Fontan or pulmonary valvotomy repairs.

Rewarming and weaning from bypass

When the congenital heart defect has been repaired, the heart is rewarmed, normally resulting in sinus rhythm or, if fibrillating, defibrillation is performed[220]. Bypass is weaned by reducing venous return and arterial flow[220]. The heart is filled with blood by inflating the lungs with positive end expiratory pressure to aid in the removal of air from the cardiac chambers and ascending aorta. The heart is then allowed to fill slowly with blood and ventilation of the lungs is recommenced[20]. Once the cannulae are removed, the effects of heparin can be reversed by administering intravenous protamine.

Morbidity associated with cardiopulmonary bypass

CPB as a technique has improved dramatically over the years. The incidence of mortality directly associated with the procedure is very small — approximately 0.06%[220]. Morbidity associated with the procedure is, however, still significant albeit less than previously and is influenced to a major degree by the length of bypass the patient undergoes[227]. Complications directly arising from bypass can place the critically ill infant or child under enormous stress requiring high levels of nursing and medical intervention. The complications may be attributed to numerous causes including cardioplegia, anticoagulation, hypothermia and the extracorporeal circuit.

Morbidity associated with hypothermia

Hypothermia, despite having positive features during cardiac surgery, can be complicated by its negative effects. It affects major organs, namely the heart, lungs, brain, endocrine system and haematological events within the body.

- The heart is prone to arrhythmias (including bradycardias) below 34°C and ventricular fibrillation with temperatures below 32°C[220]. Additionally, the force of contractility is decreased and should the hypothermia be prolonged and severe (e.g., below 15°C), ischaemic changes occur resulting in low cardiac output and even death. Cardioplegia can depress myocardial function.
- The lungs require less oxygen to perfuse the vital organs and tissues. However, activation of surfactant is prevented.
- The brain has a decreased cerebral blood flow and metabolic rate. However, autoregulation of cerebral blood flow is lost during deep hypothermic circulatory arrest[9], but still has the advantage of good recovery postoperatively[20].
- The endocrine system responds to the stress by increasing the blood glucose due to impaired insulin release, releasing cortisol, ACTH, adrenaline and noradrenaline. The systemic inflammatory response cascade is activated.
- Haematology is affected by sustaining damage to the red cells and platelets and increasing the permeability of blood vessels.

Summary

A summary of the systemic changes that occur in response to bypass are shown in Table 8.1.

Table 8.1 Systemic changes due to cardiopulmonary bypass

System	Potential systemic changes due to cardiopulmonary bypass
Cardiovascular system	Most changes depend on the pre-existing disease and results of the surgery postoperatively: • Decreased heart rate • Arrhythmias • Decreased cardiac output (hypotension) • Ischaemic changes to the myocardium • Increased energy requirements as the heart warms up
Respiratory system	Frequent problems occur: • Impaired oxygen transportation • Reduced lung compliance • Pulmonary haemorrhage

(contd)

Table 8.1 (contd)

System	Potential systemic changes due to cardiopulmonary bypass
	• Pulmonary oedema • Atelectasis despite 100% oxygen and PEEP during surgery. This reduced expansion in conjunction with hypothermia prevents the activation of surfactant (known as pump lung) and the need for increased pressures postoperatively • Acute respiratory distress syndrome (ARDS) • Endothelial lung damage causing an increase in protein permeability resulting in increased lung water • Pulmonary endothelial damage • Microemboli formation
Neurological system	Transient brain damage is common. Uneven systemic cooling can cause: • Poor perfusion • Cerebral oedema • Microemboli formation • Fitting • Confusion • Depression and anxiety • Visual disturbances • Reduced cerebral autoregulation if deep hypothermic circulatory arrest • Basal ganglia abnormalities — movement disorders[38]
Renal system	A decrease in renal blood flow can result in: • Oliguria/anuria • Acute tubular necrosis resulting in acute renal failure • Poor perfusion is perceived by the kidneys as haemovolaemic shock thus causing an increase in renin production[38] • Vasoconstriction due to hypothermia causes the angiotensin/renin response releasing aldosterone • Haematuria due to haemolysis • Impaired metabolism of drugs especially aminoglycosides and ACE inhibitors
Gastrointestinal system	Changes that occur are related to a systemic inflammatory response cascade and hypoperfusion producing: • Microemboli • Paralytic ileus • Gastrointestinal bleed • Ischaemic bowel/necrotising enterocolitis • Liver dysfunction causing clotting abnormalities • Pancreatitis
Endocrine system/ metabolic response	The release of catecholamines causing increased: • ADH secretion affecting urine output • Activation of aldosterone–renin–angiotensin mechanism • Epinephrine and norepinephrine secretion The release of ACTH causing: • Cortisol secretion • Growth hormone secretion • Reduction in insulin secretion, thus causing increased blood glucose levels • TSH secretion

(contd)

Table 8.1 (contd)

System	Potential systemic changes due to cardiopulmonary bypass
	Metabolic responses causing: • Increased protein breakdown • Increased gluconeogenesis • Increased fat breakdown • Overall increase in basal metabolic rate
Haematology	• Haemorrhage due to incomplete heparin reversal • Increased platelet aggregation • Increased platelet consumption • Red blood cell destruction causing anaemia and haemolysis of urine • Low fibrinogen and prothrombin • White cell destruction • Low plasma proteins • Haemodilution • Increased CRP
Fluid and electrolytes/ circulating volume	• Capillary leak syndrome/increased capillary permeability causing a fluid shift and whole body oedema. This is due to an increase in total body water in the extracellular and extra vascular spaces[228]. This is particularly so in neonates and infants due to the inflammatory response and the secretion of ADH[219]. • Low magnesium • Low calcium • Low potassium • High sodium
Endothelium/ inflammatory response	Due to the insult to tissue and cells from the cardiac surgery and CPB, the endothelium is activated causing varying degrees of systemic inflammatory response syndrome. Various vasoactive substances are released (e.g., interleukins, histamines, nitric oxide, prostacyclin, thromboxane, bradykinin) changing the vascular tone and thus fluid distribution by affecting capillary permeability[219]. This cascade of events predisposes to varying degrees of multi-organ failure with associated morbidity and mortality[219]

Key management issues

The key management issues are shown in Table 8.2.

Table 8.2 Assessment and management of potential problems after cardiopulmonary bypass (for detailed management of individual problems, see Chapters 10–13)

Heart failure from poor perfusion causing:
• Arrhythmias
• Low cardiac output

Respiratory distress due to:
• Pulmonary haemorrhage
• Pulmonary oedema
• Atelectasis
• ARDS

(contd)

Table 8.2 (contd)

- Lung damage
- Microemboli

Brain damage from poor cerebral perfusion causing:
- Cerebral oedema
- Microemboli
- Fitting
- Confusion, anxiety and depression
- Visual disturbances
- Movement disorders

Renal failure from poor renal perfusion causing:
- Acute tubular necrosis resulting in renal failure
- Increased aldosterone secretion
- Haematuria
- Impaired drug metabolism

Gastrointestinal problems from poor perfusion causing:
- Microemboli
- Paralytic ileus
- Gastrointestinal haemorrhage
- Ischaemic bowel/necrotising enterocolitis
- Clotting abnormalities from liver failure
- Pancreatitis

Stress response causing:
- Increased ADH secretion and therefore increased water and sodium retention
- Increased blood glucose levels

Haemorrhage due to anticoagulation and CPB causing:
- Platelet consumption
- Platelet aggregation
- Anaemia from red blood cell destruction
- Haemodilution
- Increased CRP

Fluid and electrolyte imbalances causing:
- Low magnesium
- Low calcium
- Low potassium
- High sodium

Capillary leak syndrome with:
- Ultrafiltration when weaning from CPB. This is the process of fluids passing across a membrane where a transmembrane pressure gradient exists. The higher the gradient, the more fluid is pulled off[219]. It differs from haemofiltration in that no fluid is transferred back into the patient to replace that lost from the ultrafiltration process[219]
- Peritoneal dialysis
- Diuretics

Tissue damage and cell death due to a systemic inflammatory response syndrome causing:
- Exudate release from damaged tissues
- Endothelial activation
- Multi-organ failure, septicaemia, platelet aggregation and vasodilation

Chapter 9
Elective admission for cardiac surgery

Preoperative management

Physical care preadmission

For the majority of children with a congenital heart defect, surgery will be planned in one or several stages depending on the actual lesion present. Preparation for the planned surgical event starts in the preadmission clinic. Here the child will undergo several tests ascertaining a baseline or highlighting abnormalities which need to be corrected before surgery. The child and parents can visit the ward to meet the play specialist and cardiac liaison nurse where discussion of the admission, pre- and postoperative care is undertaken. Social and domestic problems can be highlighted and referrals made where necessary to the social work team, psychologist, dietitian or other relevant members of the multidisciplinary team. See Table 9.1 for details of preoperative assessment and tests.

Table 9.1 Preoperative assessment and tests

Area of assessment	Details
Size	Weight Height Centile plotted Body surface area calculated
Laboratory	Nose, throat and rectal surveillance swabs Stool if rectal swab not taken Full blood count Urea and electrolytes Clotting profile Cross match for the appropriate number of units of blood, fresh frozen plasma, platelets. Blood products must be irradiated and cytomegalovirus negative if Di George syndrome present or suspected

(contd)

Table 9.1 (contd)

Area of assessment	Details
Cardiac	ECG Echocardiogram Chest x-ray
Observations	Temperature Heart rate, regularity, volume of peripheral pulses Blood pressure — four limb to exclude coarctation of the aorta Respiratory rate and character Evidence of cyanosis and clubbing of fingers and toes Oxygen saturations
Pain	Pain assessment can be made in the preadmission clinic and the management of pain discussed with the child and parents

Admission to the ward

On admission to the ward the child and family are met by their named nurse and shown the ward layout and their bedspace. An initial nursing assessment will be made from the child and family establishing a picture of their normal routines, likes and dislikes. The areas nursing care should cover are shown in Table 9.2.

Table 9.2 Areas the nursing care plan should cover

System	Observation
Cardiovascular system	The child's condition Initial assessment Cardiovascular status Activity level
Respiratory system	Assess respiratory status Any signs of respiratory distress Oxygen dependent Other respiratory disease — e.g., asthma, bronchiolitis
Neurological	Perform developmental assessment Development milestones being met History of fitting, abnormal movement Pain history and pain service provided in the hospital
Diet and feeding	Weight, height, head circumference, centile chart Establish the baby's or child's routine Types of drinks/food ingested Is the baby breast fed or formula fed?

(contd)

Table 9.2 (contd)

System	Observation
	• Likes and dislikes • Can the child feed him or herself? • Is the baby fed nasogastrically? • Are calories added to the diet? • Are fluids restricted if the baby has been in heart failure?
Communication	Assess the level the child is at developmentally • Special words used for objects, etc. • Provide information for the child and family appropriate to their needs
Sleep	Establish the child's sleep pattern
Play	Comforters Favourite toys Introduce to play specialist
Religious/cultural needs	Ensure religious and cultural needs have been addressed
Family needs	Ensure information has been given — e.g., booklets, glossary of terms, heart file, help groups Provide postnatal care for newly delivered mothers Contact the accommodation officer for the family's room Establish the role they would like to play in their child's care Discuss integrated care pathways if appropriate
Medications	History of medications the child is currently taking
Referrals to make	Cardiac liaison nurse Physiotherapist Cardiac social worker if appropriate Dietitian if weight below the third centile Health visitor/school nurse

Psychological care

Parents' experience

Finding out that a child has a congenital heart defect is a very frightening experience for parents, one which staff can only ever imagine and not truly understand. Discovery of the problem may be prenatally during ultrasound scan, at birth, at several days old or weeks later. Initially the family needs time to grieve about not having a "perfect" baby as feelings of shock, anxiety and fearing the baby's death may occur[11]. If the defect is one requiring years of intervention, it can place a serious strain upon family relationships:

- Mother
  Guilt feelings may occur related to giving birth to a "deformed" child.
  What did I do wrong when I was pregnant?
  Is this a punishment?
  There is all the added strain of looking after the ill child, plus the rest of the family[11].

- Father
  Feelings of inadequacy and neglect as his wife concentrates on the sick child.
  Can feel resentful, frustrated, angry, guilty.

- Siblings
  Deeply affected.
  Feelings of resentfulness and jealously as the sick child is getting all the attention.
  Can become withdrawn and isolated.
  Frightened of becoming ill themselves[11].

A father whose son was born with a bicuspid aortic valve and critical aortic stenosis describes his feelings on discoving his son's heart defect and the initial contact he and his wife had with the specialist heart centre.

Be good wee man

Tuesday 25th November 1997

The runaway train went over the hill

6 a.m.
It was a bad night. A fitful sleep followed by an early rise. Somehow I did not feel tired, my mind was working overtime as I tried to come to terms with my thoughts. Sleep could wait however because this day was to be different, another big day, the day before the biggest day in Edward Stenhouse's short but eventful life.

Edward was born kicking and screaming at 10 minutes to 9 on Thursday 6th November 1997. Like one of the many fireworks set off the night before, he seemed to jump and crackle as he proceeded to fight his midwife every step of the way. His scrawny arms pushed straight out, his long skinny legs rigid, each toe separated like a second set of fingers, he cried as the midwife gently checked, cleaned and weighed him.

"Nothing wrong with him," the midwife said.

"Fine set of lungs," said her colleague as she carefully wrapped him in a blanket and laid him in the arms of Sandra my wife. Soppy dad was already in tears. My son, I thought. Get a grip you big Jessie as my sniffles began to get out of control.

The paediatrician was called. Six weeks earlier, a skilful prenatal scan operator had noticed that Edward's heart was enlarged. Since then, Sandra had been given careful monitoring three times a week and regular scans, all had shown the signs of a normal baby. I was the hopeless optimist while Sandra was more cautious, her instincts were telling her something different, perhaps protecting her from what was to come.

The doctor was happy, a lovely baby, a slight heart murmur but that is common in new babies, she said, and then she was gone leaving Sandra, myself and Edward alone for the first time. Annabel, our 2-year-old daughter was staying with her grandma and granddad. We rang them and my family with our news and I drove home feeling overjoyed. A bottle of beer to celebrate and then bed.

Sandra slept that night with Edward in her bed. He suckled at her breast and they cuddled. Sandra slept badly but did not care. It was if she somehow knew this time was precious and as it turned out it was the only night they slept together for a very long time.

And he blew

6.30 a.m.

After a quick cup of tea, I walked over to the ICU as they say once you are in the know. Before the 8th November I would have had no idea that it meant the Intensive Care Unit but you learn quickly when you have to. I entered through the security door and walked inside the unit towards Edward.

"Morning," I said to his nurse.

"Morning." She fills me in on his night. "Quiet, been asleep most of the night," she reported.

"Has he had his fruesilide?" I enquire.

"You mean frusemide, yes and his digoxin."

Damn! I could never remember the name of the drugs.

Edward looked serene, His little face obscured by the green plastic hose that protruded from his nose connecting him to the hi-tech ventilator that was keeping him alive. He's a bonny lad, I thought as I stroked his fine brown hair. His angular face shape pure Stenhouse, his dark round eyes, now closed and slightly swollen, pure Higham. The ventilator hose only seemed to add to the contrast between his soft tender face and the man-made machines that surrounded him.

At 7 a.m. Edward was passed on to the nurse responsible for his next 8 hours while her colleague prepared herself for the drive home, window open and the radio blaring to stay awake, then a few hours in bed. All the lights came on in the unit, it was now officially day.

I had woken up at 7 a.m. the day after his birth, surprisingly sleeping well. Better a good night's sleep now I thought selfishly as I dressed. It was too early to ring everyone but I found Sandra's list, my memory is notoriously bad, and began ringing friends and relatives around 8 a.m. Everybody was overjoyed, their reaction fantastic as they transmitted their good wishes. I ate breakfast trying to plan my day ahead briefly toying with the idea of a fry up at the local café but declined. Things to do, people to see. I collected a card and some flowers and then headed back to the hospital

"No spouses before 2 p.m.," said the nurse, "so be quick," as I deliberately flouted the rules to deliver the flowers to my wife and newborn son.

Sandra, despite all, looked well. The consultant in charge of her pregnancy had visited and had left, his job done. Sandra's named midwife was confident all was well.

What is it about a mother's instinct? How can perfectly rational people know when things are not quite right? Our earlier conversations had ended in tears as I steadfastly refused to be concerned.

"Don't pre-judge," I would say. "He'll be fine, you'll see."

Why did I feel uneasy? My own Maginot wall was easily rounded by reasoned argument.

"Why is the heart enlarged then?" she would question.

"Look, all the traces you've had done show it's fine," I would say. " All the scans are normal, if there was a problem, they wouldn't let you go through a normal labour, would they?"

"Yes, but the heart is enlarged," she would repeat.

Whoo! Whoo!

7.30 a.m.

I left Edward in the capable hands of his ICU nurse and walked down the long corridor that links up the hospital wards. I wandered towards casualty. The hospital had become such a large part of our lives. How long had we been here? It seemed like forever. I headed back to the communal kitchen in McDonald house for a bowl of Alpen. Better to let the milk soak in I thought.

The ward round started at 8.30. I took a particular delight in being there for the doctor's round. I would listen to what they said about Edward but I would also be watching the reactions, the pecking order. I noticed that junior doctors do not look directly at the patient's relative, consultants do. The round always started at the same cubicle going from patient to patient clockwise in a predetermined route.

Nobody moved away from the patient before the others, it is as if a collective decision is made to all move at once. Doctors, surgeons, anaesthetists and hangers on looking for a predetermined signal, a twist of the hips, a soft shoe shuffle, not too fast, don't want too get there to soon and then like a small herd of wildebeest they move off as if as one onto the next patient. The doctor in charge of the patient reads out the notes. Gradually, I have learned the terms and codes used in the patient's notes and I get a pretty good idea of what is going on. The doctor, who has been up all night, is asked a question or two about Edward's condition — quiet peaceful night. A few wise words from the consultant, a nod of acknowledgement maybe even a word or two. Once we even got a joke about building Edward up with a pint of Guinness and a egg nog but today my reasons for being there were different, today the chief surgeon, would be there and I wanted to talk to him.

Returning from the maternity ward, I rang through to my work with the news and everyone was delighted. I arranged the next week off on holiday as Sandra would probably be out with Edward by then. It was 1.40 p.m., must get a move on.

Sandra's mum and dad had just arrived when I returned to the ward. They were at the main door with our daughter Annabel who was dressed in a way only grandmas could think of. Sandra will go mad I thought. Annabel looked as gorgeous as ever. Thick strawberry blonde hair tied back off her face, her mother's bluey-green eyes in a round face with an infectious smile.

"Edward looks just like her as a baby," I said to her granddad, his hands full with flowers and cards while trying to keep a hold on to Annabel's hand.

"We can't wait to see him," he replied as we buzzed the front desk to be allowed in.

We were met by a very distraught Sandra.

"There's something wrong with his heart."

" What?" I asked.

Sandra's mum went a funny colour.

"I don't really know but he must have an x-ray. The paediatrician will be back in a minute."

The murmur noticed at birth had not gone away, in fact it was probably stronger. We did not know it then but we were effectively starting the longest and scariest journey of our lives.

Things happened quickly. The doctor returned, an ECG scan was called for. A porter arrived with a wheelchair to take Sandra and Edward to x-ray. Annabel, blissfully unaware of what was happening stayed with granddad while grandma, Sandra and Edward and I set off towards the x-ray unit.

Hospitals are always a funny shape. This one was no different as we travelled through the long chilly corridors that connected buildings of different styles from different decades. The x-ray department was ready for us as our entourage arrived.

"Who wants to hold him?" asked the operator. "You do it Dougie," said Sandra as I was handed the heavy protective shield to wear. Why do they cover your body and not your head? My thoughts gathered quickly as I held little Edward's thin arms. The operator targeted his tiny chest with her machine. Edward was not happy, I had a great view of his tonsils as he screamed. Outside, with her mother comforting her, Sandra was now distraught, her worst fears confirmed. What could I say? For weeks I had poo-pooed her arguments.

"To me," I would shout, I always shouted. "When I see a glass of water it is always half full, to you, it is always half empty. Let's worry about it if it happens, okay? You'll see I'm right."

We made our way back to the maternity unit in a bit of a daze. We couldn't really believe all this was happening. We met the senior registrar.

"He could have a small hole in the heart," she said. " The murmur is consistent with a hole to the lower left ventricle or chamber allowing the blood coming into the heart to mix with the oxygenated blood being pumped out making it work harder which would probably account for the increase in size."

"Will he be okay?"

" A hole in the heart in babies does happen from time to time," she sought to reassure us." You should try not to worry too much, we will have to do more tests and the paediatric consultant will want to see you. In the meantime, I think it would be better to move you to the special care unit."

Special care, the words began to sink in and then begin to eat into my mind — special care.

The maternity ward had its own unit designed to cope with the premature or babies born with breathing difficulties. On the way to the birthing rooms, it has its own security door and nursing team. You sometimes wondered what went on inside it. We were about to find out.

The Stenhouse family were welcomed with a cup of tea. The SCU was very neat and tidy. The longstay babies were kept in incubators hooked up to monitors. Sandra was given a small room with her own bathroom. A small table was soon covered in flowers sent by well-wishers. Edward was given a small cot, and for the first time, a little monitor with a flashing light and bleeper every time he breathed.

"Something we do with all our babies," explained the nurse. "Just ignore it."

Ignore it? The little flashing light seemed to fill the room, the bleep — bleep — bleep seemed to be so loud. My eyes were transfixed on that flashing light, watching his every breath being counted by a machine, waves of panic occurred every time the light was a nano-second later in flashing.

The runaway train

8.40 a.m.

"It is clear we must now do surgery." The surgeon was very serious. He had dark eyes, staring, unblinking through his large black framed glasses.

"As with every operation, we must go in with more than one option because we do not know what we will find. The first option is to repair the valve if we can. That would be the preferred one. If we cannot, then we must think of replacing the aortic root. At the moment we do not have one so small so we must see if we can use one of the ones we have." I tried to find an intelligent question but all I could do was nod, as if in agreement. The doctor spoke calmly, precise with no frills — just like his job I suppose.

"The third and therefore the most dangerous option is to use his own pulmonary valve to replace the aortic valve and use a donor valve on the other side as this is less important."

"The Ross procedure?" I had heard the name from the cardiologist.

" Yes but this would only be the last option, we will repair the valve if we can. You must understand an operation such as this on such a small baby carries many risks. To do the operation his heart must be stopped and a bypass machine used. We would be concerned his heart might not restart. He is very small. Just one more kilo would make a difference." He stared at me as if to say did I realise just how serious it was. I looked at him, mumbled my thanks for his time. He spotted where the ward round had got to, nodded, then left.

On his second night in the world, Edward slept in the same room as Sandra to begin with. During the night, she had watched his breathing become more laboured, the light flashing irregularly. The sister came and moved Edward into another room. I was woken at 6 a.m. on Saturday morning with a phone call from the her telling me not to be alarmed but to make my way to the unit as Sandra was very upset.

By the time I got there, she was more in control. The nursing staff were concerned enough to have called out the paediatrician and Edward had been moved to allow Sandra to get some sleep. No chance of that.

The day before, urgent phone calls had resulted in a quickly arranged echo-vascular scan to be done on Edward that morning. The cardiac consultant was to meet us at the ECG unit. We had met the paediatric consultant the night before. He was also of the opinion Edward had a hole in his heart.

We set off down the long corridors towards our appointment, with Sandra in a wheelchair holding Edward and me pushing. Hospital wheelchairs were big and heavy and difficult to steer. On a number of occasions I nearly hit the wall as I wrestled to keep control of my passengers.

We met the cardiac consultant outside the unit. Once inside, little Edward, bright as a button, had his chest smeared in jelly as the portable machine that looked like a large computer was allowed to warm up. With a probe connected to the machine, the doctor took a sounding of Edward's heart. We had at that time no idea what he was looking for, luckily, the consultant did. Within five minutes he had identified the problem. He worked on in silence. He finished and we put Edward's babygrow back on.

"Do you know anything about the heart?" he asked.

"Not really."

He went on to explain the workings of the heart.

"The heart has four chambers, the two on the right side take the blood returning from the body and pump the blood into the lungs." He drew a diagram as he talked. He was a slightly built man of Indian origin. He talked to us in a gentle manner, trying not to be too technical.

"The two chambers on the left collect the blood from the lungs and pump it out through the aortic arch to the brain and the rest of the body. Sometimes a hole appears between the two sides allowing the blood returning from the body to mix with the outgoing blood. This is not the case with Edward. Each chamber is connected by a valve. The valves open and close when the heart pumps allow-ing the blood to flow around the heart and out into the body. In Edward's case, the aortic valve, the outlet valve, is restricted somehow. This means the blood pumped out of the heart is under a lot of pressure making the heart work harder and that is why the heart is enlarged. This condition is called aortic stenosis." We were to hear those two words again and again, aortic stenosis. The consultant went on to explain what Edward's treatment would be.

"The valve needs to be opened. One of the ways to open it is by means of a catheter." He looked at us as if to see if we recognised the word. "A wire is inserted into his vein, probably from the groin and passed up into the valve. A small balloon is inserted and blown up in the valve to stretch it and release the blood flow. An operation like this carries risks. His veins are very small and thin, the wire could pierce the vein or even the heart as it is difficult to know exactly what is happening. The blood vessel used could become clogged and stop the circulation to the leg.

"Because of the risks and the chance that surgery might be necessary, it would be better that he is taken to a special paediatric cardiac unit."

"When?" I said, my eyes like swimming pools, Sandra in tears. We were holding Edward who was still awake and looking round wondering what all the fuss was about.

"The sooner the better, I will ring straight away, possibly this afternoon. Have you any questions?"

"Will he live?" meaning will he die.

"He has every chance but there are no guarantees."

"Will he be able to live a normal life?" asked Sandra

"Yes, but he couldn't do any competitive sport like cross country running or judo."

"Will he need special care or schooling?"

"No, he should be able to go to a normal school."

We thanked him for coming to see little Edward and left to prepare ourselves for the journey.

Went over the hill

I walked back to Ronald McDonald house in a bit of a dream. The pavements and road were damp with rain. The grey clouds low and heavy as the hospital came to life with people scurrying to work. It seemed to have rained every day since we came here or had I imagined it? The house, our temporary home for nearly three weeks now, was built with the help of McDonald's Restaurants. It provided accommodation for the families of the sick children of the hospital. Without its comfortable rooms, communal kitchen and sitting rooms, life would have been much more difficult. Already, the surgeon's words were becoming distant — try and repair it, replace it, the Ross procedure — heavy stuff. Could I remember it all? Would I forget some crucial part? I walked into reception where there was another letter in our tray. We had received letters and cards nearly every day. They were a great comfort. Our families and friends had been superb. They had come to see us, sent flowers and cards or just sent their good wishes. We knew of at least four different churches and faiths who prayed for us and Edward. I ran up the stairs and through the lounge. Each room was named after an animal, ours was the Hippo room.

· Sandra had finished expressing her milk. "Well?" she enquired.

"I spoke to the surgeon."

"What's he like?"

"He's okay," I said not really knowing how to describe him.

"What did he say?"

I went through his description of how our son might die as Sandra listened and Annabel jumped on the bed asking for her breakfast. Sandra was a good listener. Did I remember it all? How did all this happen? Things like this don't happen to people like us.

Two days earlier, we had walked through Sainsbury's car park.

"You don't talk to me," she had started, "You don't touch me or hold my hand any more. I feel like I'm going through this alone."

"What are you going on about?" I shouted back as I pushed Annabel along in her pushchair, "I'm looking after Annabel!"

"No, you just seem to ignore me. You don't even want to sleep with me."

"We've got two single beds," I answered slightly confused. Annabel had gone very quiet.

"You never reach for me. I always have to make the first move, it's like I'm here on my own."

"I'm tired out," I retorted. "I'm not ignoring you. I'm just as worried as you, you know." I was beginning to get even louder. "Why do you always think I don't want you? You say I'm selfish, you're selfish, I'm only thinking of my son — my daughter!"

"Right I'm going back." She turned on her heel and headed out of the car park.

"You're driving us apart!" I shouted for no apparent reason and for the first time noticed all the shoppers loading up their cars with shopping trying not to look at us but failing miserably. Sheepishly, I pushed Annabel into the store.

The following morning Sandra was planning as we washed and dressed.

"Okay, we will both go and see him and then take Annabel to Fleetwood to stay with Grandma and Granddad," she said

"And Ben de dog," chipped in Annabel.

" We must be back for three, the consultant wants to see us and we have the forms to sign."

" If we go now, we can be back for three."

Sandra had it all sussed. Walking was a lot easier for her now. Edward was only three weeks old but she had already got her figure back and she had her jeans on.

"They are too big for me normally," she would say but I was genuinely proud of her. No one I have ever met has her commitment to looking after her figure.

We went to see Edward together. Our perfect little boy being helped to breathe by the ventilator. I studied him again as I had many times before. He was so thin, he had lost all of his weight again. You could just make out his little heart pumping away against the odds beneath the skin of his chest. Soon they would be opening him up. Morbidly, my thoughts wandered off in a tangent. I wish they didn't have to operate. I remembered a *Star Trek* film where the main characters travelled back in time to save a whale. Checkov fell off a ship and hurt his back and the 20th century surgeons wanted to operate. McCoy was horrified as he had some sort of light laser healing tool that meant that an operation was unnecessary. How I wish he was here now.

"What is it Doctor McCoy?"

"It's a valve Jim but not as we know it."

"Spock?"

"Hmm interesting, the valve seems to be obstructing the blood flow, causing the heart to work harder and therefore become enlarged. Highly illogical, Captain."

"What are his chances?"

"Hard to say, it will depend on how much power he can raise."

"Scotty, Warp factor 9."

"I'll try Captain but I dinnie think his engine can take it!".

We were still reeling from what the paediatric cardiologist had told us as we arrived back on the maternity special care unit. The consultant in charge of the unit explained to us what would happen next. He would write to the consultant at the specialist unit and Edward would be taken by ambulance to the hospital. We could have travelled with him but decided instead to follow on behind in the car, we would need transport when we got there. I quickly returned home to pick up some clean clothes for Sandra. We rang her parents with the news who, as well as looking after Annabel, were our communication to the outside world. The couple of hours before the ambulance arrived passed fairly quickly. One of the nurses had shown me Edward's heart x-ray. The heart seemed to fill his chest. I could just make out the lungs behind this huge dark shape that was his heart muscle. For the first time, I was really scared.

The ambulance arrived. Edward, in a travelling incubator was loaded into the vehicle ready for his trip to..., to what? We had absolutely no idea.

Sandra, still only two days after giving birth, walked steadily to the car. We followed the ambulance with its precious cargo as it made its way to the paediatric unit. Sandra was pleased to be out of a hospital environment for the first time in four days. We did not know it then but the hospital way of life was to become our way of life too.

The last we heard

11.30

We made ready to take Annabel to her grandparent's house in Fleetwood. She loved to stay at Fleetwood with its promenade and beaches. She loved to watch the big Pandora ferries as they made their way back and forward to Ireland. She knew all their names; the Puma, the Bison, the Leopard, she always hid her face when the boat's horn gave an almighty blast.

Sandra's parents had been a great help. They visited us every second day and looked after Annabel during Edward's first operation. At first, they had been very optimistic.

"So he's off the ventilator, that's good," granddad would say hopefully.

"Yes, but he has still got a long way to go," we would answer.

"He's making progress though," he would insist.

We had to be careful not to hurt their feelings without getting carried away ourselves. The pain and anguish was still very fresh in our minds. Even I, after Edward's first operation, thought we would be home in a few days and live happily ever after. But then I had spent five awful days watching Edward struggle to breathe unaided with oxygen pumped into his incubator. I would watch for hours, my head resting on the plastic surround, my hand holding his through the small service hole on the side of his artificial home. I looked on as he panted and struggled to get into a regular breathing pattern. Short breaths, sometimes reaching over one hundred a minute. I knew, deep in my heart then, that he was not going to recover. He had tried so very hard.

We stopped at the local supermarket in the car and bought some sandwiches for the journey. After we had eaten our food, the rest of the hour-long journey was held very much in silence. Sandra's parents were also fairly quiet when we arrived. We stayed for an hour not mentioning the unmentionable then said our goodbyes to Annabel, thanked them once again and left promising to let them know as soon as there was any news. We scoffed a huge bag of chocolate raisins on the way back but didn't speak much. Our thoughts were elsewhere as we drove back to the hospital to meet the consultant in charge of Edward's care.

We drove into the gates of the children's hospital, what would we find? The entrance was not what we expected. Squeezed between the cardiac day unit, the operating theatres and the older part of the hospital, it seemed like the back door. The porters lowered Edward inside his incubator and took him into the hospital to the cardiac ward. The place seemed a hive of activity with a long ward full of beds on the left and a squarer room with cots and incubators on the right. We were allocated a place next to the nurses' station. We met the nurse assigned to Edward who always looked really sad and worried but was extremely kind. Edward was crying. He was placed into his new cot bed and a new monitor was hooked to his foot. Bleep, bleep, bleep. The midwife and the ambulance people said their goodbyes and we were in.

"Shall I feed him?" enquired Sandra, a little unsure.

"Let me see," said the nurse as she scanned his notes. "I don't see why not."

The curtains were pulled around us and Edward fed. As it turned out, it was his last feed for a very long time.

The ward sister came over. "The cardiology consultant will see you now."

We made our way back downstairs. A tall man waited by a door near the entrance we had just come in. He seemed young for a consultant cardiologist, not what I imagined at all. Surely consultants should look like the big bloke with the beard in *Carry On Doctor*. He invited us into the echo-vascular scan unit. He introduced himself and began to tell us what he planned to do. He had spoken to his colleague from the maternity unit and was fully aware of Edward's condition. He quickly read the notes and set about spreading a lump of gel on Edward's now bare chest. His machine was already up and running and he quickly keyed in Edward's name. He worked quickly and described to us what he could see. Edward, unblinking watched as this man poked about his upper rib cage with a probe shaped like an electric shaver. We did not know it but Edward was very ill, another two days and he would have died.

The cardiologist turned to us and said, "The pressure through his valve is too high. The valve is restricted and must be opened, has anyone explained to you about a catheter?"

"Yes," we sort of nodded in unison.

"I think it is the best option, I will check with the surgeon but we will need to begin very quickly."

The cardiologist thought for a moment. "We need to begin very soon, his ductus is closing, make arrangements, while I talk to the surgeon."

The ductus is a bypass valve and the connection between a mother and the unborn baby. If Edward's had closed, his heart would have failed and he would have died.

The cardiologist returned, "I have spoken to the surgeon and he agrees the best option is to balloon the valve. We will have to empty his stomach and administer prostin to keep the valve open."

Poor Edward, he could have just had his last meal and here he was about to give it all back. The cardiologist again emphasised the risks of the operation then left to prepare.

He was going still

3.00 p.m.

"What shall we do tomorrow?" asked Sandra as we made our way to the ICU to see the consultant. She answered her own question. "We need to get away from here, I can't just sit around while they operate. Shall we go to the cathedral?"

"Tell you what," I countered. "You need a new coat, let's go down to the town centre, buy you a coat then we will go up to the cathedral."

"The Anglican one?"

"The big brown sandstone one, I think that's the Anglican."

"Okay."

"If we have time," I went on. "McDonald House need some Christmas cards delivered, we could volunteer to do that if you like."

"Okay."

We had agreed. The thought of tomorrow was just too much to contemplate. Now we had something to do, to aim for. We were positive. Inside, was a different matter.

The intensive care consultant took us into his office. It was quite small with lots of paperwork and memorandums scattered about the desk. A computer was on the desk.

The ICU consultant was very serious. He talked us through the aftermath of the operation. The risks were many, the good things were few and far between. It must have been difficult for him, he was basically telling us our son was going to die tomorrow or if not could become an invalid or suffer brain damage. He emphasised that Edward's heart would be stopped and may not start again after the surgery. He painted a very bleak future. Sandra was very upset but in control. The doctor had a scared look about him and a very nervous smile as he tried to be kind but also realistic. The nurse assigned to heart patient families to help them come to terms with their problems joined us. Sandra started to cry.

"Be brave," I said.

"No, let it out, you will feel better," argued the nurse.

I shut up, she knew best.

We left the meeting feeling worse than ever. Heart failure, the heart might not restart, death. Morbid thoughts began to take over. I imagined myself picking up his body from the mortuary.

"Challenge!" Sandra interrupted my thoughts.

"What?"

"Challenge," repeated Sandra. "He said Edward would be a challenge. He could have picked a better word."

I was silent for a moment. "Perhaps he means they will work to get him better," I tried to defend him. "You know, with the help of his medicines like captril."

"Captopril!" said Sandra with a smile, I still could not get to grips with the names of his drugs.

We walked back through the ward towards Edward. We had another meeting to look forward to, this time with one of the registrar surgeons.

One of our favourite nurses was with Edward. She smiled as she saw us approach. Edward looked very comfortable. Some of the nurses went that extra bit for Edward, little things that just made his life a tiny bit better. She had found a fake sheepskin underblanket for him and he had a clean nappy on.

"How are you?" she asked.

"Okay," we lied. "Has the surgeon been round?"

"You mean the registrar surgeon, the surgeon's assistant?"

"Yes."

"No, I will try to find him." She turned to the nurse who was looking after little Alex over the way and asked her to look out for Edward as she disappeared into the operating theatres. The nurses often covered for each other when they needed to fetch something or have a break but most of the time the little patients had a 24-hour carer to chart their progress and administer their medicines.

While we waited, I looked round the unit. It was quieter than usual. We had got to know everybody who worked there, the doctors, nurses and ward assistants. Other parents sat by their children. Some of the patients were newborn babies like little Liam, whose heart kept stopping, causing waves of panic. Others were older. We had been here so long we would see them being wheeled out of the theatre surrounded by lots of doctors, nurses, technicians and anaesthetists. They would all head for a predetermined cubicle and close the curtains. Twenty minutes later, the curtains would open and there would be another heart child hooked up to the monitors being helped to breathe by the ventilator. The alarms would go off regularly as the nursing staff fought to stabilise their little patient. A constant bleep, bleep, bleep sound that became very familiar. The new arrivals are out for the count with their chest wounds dressed. From the wound, two pipes lead to plastic vessels under the bed. The vessels collect fluid from the wound, horrifying at first glance but necessary. The nurse in charge, sometimes two, work beaverishly to stabilise the child. The older kids seem to recover within days, often up and walking in 48 hours. Babies were much more volatile.

Our nurse returned. "He will see you at seven."

We were back on the cardiology ward trying to come to terms with what the cardiologist had said. We had so little time to prepare for Edward's operation. We filled out the consent form and began to get more than a little upset. The nurse showed us to a little room near the entrance to the ward. Inside were two funny looking pumps covered in clear Perspex. "What are they?" asked Sandra.

I had my know-it-all head on. "It's a model of a heart and lung machine to show you how they work. These pipes must connect up to the veins." I was interrupted by the nurse entering the room.

"Have you used a breast pump before?" She enquired pointing at the machines.

Sandra started to laugh, "Doug thought it was a heart and lung machine," she giggled. The nurse nearly smiled and began to show Sandra how to express milk using the pumping machines. I left Sandra as she began to express her milk, something she managed to keep up throughout our stay in the hospital, and I headed back to the ward to be with Edward.

And he blew

5.00 p.m.
We left Edward in the ICU nurse's capable hands and headed back to Ronald Mcdonald house. Entering the large diningroom area, we met Jack's mum. Every meeting between parents of sick children always started the same. "How is he/she? Any news?" We told her of our meeting with the ICU doctor.

"Shall we go for something to eat?" she continued.

"Must we, the food's horrible."

Sandra received free meals in the hospital's restaurant. "Yes come on, it's not that bad," she laughed.

Sandra ate while I observed what seemed like an endless line of patients' relatives head into the designated smoking room. It must be awful in there, like a smelly Turkish bath. I supped my coffee. On the third day here, I had a touch of Delhi Belly. Other people had said that they too had suffered.

Edward had been given more monitors and his little hand had been bandaged to protect the tubes that had been inserted into his vein. I stood over him trying to gather my thoughts. In the next bed, I watched a couple administer what I thought was medicine through a tube to their son, in fact he was being fed. The little boy, called Jack, was breathing very heavily with loud rasping breaths. His chest was pumping while mum and dad worked diligently to feed and take care of him. I noticed Jack's scar still quite red down the middle of his chest. At least Edward will escape being cut open I thought as I concentrated on my own sick child.

Blew, blew, blew, blew

7 p.m.

The registrar surgeon was a tall man. He was new to the department. He sat down next to us near Edward's cot bed. "I will now tell you what we plan to do in the operation tomorrow," he said in his perfect English with a slight Indian subcontinent accent. He started "The heart has four chambers…" We sat patiently as he described in the simplest terms how the heart functioned. Had this been Edward's first operation, had we been new arrivals, his description and very basic lecture would have been useful. As it was, we had just sat through a very graphic description of how our son might die and we struggled to be patient with this man's very slow and basic lecture. We sat through 20 minutes of what we had heard before and thanked him for his time. We signed the operation consent form and he left us.

"Bloody hell!" exclaimed Sandra. "It's a wonder he didn't start with everybody has a heart except for the Tin Man!" Just loud enough for the nurses to hear. For all we know, he may still be called the Tin Man.

We returned to our room in McDonald house. It was time for Sandra to express her milk as she had done every day during our three week stay. She expressed her milk for Edward three or four times a day. It kept her going through the bad times as it gave her hope, something to aim for. "When he gets better, we will take the milk home with us and you can feed it to him in the night while I get some sleep," she promised me.

Our whole life revolved around her being linked to the electric powered pumping machine. She had kept going being supplemented by the stodgy food served up by the restaurant. At times little Edward was fed only one millimetre of milk an hour — just 24 mls a day. Sometimes, he only received the saline fluid from a drip feed. As a consequence, the freezer in the special feeds unit was full of little plastic bottles filled with her breast milk. The unit staff knew us both by name as we deposited the milk there on a regular basis.

By now, Sandra had seen Edward for the last time before his operation. She was too upset to return. it was as if her defensive mechanism was setting in, trying to distance herself from the pain and anguish we both felt. I made the effort to try and talk to her. It was difficult. I have a problem in that when things go wrong, instead of talking it through, I go into my shell. This infuriates Sandra and has caused umpteen arguments between us but how do you change? How do you adapt to situations you have never faced before? What are the rules when you face death or impending doom? My father had died on a Friday and my family had gathered in mourning over the weekend. I heard the story of his death on three or four occasions and it was just too much to bear. I went out to a football match on the Saturday. Why? I don't really know, perhaps to shut it out — to hide my feelings. Was I unthinking? Cruel? Perhaps, I only know by burying the anguish, the suffering deep inside, I coped. I must learn to cope with others but it's difficult.

I started to cry. I wept openly as I rested on Edward's incubator. Tears rolled down my face and dripped onto the floor. My nose began to run but I did not care. The ward was full of people but I was oblivious to it all. Sandra joined me at his side. I love her so much. We hugged as it was time for Edward to go to theatre. I had thought about how I would say goodbye to him, to tell him to be brave, to know we would be thinking of him and praying for him, so many things needed to be said. When the time came for us to go, the words seemed to come from somewhere else. I looked for one last time and said "Be good wee man," and left — the waiting had begun.

Whoo! Whoo!

9.30 p.m.
My favourite time on the ICU, if there could be such a thing, was late evening. With less people about, the lights were dimmed, the unit so full of pain and suffering became almost homely. The highly trained nurses never letting up from observing and recording every change in their little patients, their conversations were muted and even the bleep of the alarms seemed to be an octave lower.

As I walked down the long corridors on my way to see Edward, as I had had done so many times before, I thought of what I would say to him this time, how I would feel if he did not pull through. His second operation and he was still only three weeks old. We did not really know him yet, our little son with his pert nose and scrawny limbs. He knew only hospitals, ventilators, drugs with funny names and the bleep, bleep, bleep of the alarms. I walked into the intensive care unit determined to give him a good talking to.

Pulling up the high stool next to his bed, I held his hand and talked. I spoke of him, his life, our life together. I told him about his sister, so full of beans; his beautiful mother whose breast he had suckled on when he was born. I told him about his grandparents, about our friends and their children and how we all prayed for him. I talked about what we would do together, how we would be when he got better — if he got better. My eyes were filled with tears but I did not cry. I had too much to say. All around, nurses and unit staff got on with

their job but I was oblivious to it all. All that mattered was Edward. For a brief
moment, I felt I knew him — like I had got through to him and he had listened.
The tears began to flow as I began to get up to go. The words seemed to come
from somewhere else. I looked at him for the last time and said, "Be good wee
man." I turned and left the unit, my tears as if released from an imaginary dam,
flowed freely and splashed onto the floor. The waiting had begun once more.

Douglas Stenhouse 1998

Helping the family cope

Each family member, no matter how old or young must be helped
individually so that they can provide support for each other and the ill
child. Communication is vital and accessibility to information is very
important. To assist parents with this ordeal, information must be readily
available to help them make informed decisions about their child's
management. Questions must be answered at a level appropriate to their
understanding. The two main aspects that worry parents the most tend to
be the surgery to be performed and the prognosis[229]. They must be seen
by various members of the team including their named nurse, cardiologist, cardiac surgeon and anaesthetist not just on one occasion, but as
often as the parents require. Visits to the ward and the intensive care unit
should be arranged as they often help allay fears, although at the time it
will heighten awareness of the forthcoming operation. The intensive care
visit should show the child only what he or she will come into contact
with, for example, noises from the monitors, chest drains, a wound dressing, urinary catheter, breathing tube and machine. Children must be told
their mum and dad can stay with them and that they can bring their
favourite toy and comforter. Parents can be given a more detailed explanation should they require it.

Self-help groups, booklets, the Internet and staff are all excellent
sources of information, and support, but the family must also be given the
opportunity to discuss the impact on themselves as a family unit and the
effects on work, finances, relationships, the marriage and so on[11].
Psychologists, cardiac social workers and pastoral support may all help
with these aspects.

Impact on the child

Obviously, the impact of the discovery of a heart defect depends on the
child's age and level of cognitive development.

- Neonate/infant: Newborn or infant children will be unaware of having "something wrong" as they have known nothing else. However, this is a time when building of trust between the child and the family is important, a healthy relationship being paramount. Equally, parents may be having problems bonding, which will also affect this critical period of their relationship.
- Toddler: Children entering the toddler period will be developing autonomously[230], wanting to be independent and do things for themselves. Confronted with illness, the toddlers' need for dependence will render them passive and clinging[231]. Regression, that is relying on parents to carry out tasks they were capable of doing before, may occur.
- Preschooler: Preschool children have a strong imagination in which a conscience and feelings of fear develop[11]. They may react to illness by blaming themselves and feeling guilty for the illness which can have a profound effect on self-esteem[11].
- School age child: School aged children are at an industry versus inferiority stage[230]. They want to achieve by completing tasks and can experience inadequacy and inferiority if not competent. Faced with illness the children may withdraw as they feel different from their peers or rebel, refusing any medications, special diets and so on[11].
- Adolescent: Adolescents are going through an identification stage[230], worried about how they appear to others, and especially wanting to be normal and fit in[11]. Teenagers facing open heart surgery are particularly frightened of body mutilation and loss of control.

Help for the sick child

- Neonate to toddler years: The family are encouraged to participate in the baby's care thus allowing bonding and for the development of the trust relationship necessary between the sick child and the family.
- Preschool and older: The nurse must establish what the child knows and understands about the illness and how he or she copes, both physically and psychologically. Children who feel well will not understand staff who say they are going to make them better when in fact they will feel worse immediately after surgery[10]. If children are unable to verbalise how they feel, the use of play may help enact the situation whilst enabling feelings to be exposed[11]. Children must be given information about the forthcoming hospitalisation and surgery in a manner appropriate to their age and level of understanding. Opportunity for children to ask questions is very important, the answers again should be simple, but truthful. Discussing

fears such as being in pain can be made more manageable by offering solutions such as use of the pain team and patient-controlled analgesia. Adolescents will need reassuring that their dignity and privacy will be maintained. Although the legal age of consent in the UK is 16 years old, children under this age must have their feelings taken into consideration when obtaining consent from both parents and health care professionals. Adolescents should be allowed to choose who they want to visit them as peer support is often of more value to them than great aunty Margaret!

Day of surgery

Certain routines have to be performed to ensure the safety of the patient prior to surgery. These include the following:

- Baseline observations: To ensure the child is in a fit state for surgery.

- Nil by mouth: Follow individual hospital policy. However, the following can be used as a guide:
  6 hours preoperative for food.
  4 hours preoperative for formula milk.
  3 hours preoperative for breast milk.
  2 hours preoperative for clear fluids.

- Administration of the prescribed preoperative medications and local anaesthetic creams for intravenous needle insertion. Ensure bedrest is undertaken once premedication has been taken and that the parents are aware of the need for rest. Use of cot sides to prevent self-injury is important.

- Patient safety: The following must be checked:
  Armband with name, date of birth, hospital number.
  Removal of jewellery, braces, contact lenses, nail varnish, etc.
  The consent form is signed for the relevant procedure. If the parents are not married, legally the mother has to sign for consent to operate.

Preparation in the intensive care unit

The bedspace for the child following open heart surgery can take 30 minutes or so to prepare properly. This is fundamental in ensuring the maintenance of a safe environment once the child has returned from theatre. The equipment chosen by the nurse depends on the age of the patient and the operation undertaken. The bedpace should contain only relevant equipment as a cluttered cubical is potentially unsafe. See Table 9.3.

Table 9.3 Equipment necessary to set up a cubical for a postoperative cardiac patient

System	Equipment
Cardiovascular	Heart monitor ECG leads and electrodes Pacing box and leads (especially for the patient who has undergone septal surgery, Fontan procedure, etc.) Transducer and flush system to measure arterial blood pressure, left atrial pressure, pulmonary artery pressure, central venous pressure Core and peripheral temperature monitoring Cooling mattress for major surgery Appropriate bed for the type of surgery — if a Fontan procedure is being performed, the bed must be capable of sitting the child upright
Circulating volume	Blood bottles and cards to assess full blood count and clotting profile Chest drain stands and connections to low grade suction device Chest drain rollers and clamps Blood products and delivery systems Protamine to reverse effects of heparin from bypass
Respiratory	Oxygen saturation monitoring Respiratory rate monitoring Arterial blood gas analysis Appropriate ventilator and tubing Humidification device Hand ventilation equipment Appropriate face mask Oxygen delivery system if the child is likely to be extubated early Appropriate suction catheters and Yankeur Suction receptacle and tubing Appropriate preset suction pressures Distilled water to clean suction tubing Sterile gloves for suctioning Stethoscope Oxygen, air or oxygen/air mixer cylinder
Neurological	Pen torch to assess pupillary reactions
Renal, fluids and electrolytes	Blood bottles and cards to assess urea and electrolytes Syringe and infusion pumps with appropriate delivery systems Selection of crystalloid fluids and electrolytes
Gastrointestinal	Nasogastric aspirate/feeding equipment Appropriate enteral feed Tape measure to assess girth measurements Accurate weight/height

(contd)

Table 9.3 (contd)

System	Equipment
Skin and nursing care interventions	Appropriate bed/cot Pressure relieving devices Nappies Toothbrush/paste Oral and eye care Inconti sheets
Drugs	Emergency drugs Inotropes Vasodilators Sodium bicarbonate Sedatives Analgesics Naloxone Paralysing agent Anti-arrhythmics Electrolytes Diuretics Glucose Prophylactic antibiotics Saline Water for injection
Record keeping	Charts/electronic recordings of: Vital signs Fluid balance and IV pump pressure monitoring Blood results Drugs prescription and administration Blood product prescription and administration Patient care plan Special intervention charts — intra-aortic balloon pumping, PD therapy, haemofiltration, high frequency oscillation, nitric oxide therapy Daily/weekly safety checks Patient summary/event details Patient information board (name, age, date of birth, hospital number, diagnosis, endotracheal tube make, size and length, weight, names of consultant, nurse and registrar, names of parents and contact numbers)
Child	Favourite toy/comforter When the child's condition allows, consider sensory toys
Environment	Sharps box Yellow and black bags Hand soap, alcohol rub and detergent Paper towels

The ward staff liaise with ICU regarding documentation and information acquired on admission. The parents are advised not to leave the hospital grounds during their child's surgery and are issued with a pager so staff can contact them when required.

Receiving a postoperative cardiac patient

The patient is transferred from theatre to intensive care with the theatre team who will continually monitor haemodynamic and respiratory signs for the albeit short but potentially dangerous journey. The staff provide a full handover of information on the lesion, the operation performed, the cardiopulmonary bypass time, intra-operative problems, inotropic and vasodilator support, optimal filling pressures and the most recent vital signs, arterial blood gas and packed cell volume.

Two nurses and an intensivist are required to receive the patient, the roles of each clearly distinguished to provide a thorough assessment and management of the postoperative patient. The intensivist, in conjunction with the surgeon, outlines a plan of management, stating acceptable parameters and the desired outcomes for the patient. The nurses' roles are shown in Table 9.4.

Table 9.4 Roles of the nurses in the care of the postoperative patient

Nurse looking after patient	Assisting nurse
Perform nursing assessment of cardiovascular and respiratory status	Ensure inotropes up and running Plug into mains

Chest drains:
  Untangle, support tubing
  Put down on floor
  Check tube is lower than water
  Mark prime level
  Label 1,2,3, etc.
  Unclamp as soon as possible
  Milk until movement of blood
  Connect to low grade suction
  (max 5 kPa)
	Ensure enough blood products are available for now and later
	
	Replacement of chest drain losses:
	  Assess filling pressures (CVP/LAP)
	  Assess core: peripheral temperature gradient
	  Assess blood pressure
	
	What to use:
	  PCV 35% use half blood/half plasma

The drains are the most important role when the patient first gets back from theatre, Ensure the drains are promptly attended to and frequently reassessed	PCV less than 34% use blood PCV greater than 36% use plasma If the patient is bleeding use fresh frozen plasma Change to manufactured plasma once the clotting is normal and the patient is not bleeding

(contd)

Table 9.4 (contd)

Nurse looking after patient	Assisting nurse

Signs and symptoms of cardiac tamponade:
  Rising CVP/LAP
  Chest drainage stopping
  Pulsus paradoxus on arterial tracing
  Cooling peripheries
  Low urine output
  Late signs affecting HR and BP,
  may happen over minutes or
  progressively
	Volume replacement:
	  In a neonate or child who is bleeding, the
	  drainage may need to be assessed every 10–15
	  minutes and drainage replaced at these
	  intervals if indicated
	Acceptable blood losses for the first 4 hours:
	  Less than 3 ml/kg/hour
	  3–10 ml/kg/hour contact surgeon who may
	  want fresh frozen plasma, platelets, protamine
	  Above 10 ml/kg/hour the chest may need to be
	  re-explored

Empty urine burette, starting the fluid balance from now	Untangle invasive lines
Check and milk drains	Plan where infusions are to go
Record observations noting any change from when patient came back from theatre. Assessment of girth, neuro, toe and rectal/bladder temperatures	Make infusions up ensuring excess taps and lines are removed Enoximone is incompatible with three-way taps and all other drugs except saline/water for infection
Take U&E, FBC, clotting, arterial blood gas, throat/rectal swabs	Total of infusions must be 1 ml/kg/hour so consider doubling, quadrupling infusions
Check and milk drains	
Ensure chest x-ray done	
Physical care – suctioning may require bagging and saline instillation early on as plugs of mucus and atelectasis may have formed in theatre, positioning the patient to mobilise secretions and relieve pressure	
Psychological care – talking, reassuring and touching the patient is most important orientating him or her to time and place (age appropriate)	
Allow parents to visit as soon as possible	
Paperwork when time permits	

Assessment and management

The assessment and management of the patient must commence with an assessment of the airway, breathing and circulation.

Respiratory assessment

- Endotracheal tube type, oral/nasal, size, cuff and length.
- Ensure the tube is securely taped and supported with a tube support.
- Is there a leak?
- Arterial blood gas.
- Oxygen saturation.
- Attach to age-appropriate ventilator.
- Set appropriate mode, alarms and other parameters.
- Auscultation of breath sounds.
- Chest movement equal and adequate.
- Assess lung compliance and resistance.
- Any signs of respiratory distress.
- Perform chest x-ray, note for atelectasis, pneumothorax, pulmonary vascular markings, heart size, lines, drain and endotracheal tube positions.

Cardiovascular assessment

- Heart rate and rhythm.
- Is the patient paced? Identify atrial and/or ventricular pacing wires, mode of pacing, pacemaker settings, secure pacing wires.
- Pulse volume.
- Presence of peripheral pulses.
- Arterial blood pressure/four limb if coarctation surgery has been performed to assess for residual coarctation. Check cuff BP to ensure it is consistent with arterial blood pressure.
- If receiving inotropic and vasodilator therapy, establish the dose and route of administration.
- Heart murmur/heart sounds/shunt.
- Precordium (hyperdynamic).
- Core: peripheral temperature gradient — a greater than 2°C difference is associated with a severely compromised cardiac output[38].
- Capillary refill/peripheral perfusion.
- Filling pressures LAP/CVP.
- Pulmonary artery pressure.
- Chest open with/without stent or closed?

Circulating volume

- Assess losses from various drains (mediastinal, pleural, peritoneal, chest dressings).

- Assess need for colloid replacement (remember a cyanotic child may bleed more in response to the polycythaemia). Neonates with a pre-existing coagulopathy will need close observation.
- Administer prescribed colloid depending on PCV, the presence of a coagulopathy and filling pressures.
- Clotting profile and its interpretation.
- Ensure adequate units of blood, fresh frozen plasma and platelets if required.

Neurological assessment

- A full assessment can be made when the child is more awake.
- Modified Glasgow coma scale.
- Assess pupillary reactions with a torch.
- Appropriateness of movements.
- Fontanelle.
- Assess pain and sedation level with scoring system.

Gastrointestinal assessment

- Liver size — take liver function tests if hepatomegaly or jaundice present.
- Blood glucose.
- Abdominal girth, is abdomen distended or soft?
- Presence of bowel sounds/bowels opened.
- Nasogastric aspirate (character, colour and amount).
- Commence enteral feeding within 4 hours if extubation is not predicted or the patient has not had prolonged periods of hypoxia preoperatively.

Renal assessment

- Urine output — 1–2 ml/kg/hour post bypass.
- Diuretics given at the end of bypass.
- Haematuria and haemolysis if prolonged bypass.
- Catheter size and type.
- Degree and site of oedema.

Fluid and electrolytes

- Check urea, electrolytes and acid–base balance.
- Assess potassium, magnesium and ionised calcium at regular intervals as they affect the contractility of the heart.

- Restrict fluids to 1 ml/kg/hour or 2 ml/kg/hour if closed heart surgery. Minimise rate of infusions by increasing their concentration. Calculate the additional boluses of flush solutions and intermittent or bolus drugs.

Skin assessment

- Turgor.
- Colour (normal colouration, cyanosed, grey, mottled).
- Presence of pressure areas if poorly perfused.
- Temperature: Normothermia should be aimed for although caution with artificial rewarming is necessary as vasodilation can occur requiring colloid replacement. Hypothermia in an older child will cause shivering thereby increasing the metabolic demands so if cooling is required the child must be adequately sedated and paralysed to prevent shivering. Conversely, each 1°C rise in body temperature will increase the insensible losses by approximately 10%[38].

Sepsis/inflammation

- Possible from invasive lines, surgical procedure, poor nutritional status.
- Prophylactic antibiotics.
- Selective decontamination of the gut if the chest is left open or there are prolonged periods of hypoperfusion.
- Assess pyrexia — establish whether inflammatory or infected with white cell count and septic screening. The CRP is not an effective infection marker immediately postoperatively as the inflammatory response to CPB is vast.

Family assessment

- Ensure the family is allowed to see the child as soon as convenient.
- Provide contact with the surgeon and intensivist.
- Encourage questions and answer honestly.
- Allow them to participate in the care of their child.

Daily progress

The child is continually assessed for improvement in vital organ function. When there is improvement, progress can then be accelerated in areas

such as the weaning of ventilation and drugs, increasing fluid requirements, removing invasive lines and drains and so on.

The physiotherapist ensures a plan of mobilisation is followed according to the cardiovascular and pulmonary limitations of the child, thus
preventing the complications of bedrest. Should enforced bedrest be
necessary, passive exercises are commenced to prevent venous stasis and
promote adequate circulation. Older children should have antithrombo-
embolic stockings and subcutaneous heparin. Good pain management
must be given prior to exercise to help encourage the child to start
mobilising.

Integrated care pathways

Integrated care pathways (ICP) provide a framework with which quality
care can be continually assessed and evaluated to see if it is delivered in a
time and cost-effective way[232]. This critical appraisal of clinical practice is
utilised when patients with similar conditions undergo a period of hospitalisation and follow the same course of treatment. For example, a patient
admitted preoperatively for tetralogy of Fallot has a pathway stating the
required interventions necessary to meet the desired outcomes of the
treatment[232]. When the patient deviates from the desired outcome, it is
recorded as a variance and the intervention altered accordingly[233]. This is
achieved by collecting data from the pathway, so the co-ordinator can
analyse the variance and amend it to ensure practice is current and the
most appropriate for the patient. Variance can be to the detriment or
benefit of the patient.

Advantages of ICP

- Cost effective: it is proven to reduce length of hospital stay[234], phar-
  macy costs, therapy costs, duplication of care[235], errors and ineffective
  practice.
- ICP teaches the multidisciplinary team (MDT) about the care
  required for certain conditions[235].
- Develops an MDT approach, encouraging communication[235].
- Educative tool.
- Maximises the quality of care given[234].
- Structured, co-ordinated daily plan of care[232].
- Care is continually assessed and evaluated, thus improving clinical
  outcomes.

- Reduces documentation as it may be the only document used in investigations such as cardiac catheterisation[235].
- Should a patient deviate from the pathway, analysis of the variance can be undertaken and prompt appropriate intervention taken[235].
- ICPs reduce unnecessary variation from the pathway[234].
- The pathway can be used from admission to discharge.
- Benchmarking — pathways that have superb results can be used as a form of benchmarking[234].
- Pathways implement the audit process[235].
- Involves the child and parents in the management of care.
- Assesses family contentment with the process[235].

The ICP for a patient with tetralogy of Fallot

The ICP for a patient with tetralogy of Fallot admitted to the ICU is shown in Table 9.5.

Table 9.5 An example of an ICP

Name	Day of operation		Variance analysis
Cardiovascular system	Returned to theatre at	.....	e.g., Chest drainage 6ml/kg/hour for 3 hours despite FFP, platelets and protamine. Re-explored chest ICU – bleeding point
	Chest drainage less 3 ml/kg/hour for first 4 hours	Y/N	
	Notes written by doctor on return to intensive care	Y/N	
Drugs	Inotropes weaned	Y/N	
	Antibiotics	Y/N	
Temperature	Core: peripheral temp difference less than 2˚C within 2 hours	Y/N	e.g., Temp difference 9˚C until bleeding point cauterised. Now 1.5˚C
Respiration	Extubated within 8 hours on ICU	Y/N	Not extubated due to bleeding
	Coughing post-extubation	Y/N	
Gastrointestinal tract	Feeding started within 4 hours of extubation or 4 hours postoperative if extubation not possible	Y/N	Nil by mouth due to the re-operation for bleeding
	Time of first feed	.....	
Fluids	1 ml/kg/hour	Y/N	
	Change from FFP to HAS when clotting normal	Y/N	
	Urine output greater than 2 ml/kg/hour	Y/N	

(contd)

Table 9.5 (contd)

Name	Day of operation		Variance analysis
	ml of urine from theatre	..... ml	
	ml/kg/hour of urine during first 4 hours	..... ml	
Laboratory tests	Tests done within 30 mins of arrival on ICU	Y/N	
	Tests as listed – ABG with PCV and electrolytes	Y/N	
	Full blood count	Y/N	
	Full urea and electrolytes	Y/N	
	Clotting profile	Y/N	
	Throat and rectal swabs	Y/N	
	Chest x-ray within 1 hour of arrival	Y/N	
	Repeat ABG at: 4 hours	Y/N	
	Pre-extubation	—	
	Post-extubation	—	
Skin	Incision covered, not oozing	—	*Oozing, gauze dressings weighed*
Pain/sedation	Pain scoring, analgesia and outcome as per analgesia pathway	Y/N	
Activity	Responding to stimuli within 4 hours	Y/N	*Remains paralysed until bleeding under control*
Family	Surgeon to speak to parents	Y/N	
	Reassure parents and assess parental concerns	Y/N	
	Explain plan of care to family	Y/N	
	Pathway reviewed by medical staff	Y/N	
	Pathway completed by nursing staff	Y/N	

Cardiac Unit, Royal Liverpool Children's NHS Trust, Alder Hey, UK (reproduced with permission)

Discharging the child home

Discharge planning must be commenced before the child leaves intensive care and goes back to the ward to convalesce. Numerous factors have to be taken into consideration including the individual needs of each family unit. See Table 9.6.

Table 9.6 Discharge planning

Personnel to be contacted prior to a cardiac child's discharge	Reason for contact
Family of the child	To ensure they can make appropriate plans in the home environment
District general hospital (DGH)	Should the child need further convalescing, it may be done nearer home. Liaison with the DGH to arrange a transfer date and time plus outlining the child's history and requirements is important
Cardiac liaison nurse	Can support the family at the time of discharge providing home visits for many patients. Education is given about the care for the child's condition especially if life threatening or complex
Cardiac social worker	Can provide help with finances, information on benefits available from the government and a general form of support
Dietitian (probably already involved)	Special diets/feeds need to be discussed prior to discharge and the appropriate supplements given
Health visitor/school nurse	Informing the HV and school nurse of the discharge of a cardiac child into the community so special provisions can be made
District/community/paediatric nurse	As above plus any clinical practical issues such as removal of sutures, help with nasogastric feeding, wound care, etc.
GP	Informing the GP of the patient's discharge and the care needed whilst at home
Outpatient department	10 day follow-up appointment to be made
Take-home drugs	The first week's supply to be arranged
Transportation	Ambulance with/without escort, hospital taxi, taxi, private arrangements

Parental teaching and paperwork

- Parental discharge advice booklet — see below.
- Teaching about the importance of meticulous dental hygiene and antibiotic prophylaxis when visiting the dentist, having ears pierced and so on.

- Resuscitation training if appropriate.
- Teaching of nasogastric feeding and passing of the tube.
- Teaching how to administer medications.
- Teaching about anticoagulation and how to manage the child.

Parental discharge advice booklet

Written information regarding discharge advice is necessary so there is something concrete for parents to refer to. Contact numbers should be included in case of any queries. The following issues need to be addressed:

- Wound care
  When the child can be bathed or showered.
  Report any redness, tenderness, hotness, swelling, discharge from the wound to the GP or hospital staff.
  Report the development of a temperature.
  Advice on when stitches are to be removed.
  Dissolving stitches may show a brief inflammatory response at 10–14 days.

- Feeding the baby
  Inform that the baby is likely to tire quickly when feeding.
  May require initial oral feeding, topped up with nasogastric feeds to prevent exhaustion.
  Added calorific intake may be necessary.
  Advice regarding excessive vomiting and diarrhoea.
  Attendance at baby clinics for regular weight analysis.

- Diet/fluids
  Follow advice given by the dietitian.
  If cyanotic, ensure plenty of fluids are given, especially during hot weather.
  If diarrhoea and vomiting, contact GP or local hospital particularly if taking diuretics.

- Pain relief
  Pain/discomfort may continue after discharge.

Paracetamol should manage the pain in conjunction with diversional therapy.

- Medication
  Contact GP early after discharge to ensure a prescription is available for child's medications.
  Ensure drugs are stored safely.
  If medicine is in syrup form, encourage child to have a drink afterwards as it is likely that the drugs have a high sugar content and will cause tooth decay.
  Advice on action if the child vomits after taking drugs. Medications should never be repeated as it is hard to say how much has been absorbed initially.

- Dental treatment
  Advice on seeing a dentist regularly.
  Carry an antibiotic prophylaxis card.
  Importance of brushing teeth regularly and after eating.
  Avoidance of added sugar.

- Immunisations
  May resume the normal immunisation plan 4 weeks after surgery unless the child has Di George syndrome, asplenia or is on steroids.
  If the child is taking warfarin, the immunisations should be given subcutaneously, not intramuscularly.
  If the child is due to come in for surgery, he or she must not have had the polio vaccine for 8 weeks prior to the surgery.

- Day to day
  Activities — go by the child's limitations. Don't overprotect.
  Consultant will see in 10 days to advise on school and sport activity (normally 4–6 weeks).
  Swimming can take place 4 weeks after surgery.
  Holidays abroad — notify the consultant.
  Avoid people with coughs, colds, infectious diseases for 4 weeks after the operation.
  The child must wear a car seat-belt despite the wound.

- Contact staff if:
  Increasing shortness of breath, change in colour, more sweaty.
  Off foods or feeds.
  Change in behaviour (irritable, lethargic, quiet).
  Wound problems.
  Chest pain.

This advice is given to all parents upon discharge of their child from the Royal Liverpool Children's NHS Trust, Alder Hey, UK (reproduced with permission).

Chapter 10
Respiratory management

The cyanotic child

Definition

Cyanosis is manifested as the presence of a dusky blue/grey colour around the mucus membranes, sclera, skin and nail beds being central or peripheral in nature. In congenital heart disease, cyanosis occurs as a result of deoxygenation (desaturation) of the haemoglobin when the deoxygenated blood mixes with the oxygenated blood of the systemic circulation. It results in hypoxaemia. Other causes not related to congenital heart disease include lung disease, central nervous system depression and pulmonary arteriovenous fistula[4, 20].

Grades of cyanosis

Ross et al.[20] describe four degrees of cyanosis:
- Grade I: Cyanosis on exertion.
- Grade II: Mild cyanosis at rest. Oxygen saturations approximately 85%. Difficult to detect.
- Grade III: Obvious cyanosis with oxygen saturations approximately 75%.
- Grade IV: Extreme cyanosis.

Signs and symptoms

Respiratory signs and symptoms

- Peripheral cyanosis: Blueness around the mouth and extremities.
- Central cyanosis: Blueness present around the nail beds and mucus membranes.

- Decreased cyanosis when crying is usually respiratory in nature, as it responds to the increased tidal volume[10].
- Pulmonary vascular obstructive disease.
- Respiratory distress.
- Low oxygen saturations.
- Hypoxaemia.

Cardiovascular signs and symptoms

Cyanosis which usually increases when crying is usually related to cardiac causes and does not improve with oxygen administration due to the intracardiac shunt[10].

Haematological signs and symptoms

Chronic hypoxia and cyanosis cause polycythaemia. This results from an increase in red blood cell production due to increased erythropoietin secretion. Polycythaemic patients with a haematocrit above 0.6 can present with thrombocytopenia, platelet aggregation and coagulopathy due to a reduction in clotting factors. This predisposes to haemorrhage, development of thrombus/emboli causing CVA and microcytic anaemia.

Sepsis

- Rarely, brain abscess.

Other signs and symptoms

- Digit clubbing, although this is rare nowadays due to early intervention of treatment.

Diagnosis

To establish whether cardiac or respiratory in nature, the patient breathes room air, then 100% oxygen. Arterial blood samples are taken during both aspects and the results analysed. If the partial pressure of oxygen is high then the cause of the cyanosis is probably respiratory in origin[10].

Key management issues

The key management issues for a child with cyanosis are shown in Table 10.1.

Table 10.1 Assessment and management of potential problems in a child with cyanosis

Establishment and maintenance of a PDA if there is a duct dependent circulation

Management of profound cyanosis:
- Oxygen administration which, although it will not increase the partial pressure of oxygen, will increase tissue perfusion of vital organs and peripheries. An increased oxygen level will increase pulmonary blood flow by lowering the pulmonary vascular resistance which may or may not be advantageous depending on the underlying condition
- Provision of respiratory support
- If untreated congenital heart disease with chronic cyanosis, blood is removed periodically to help lower the packed cell volume and associated respiratory distress

Management of hydration:
- Prevention of dehydration is a priority during periods of "nil by mouth" and diarrhoea and vomiting. The polycythaemic child who becomes dehydrated will exhibit increased blood viscosity thus predisposing to the development of thromboembolic formation. Intravenous fluids may be necessary if oral intake is not possible. Diuretics should be reduced or omitted during periods of prolonged "nil by mouth" and diarrhoea and vomiting until intravenous therapy can be established or oral intake tolerated

Management of haemostasis:
- Assess for the formation of emboli at times when most at risk (e.g., dehydration)
- Monitor coagulation and full blood count at regular intervals
- Administer prescribed fresh frozen plasma and other blood products if clotting very deranged

Management of intravenous therapy:
- When giving an intravenous bolus or infusion, *no air* must be allowed to enter the line as when the patient is cyanosed due to a congenital heart defect, there is mixing of both systemic and pulmonary circulations which will predispose the patient to air emboli and the possibility of CVA

Detection and management of a brain abscess:
- This is a rare complication of cyanosis and is not now seen very often due to early surgical intervention of the underlying lesion. However, a cardiac child presenting with neurological symptoms should be considered for the presence of a cerebral abscess

Management of anaemia:
- The child should not be allowed to become anaemic as this will further decrease the oxygen carrying capacity of the blood. The haemoglobin should be maintained around 15 g/dl and certainly not less than 12 g/dl

Management of the underlying condition:
- Early surgical intervention in most instances will prevent the chronic effects of hypoxaemia. An example being tetralogy of Fallot whereby surgeons now commonly operate before the age of 12 months. Up until several years ago, children with tetralogy of Fallot were not admitted for corrective surgery until 18 months or 2 years of age, by which time the chronic effects of cyanosis had become well established

Pulmonary hypertension

Definition

Pulmonary hypertension is defined as raised blood pressure in the pulmonary vasculature. The normal mean pulmonary artery pressure (PAP) is approximately one third of mean arterial blood pressure.

Classification of pulmonary hypertension

Several classifications exist depending on when the signs present and any non-cardiac causes. Related pulmonary hypertension and cardiac disease tend to be classified as secondary pulmonary hypertension, which is subdivided into three types:

Passive pulmonary hypertension

Raised pressure in the pulmonary vasculature results from a back pressure in the pulmonary veins and left atrium. Right ventricular pressure is therefore raised pumping blood into the lungs at high pressure in an attempt to compensate for the left sided obstruction[20].

- Causes: Pulmonary vein stenosis, pulmonary vein obstruction, e.g., TAPVD, cor triatriatum.
- Treatment: Treatment of the cause.

Active pulmonary hypertension

Raised pressure in the pulmonary vasculature results from increased flow or pressure in the pulmonary vascular bed[20]. The increased pulmonary artery pressure causes changes to the lung arterioles resulting in increased pulmonary vascular resistance reversing the shunt to right to left (Eisenmenger's syndrome). This is due to the right ventricular pressure being equal to or greater than the left ventricular pressure and results in cyanosis.

- Causes: Left to right shunts — ASD, VSD, AVSD, PDA.
- Treatment: Treat the lesion before permanent damage to the vasculature occurs.

Reactive pulmonary hypertension

Raised pressure in the pulmonary vasculature results from an increase in pulmonary vascular resistance.

- Cause: Constriction of the pulmonary arteries[3] due to hypercapnia, acidosis, Eisenmenger's syndrome.

Changes to the pulmonary arteries

After a period of time changes occur to pulmonary arteries that have been under high pressure. Heath and Edwards[269] classify the changes into six categories:

- Grade I: Hypertrophy of the media lining of the artery (reversible).
- Grade II: Proliferation of the intima (reversible).
- Grade III: Fibrosis of the intima (reversible).
- Grade IV: Dilatation of the pulmonary arteries (irreversible).
- Grade V: Thrombosis formation (irreversible).
- Grade VI: Necrosis of the intima and media (irreversible).

If treatment is instigated before the changes to the pulmonary arteries become irreversible, it will avoid the need for a heart–lung transplant at a later date or even death. It is therefore vital that measures are taken as soon as possible to prevent these changes from occurring.

Pulmonary hypertensive crisis

A pulmonary hypertensive crisis results in a sudden rise in PAP causing a drop in oxygen saturation, bradycardia, reduction in cardiac output, mottled appearance and generally a very unwell looking child. The PAP can equal or be higher — suprasystemic — than arterial blood pressure. Prevention of these episodes must be achieved by managing nursing care and other interventions as events can rapidly cause a downward spiral in the patient's condition, often culminating in cardiac arrest and death.

Signs and symptoms

An increase in pulmonary vascular resistance and PAP cause dramatic cardiovascular and respiratory effects.

Cardiovascular signs and symptoms

- Increased right ventricular afterload.
- Bradycardia.
- Reduced cardiac output.

Respiratory signs and symptoms

- Increased pulmonary vascular resistance.
- High PAP.
- Reduced pulmonary blood flow.
- Low oxygen saturations.
- Hypoxaemia.
- Acidosis.
- Hypercapnia.
- Reduced lung compliance.
- Increased airway resistance.

Key management issues

The key management issues for a child with pulmonary hypertension are shown in Table 10.2.

Table 10.2 Assessment and management of potential problems in a child with pulmonary hypertension

Prevention of hypoxia, acidosis and hypercapnia:
- Positive pressure ventilation releases prostaglandin which vasodilates the pulmonary arterioles[4]
- Maintain the pCO_2 at approximately 30–35 mmHg
- Commence fentanyl infusion as it blunts the stress response to the highly reactive pulmonary circulation that predisposes to pulmonary hypertension[150]
- Paralyse the patient until pulmonary artery pressures are half the mean arterial pressure
- Frequent blood gases to assess the parameters

Management of the pulmonary hypertensive episodes:
- Hand ventilate with 100% oxygen to vasodilate the pulmonary vasculature
- Consider the use of inhaled nitric oxide to vasodilate if hyper-reactive pulmonary vasculature
- If nitric oxide not available, administer prescribed prostacyclin. This may also be used in conjunction with nitric oxide in very unstable patients. It has the disadvantage of vasodilating systemically which may compromise the already critically ill child
- Vasodilate to reduce the afterload
- Administer inotropes to increase cardiac output
- Minimal handling of the patient with co-ordinated cares
- Preoxygenate and administer a bolus of fentanyl before physiotherapy and suctioning to avoid hypoxia and vasoconstriction
- Hand ventilate with fast, small inflations to encourage carbon dioxide removal

Pleural effusion

Aetiology

Pleural effusion may be due to several factors producing either:

- Exudate due to infection (empyema), malignancy, trauma and inflammation (post pericardiotomy syndrome).
- Transudate due to fluid overload, increased systemic venous pressure, congestive heart failure, hypoalbuminaemia and chylothorax which is discussed later.

Definition

A pleural effusion is an accumulation of fluid in the pleural space.

Signs and symptoms

Respiratory features

- Pleuritic pain.
- Increasing respiratory distress.
- Decreased lung compliance.
- Atelectasis.

Diagnosis

Chest x-ray, echocardiogram, chest aspiration and analysis of pleural fluid.

Key management issues

The key management issues for a child with a pleural effusion are shown in Table 10.3.

Chylothorax

Definition

Chylothorax is an accumulation of lymph fluid in the pleural space. It is a cause of pleural effusion and results from a fistula connecting the pleural space and thoracic ducts[172]. The fistula commonly develops from direct

Table 10.3 Assessment and management of potential problems in a child with a pleural effusion

---

Management of respiratory distress:
- Supportive measures are employed until a chest aspiration/chest drain insertion is performed. This should relieve the respiratory embarrassment

Assist with chest aspiration or chest drain insertion

Establishing the cause:
- The aspirate should be sent for analysis so appropriate treatment can be started

Management of the cause — see appropriate section for treatment:
- If infection is found to be the cause, antibiotics and chest drainage are required
- Post pericardiotomy syndrome can cause an inflammatory response predisposing to pleural effusion
- Congestive heart failure
- Fluid overload
- Chylothorax

---

injury to the thoracic duct, the incidence of which is higher when surgery is undertaken near to the thoracic ducts, e.g., modified Blalock–Taussig shunt, coarctation of the aorta and patent ductus arteriosus. Other causes include a congenital abnormality of the lymphatic system, certain malignancies or if very high venous pressures are present, for example, post-Fontan procedure[270].

Signs and symptoms

Chylothorax usually presents several days postoperatively when the child starts to ingest the fat present in a normal diet. If the chest drains have been removed, the features are the same as a pleural effusion. If drains are still present, drainage will increase once the child starts eating or the baby ingests milk. The drainage has a characteristic opaque milky/amber appearance and separates from less fatty drainage in the collection bottle.

Diagnosis

Chest x-ray and echocardiogram will show an effusion. Aspiration and examination of the fluid will show the presence of triglycerides, lymphocytes and cholesterol.

Key management issues

The key management issues for a child with chylothorax are shown in Table 10.4.

Table 10.4 Assessment and management of potential problems in a child with a chylothorax

Management of the chylothorax:
• Same as for pleural effusion plus:

Management of the fat intake:
• A medium chain triglyceride diet, i.e., low fat, is required[271] for around 3 weeks[270] to ensure the thoracic duct has had time to heal. The chylothorax drainage additionally causes a reduction in protein, electrolytes and fat soluble vitamins so help from the dietitian is required to provide the balance of nutrients throughout this period. If after 1 week the drainage is still greater than 10 ml/kg/day, TPN will be required. After 3 weeks of TPN, a medium chain triglyceride diet can be given for a further 2 weeks. Should drainage still be greater than 10 ml/kg/day after this regime, surgical ligation of the thoracic ducts will be required or a pleurodesis performed[270]

Replacement of clotting factors and immunoglobulins may be required

Pneumothorax

Definition

A pneumothorax can be defined as the presence of air in the pleural space caused by perforation of the chest wall. A postoperative pneumothorax is normally attributed to barotrauma from mechanical ventilation, chest drain removal whereby air re-enters the pleural space, inadequate drainage of air from the chest drain or insertion of a subclavian central venous line. Air can accumulate slowly or rapidly (tension pneumothorax).

Signs and symptoms

Cardiovascular signs and symptoms

• Tachycardia progressing to bradycardia.
• Hypotension.
• Pulsus paradoxus on the arterial line waveform.

Respiratory signs and symptoms

- Respiratory distress.
- Hypoxaemia.
- Cyanosis.
- Unequal chest movement.
- Reduced air entry on the affected side.
- Reduced lung compliance.
- Increased peak inspiratory pressures.
- Tracheal deviation from the affected side.
- Mediastinal shift with tension pneumothorax.

Other signs and symptoms

- Agitation.

Diagnosis

- Auscultation: Reduced breathing sounds on the affected side.
- Chest x-ray: Shows blackened area; if tension pneumothorax, a mediastinal shift and tracheal deviation will be present.

Key management issues

The key management issues for a child with pneumothorax are shown in Table 10.5.

Table 10.5 Assessment and management of potential problems in a child with a pneumothorax

---

Management of the respiratory distress:
- If a tension pneumothorax presents and the child is unstable a needle aspiration to remove the air will be undertaken as an urgent procedure
- Chest drain insertion
- Check chest x-ray

This should alleviate other symptoms

Phrenic nerve damage

Definition

A paralysed or hemiparalysed diaphragm may result should damage to the phrenic nerve occur during thoracic surgery. The injury is likely to be due to trauma, stretching of the phrenic nerve or hypothermic damage which occurs during cardiopulmonary bypass[4]. It tends to affect small babies and is more common on the left side of the chest.

Signs and symptoms

Respiratory signs and symptoms

- Failure to wean from the ventilator.
- Respiratory failure.
- Increased work of breathing.
- Reduced tidal volume.
- Hypoxia.
- Hypercarbia.
- If hemidiaphragm is present there will be asymmetric chest movement.
- Atelectasis.

Diagnosis

- Chest x-ray: Shows elevation of the affected diaphragm. If the child is ventilated, the ventilator must be disconnected to allow spontaneous, unsupported breathing to assess the child's breathing pattern.
- Echocardiogram: Screens the diaphragm.
- Diaphragmatic fluoroscopy: Diagnostic for hemidiaphragm. The affected side will be elevated on inspiration.

Key management issues

The key management issues for a child with a paralysed diaphragm are shown in Table 10.6.

Table 10.6 Assessment and management of potential problems in a child with a paralysed diaphragm

---

Management of the respiratory failure:
- Supportive ventilation weaning to CPAP either with an endotracheal tube or nasal prongs
- This may be required for up to six weeks[4, 220]

Management of the damaged phrenic nerve:
- If the respiratory failure persists longer than six weeks, surgical ligation of the phrenic nerve will be required as a transected nerve is usually the cause. However, babies requiring surgical ligation are likely to be premature, sick infants who may not tolerate a further surgical procedure well[220]

Atelectasis

Aetiology

Atelectasis is common in children following cardiac surgery and usually results from hypoventilation, chest wall splinting if in pain, low peak inspiratory pressure if ventilated, obstructed endotracheal tube from a mucus plug, endotracheal migration into the right main bronchus or rarely the left main bronchus.

Definition

Atelectasis is whole or partial collapse of the alveoli in one or more lobes of the lung.

Signs and symptoms

Respiratory signs and symptoms

- Respiratory distress.
- Hypoxia.
- Chest infection.
- Reduced breath sounds.
- Reduced chest expansion.

Diagnosis

- Auscultation: Reduced air entry.
- Chest x-ray: Showing areas of collapse and possible endotracheal tube migration.

Key management issues

The key management issues for a child with atelectasis are shown in Table 10.7.

Respiratory intervention

Mechanical ventilation

A brief overview of the nursing management of the ventilated child will be discussed. Detailed management can be found in specific texts pertaining to paediatric ventilation.

Table 10.7 Assessment and management of potential problems in a child with atelectasis

Management of the respiratory failure:
- Supportive therapy in the form of oxygenation and mechanical ventilation if the child is unable to maintain oxygenation and excrete carbon dioxide. This may mean increasing peak inspiratory pressure and positive end expiratory pressure to inflate the collapsed area(s)
- Provision of adequate humidification of inspired gases — this plays an important role in secretion mobility
- Undergoing a physiotherapy assessment and treatment to aid in the removal of secretions and inflate the collapsed area(s) of lungs
- Encouraging the child to cough, take deep breaths and change position frequently will aid in the mobilisation of secretions
- Ensure adequate hydration to maintain thin secretions
- Control of pain to prevent chest wall splinting

Management of infection associated with atelectasis:
- Obtain a sample of mucus for microculture and sensitivity and virology analysis
- Administer prescribed antibiotics if bacterial infection present
- Management of pyrexia

The child requiring mechanical ventilation is unable to maintain adequate gaseous exchange and tissue oxygenation due to respiratory failure. The reasons for the respiratory failure are numerous but those associated directly with the cardiac patient are usually attributed to:

- Cardiovascular collapse.
- Respiratory distress.
- Closure of the PDA in a duct-dependent neonate.
- Pulmonary oedema.
- Pneumothorax.
- Pleural effusion.
- Chylothorax.
- Electrolyte imbalance.
- Sepsis.
- Postoperatively following major cardiac surgery — an ASD will only require two to four hours' ventilation postoperatively whereby a TAPVD may require days or several weeks if multi-organ failure develops.

Key management issues

The key management issues for a child requiring intubation are shown in Table 10.8.

Table 10.8 Assessment and management of potential problems in a child requiring intubation

Elective intubation:
- "Nil by mouth" four hours prior to intubation

Emergency intubation preparation:
- Ensure that the child's airway is maintained with an artificial airway, appropriate-sized facemask and bag if the child is unable to do so himself or herself
- Connect to ECG monitor, measure blood pressure and oxygen saturations
- Perform suction to clear the airway with appropriate sized catheter/yankeur
- Pass a nasogastric tube and aspirate stomach contents
- Draw up and administer prescribed sedation, paralysing agent and flush solution
- Have emergency drugs to hand
- Select appropriate ventilator
- Ensure stethoscope is available
- Select appropriate-sized endotracheal tube (ETT)/nasal or oral tube, laryngoscope blade and handle, rebreathing bag, McGill forceps, lubricating gel, tape to fix tube
- Explain the need for intubation to the child, if appropriate, and family

During intubation:
- Assist the intensivist/anaesthetist throughout the procedure
- Observe haemodynamic and respiratory parameters during the procedure and report deviations to medical team

After intubation:
- Auscultate to assess effectiveness of tube insertion and to assess the degree of leak from around the ETT
- Continually assess the child's respiratory status
- Perform chest x-ray to ensure tube in correct position
- Perform arterial or capillary blood gas
- Record the size, type and length of ETT/oral tube

Positive pressure ventilation

Positive pressure ventilation forces air into the lungs by using intervention known as the drive force[272]. The drive force creates a pressure at the opening of the airway, which is higher than the intra-alveolar pressure[10] thus forcing air from the mechanical ventilator to the lungs.

Effects of positive pressure ventilation

During cardiovascular surgery the lungs will have undergone varying degrees of trauma, prolonged atelectasis and insertion of chest drains. This may be in conjunction with the events associated with mechanical ventilation, possible pleural effusion, chylothorax, phrenic nerve paralysis, pump lung and so on. The various systems are affected as shown in Table 10.9.

Table 10.9 Effects of positive pressure ventilation

System	Effects
Respiratory	• Increased airway pressure • Increased intrathoracic pressure • Decreased lung compliance • Barotrauma • Increased ventilation/perfusion mismatch • Nosocomial pneumonia from hypoperfused gut and translocated bacteria
Cardiovascular	• Decreased venous return • Decreased cardiac output
Neurological	• Decreased cerebral perfusion
Renal	• Decreased renal perfusion • Decreased urine output • Increased water retention • Oedema
Endocrine	• Increased ADH secretion • Renin–angiotensin–aldosterone mechanism triggered due to hypoperfusion
Gastrointestinal	• Decreased hepatic perfusion resulting in coagulopathies, hepatomegaly, reduced metabolism of drugs • Gastric bleeds • Hypoperfused gut resulting in translocation of bacteria • Increased risk of sepsis if hypoperfusion affects organs

Mechanism of cycling from the mechanical ventilator

Ventilators were traditionally categorised by a mechanism which cycles ventilation from the inspiratory phase to the expiratory phase[272]. Nowadays, many ventilators combine the four cycling mechanisms providing modes of ventilation for the individual patient. The four cycling mechanisms are pressure, volume, time and flow.

Pressure cycled ventilation

In pressure cycled ventilation, inspiration ends and expiration begins when the preset inspiratory pressure is reached. Advantages of this method include the fact that it is pressure limited therefore reducing the risk of barotrauma. However there is no guarantee of adequate tidal or minute volume should the patient's resistance and compliance change.

Volume cycled ventilation

In volume cycled ventilation, inspiration ends and expiration begins when the preset tidal volume is delivered. Advantages of this method include a ventilation guarantee. However, the disadvantage is that the pressure required to deliver the volume depends on the resistance and compliance of the patient's lungs and the actual ventilator circuit. If resistance increases or compliance decreases, the peak pressure will continue to rise until the ventilator has reached its preset volume, therefore increasing the risk of barotrauma.

Time cycled ventilation

In time cycled ventilation, inspiration ends and expiration begins when the preset inspiratory time has been reached. This time period is set by a time mechanism, setting the rate and adjusting the inspiratory/expiratory ratio[272]. The disadvantage is that the gas will be delivered until the inspiratory time has been reached without consideration of the volume delivered, the amount of pressure produced or changes in the resistance and compliance of the lung[10].

Tidal volume is determined by: gas flow × time = volume.

Flow cycled ventilation

Flow cycled ventilation is achieved when the preset flow rate reaches a predetermined percentage of its peak value. It responds to changes in resistance and compliance similar to the pressure cycled ventilators.

Modes of ventilation

There are numerous modes of ventilation now available. The method of choice will depend on the type of ventilator available, the patient's condition and the need for either full (controlled) or assisted (supported) ventilation.

Control modes are only suitable for fully ventilated, sedated and paralysed patients as the ventilator will not take into account any effort by the patient. Supported modes work in varying degrees with the ventilator recognising and being triggered by the patient's respiratory effort. Increased effort allows the contribution of the ventilator to be reduced either automatically or manually after assessment. Today there are modes which combine both controlled and support modes to minimise barotrauma and make respiration easier and more comfortable for the patient.

Examples of controlled modes

- Intermittent mandatory ventilation (IMV).
- Controlled mandatory ventilation (CMV).
- Volume control (VC).
- Pressure regulated volume control (PRVC).

Examples of support modes

- Synchronised intermittent mandatory ventilation (SIMV).
- Pressure support (PS).
- Assisted spontaneous breathing (ASB).
- Volume support (VS).

Examples of mixed modes

- SIMV with VC and PS.
- SIMV with PC and PS.
- BIPAP.

Key management issues

The key management issues for a child requiring mechanical ventilation are shown in Table 10.10.

Troubleshooting for the child who is ventilated

Details of troubleshooting for the child who is ventilated are shown in Table 10.11.

Table 10.10 Assessment and management of potential problems in a child requiring mechanical ventilation

---

The child is unable to maintain the airway and needs to receive mechanical ventilation to ensure oxygenation and elimination of carbon dioxide:
- Ensure rebreathing bag, facemask, correctly sized suction and yankeur suckers are available
- Select appropriate type, size and length of endotracheal tube specific to patient's age and weight
- Select appropriate ventilator for age and weight
- Select appropriate mode of ventilation for the individual patient's requirements
- Set appropriate parameters depending on mode
- Measure the appropriately set parameters

Assess the effectiveness of the mechanical ventilation:
- Perform arterial or capillary blood gases at regular intervals acting on results of respiratory or metabolic acidosis/alkalosis
- Continuously monitor the child's oxygen saturations
- Assess and observe the child's colour, breathing pattern, evidence of bilateral air entry and equal chest movement
- Ensure the adequacy of minute and tidal volumes, peak inspiratory and end expiratory pressures which are appropriate for the child's weight and condition

Ensure the patency of the ETT:
- Assess the need for suctioning – see section on suctioning
- Provide adequate humidification of inspired gases – see section on humidification

Ensure the child has adequate analgesia and sedation to keep comfortable:
- Provide prescribed analgesia, sedation and paralysis (if necessary)
- Assess the effectiveness of the analgesia and sedation

Liaise and work with the physiotherapists to:
- Maintain bilateral air entry
- Remove secretions safely and effectively
- Encourage coughing if the patient is capable
- Change the position of the patient to help in the mobilisation of secretions

Prevention of infection due to: (1) the presence of a critical illness predisposing to translocation of bacteria from the gut causing a nosocomial pneumonia[273], (2) poor suctioning technique, (3) disruption of mucociliary function[274]:
- Perform a chest x-ray and analyse the endotracheal secretions for the presence of infection
- Protect the gut to prevent translocation of bacteria – see relevant section
- Perform suction in an aseptic manner

ETT obstruction from thick secretions, kinked tube[275] resulting in increased inspiratory pressures, decreased tidal volume, hypoxia, respiratory distress and bradycardia:
- Hand ventilate to assess whether the patient has deteriorated or there is a mechanical fault with the ventilator
- If chest expansion is poor and clinical deterioration persists, suction the ETT

(contd)

Table 10.10 (cont)

- If this fails to oxygenate the patient, call for help and remove the ETT, hand ventilating the patient via an oral airway and facemask until reintubated
- Ensure adequate humidification, chest physiotherapy, effective suctioning and frequent change of position to mobilise secretions

Prevention of accidental extubation:
- Ensure the ETT is securely taped
- Support the weight of the tubing
- Ensure the child's hands cannot interfere with the ETT or ventilator circuit

ETT complications:
- Oral intubation can cause a groove in the palate affecting speech
- Nasal intubation can cause tissue necrosis of the nose and septurn
- Both can cause damage to the vocal cords and tracheal mucosa resulting in subglottic stenosis and stridor[273]. This is normally due to too large an ETT, a mobile ETT or prolonged intubation[214]

Monitor the patient for the development of a pneumothorax:
- See section on pneumothorax

Monitor and treat the patient for other systemic effects caused by positive pressure ventilation:
- Cardiovascular effects — reduced systemic venous return and low cardiac output. Treat with appropriate fluid loading and inotropes
- Renal/endocrine effects — due to the secretion of ADH, water retention and low urine output will occur. Administering prescribed diuretics, restricting fluids and maintaining the electrolyte balance will help in the prevention of oedema formation
- Gastrointestinal effects — a poor nutritional status will predispose to a catabolic state with breakdown of tissues including wastage of muscles. It is important to prevent this by liaising with the dietitian to provide a high calorie diet. This will help prevent muscles from breaking down, especially respiratory muscles which may predispose to a longer period of ventilation. Additionally, milk feeds will help in the prevention of stress ulcers

Anxiety for the family at the thought of their child on a "life support machine":
- Explain the need for mechanical ventilation
- Comfort and reassure as required
- Involve the family in their child's care

Anxiety for the child on a mechanical ventilator:
- Explain the need for the mechanical ventilation if the child is able to comprehend
- Administer prescribed analgesia and sedation to keep the child comfortable
- Comfort and reassure as required
- Orientate the child to time and place
- Provide quiet times when the child can rest undisturbed. Inform the child he or she is having a period of undisturbed sleep whereby he or she can relax knowing only vital interventions will be undertaken
- Provide a pen/paper or sign board to communicate if the child is capable of writing

Table 10.11 Troubleshooting for the ventilated child

Increased peak inspiratory pressure:
- Ventilator:
  Is the tubing kinked?
  Is there water in the circuit?
- Patient
  Is the patient anxious?
  Has the lung compliance deteriorated?
  Has a pneumothorax developed?
  Are there secretions in the ETT?

Decreased peak inspiratory pressure:
- Ventilator
  Is the circuit cracked?
  Is the circuit disconnected?
- Patient
  Is there a leak around the ETT?
  Has the lung compliance changed?

Increased tidal volume:
- Patient — The lung compliance is improving and the patient is getting better

Decreased tidal volume:
- Patient —The lung compliance is deteriorating and the patient is deteriorating

Key management issues

The key management issues for a patient requiring extubation are shown in Table 10.12.

Table 10.12 Assessment and management of potential problems in a child requiring extubation

Prior to extubation:
- Wean the ventilator over a period of hours to days depending on the age and condition of the child, taking into account how long the child has been ventilated for
- Place "nil by mouth" four hours prior to planned extubation. If a small baby or profoundly cyanosed, ensure intravenous fluids are commenced over this period
- Draw up prescribed intravenous sedation, paralysing agent, flush solution and have emergency drugs to hand
- Ensure the same size and next size down ETT, laryngoscope, facemask and other intubation equipment is close by
- Choose oxygen delivery system appropriate to the child's age
- Explain the forthcoming event to the child and parents

During the procedure:
- Aspirate the child's nasogastric tube
- Suction the child's ETT and oropharynx

(contd)

Table 10.12 (cont)

- Place the child on his or her side
- Assist the doctor with the extubation
- Administer the chosen oxygen delivery system. Liaise with parents who may know which their child prefers

After the procedure:
- Observe the child closely for respiratory distress and apnoea
- Perform an arterial or capillary blood gas half an hour post-extubation
- Wean oxygen according to child's response
- Encourage coughing, deep breathing and movement around the bed/cot

Suctioning the ventilated patient

Suctioning the ventilated patient is an invasive procedure but is necessary to remove pulmonary secretions from the ETT thus maintaining airway patency. Although this is a commonly performed procedure on an intensive care unit, it is associated with many complications, most of which are preventable if the nurse is informed of the dangers. See Table 10.13.

Table 10.13 Complications of suctioning

Infection:
- Ensure a strict aseptic technique is performed during the procedure

Right upper lobe collapse and atelectasis due to:
- High negative pressure exertion. Ensure no more than 12–20 kPa of pressure and shallow suctioning technique is employed. Shallow suctioning technique consists of measuring the ETT length, adding on 2.5 cm for the catheter mount and 1 cm extra. This gives the exact length that the graduated suction catheter should be passed[276]
- Inadequate airway clearance resulting in hypoxia[277]

Tracheobronchial tissue injury[278]
- Deep suctioning technique causes injury to tissues which can be avoided when shallow suctioning is undertaken

Hypoxia[277] caused by:
- Deep and prolonged suctioning technique. Preoxygenating the patient prior to suctioning will help in prevention. However, remember if a neonate or duct dependent patient receives 100% oxygen, it can have deleterious effects. Preoxygenation to 10% greater than the child's baseline requirements should be adequate[10]

Laryngospasm:
- Perform quick, efficient, safe suctioning

Arrhythmias[279]:
- Atrial arrhythmias, bradycardia and cardiac arrest can result from hypoxia or increased vagal tone. Therefore, perform quick and efficient suctioning

(contd)

Table 10.13 (contd)

Increased mean arterial pressure and tachycardia:
- Increase analgesia and sedation prior to the event

Raised intracranial pressure[277]:
- Ensure adequate sedation and paralysis when a rise in intracranial pressure can be dangerous

Pneumothorax:
- Associated with the hand ventilation and hyperinflation performed when suctioning. The catheter can cause perforation of the bronchial segments predisposing to pneumothorax, therefore gentle technique is vital

Mucociliary disruption:
- This will actually necessitate suction[280] as the cilia cannot waft the mucus up the tracheobronchial tree due to the presence of the ETT, thus predisposing to infection[281]

Pain:
- Ensure adequate analgesia has been administered
- Prepare the patient for the event
- Use of diversional therapy and guided imagery may be required

Inadequate clearance of secretions:
- Instillation of normal saline is thought to help with secretion removal. However, this technique was designed before the implementation of sophisticated humidification units

Summary of considerations for suctioning

The patient should be fully prepared for the event.

- The patient should be assessed before being "routinely" suctioned. This assessment should include auscultation, listening for reduced air entry and the presence of secretions, desaturation, changes in blood gas parameters, increased respiratory effort, coughing, increased peak inspiratory pressures and decreased tidal volumes, bradycardia or tachycardia, not just because it was three hours after the previous suctioning!
- Hyperoxygenation, 10% higher than the patient's baseline will help prevent the hypoxia associated with suctioning.
- Perform a strict aseptic technique.
- Hand ventilate although this may cause hypocapnia and a reduction in cardiac output if too much positive end expiratory pressure is exerted. Hyperventilate to increase the tidal volume to re-expand collapsed areas of lungs.
- Consider the use of instillation of saline which although not proven may help mobilise secretions.

- Perform shallow suctioning technique, choosing appropriately sized catheter (double the size of the ETT diameter). The type of suction catheter is important — multiple eyelet catheters have been shown to reduce tracheal trauma[282]. Closed suction catheter systems have the advantage of not disconnecting the patient from the ventilator, thus maintaining positive pressure ventilation, minimal contamination and continuous delivery of oxygen[272]. However, it can increase the dead space changing carbon dioxide levels which in patients such as those with HLHS, may be dangerous. Ensure the suction pressure is between 12–20 kPa to reduce the aforementioned complications. The catheter should be inserted quickly, to the predetermined length, suction applied on withdrawal only, and the catheter removed without "stirring".
- Continuously monitor the patient's haemodynamic and respiratory status before, during and after the event.
- Position the patient correctly depending on where the secretions are collecting and causing atelectasis.
- Encourage the patient to cough if coherent.
- Auscultate before and after to compare the effect of suctioning.
- Leave at least 20 minutes for the child to recover from suctioning before taking blood gases.

Humidification

As the upper airway naturally humidifies the gas breathed[10], placing an ETT in the patient's airway inactivates this mechanism rendering artificial humidification of inspired gases vital.

Humidification is necessary to protect the epithelium of the lower airways and for the provision of optimal conditions for mucociliary function and gaseous exchange[284]. If gas is cold and dry, secretions will become thick and sticky and collect in the lower airways[283, 284]. This is as a result of the impaired functioning of the mucociliary transport system which is sensitive to changes in the environment.

Optimal humidification is achieved by administering 44 mg/l of water vapour via a system which heats the gas and saturates it with water vapour[283–285]. Excess humidification is equally damaging as it leads to excess water (condensation) in the ventilator circuit predisposing to bacterial colonisation[283, 286, 287], increased peak inspiratory pressure and PEEP, triggering the ventilator if the trigger sensitivity is too low and reducing the volume of gas to the patient[10].

The temperature at which the humidifier is set is equally important. If it is too high it will cause tracheal burns from condensation and increase the patient's temperature and thus metabolic and oxygen demands. If it is too low it will cause thickened secretions due to the inadequate delivery of humidified gases to the patient.

Acid–base balance

Definitions

- *pH*: The concentration of free hydrogen ions in a solution. It is represented on a scale of 1–14, the higher the pH, the lower the concentration of free hydrogen ions and the more alkaline the substance. Normal arterial blood pH is 7.35–7.45.
- *Acid*: A substance capable of releasing hydrogen ions.
- *Base*: An alkaline substance capable of buffering hydrogen ions
- *Base excess/deficit*: A reflection of the concentration of bicarbonate or acid which must be added to the blood to return it to the normal pH. It is only affected by metabolic processes. The range is +2 to –2 mmol/l.
- *Standard bicarbonate*: The bicarbonate level which has been corrected for the variables of temperature, partial pressures of oxygen and carbon dioxide. Once corrected, the figure given is due to metabolic causes. Normal level is 22–26 mmol/l.
- *Buffer solution*: A solution that can maintain the homeostatic pH in response to fluctuations in the concentration of hydrogen ions. There are three main buffers — bicarbonate, phosphate and protein systems.

Regulation of pH

The pH of the blood varies with the relative concentration of hydrogen ions. If free hydrogen ions accumulate, the pH falls and acidosis occurs. Conversely, if free hydrogen ions decrease, the pH rises and alkalosis occurs.

Three main homeostatic systems maintain the pH:

- Buffer solutions.
- Lungs.
- Kidneys.

In acidosis

- Buffer solution: Bicarbonate combines with free hydrogen ions to form carbonic acid which is broken down rapidly into carbon dioxide and water. These byproducts are excreted by the lungs.

- Respiratory system: The respiratory centre is stimulated by changes in pCO_2 in the blood, resulting in increased ventilation to excrete carbon dioxide.
- Renal system: The kidneys excrete hydrogen ions and retain bicarbonate which happens gradually.

In alkalosis

- Buffer solution: Carbon dioxide and water combine to form carbonic acid which breaks down into free hydrogen ions and bicarbonate.
- Respiratory system: The respiratory centre is stimulated by changes in the pCO_2 decreasing ventilation to retain carbon dioxide.
- Renal system: The kidneys excrete bicarbonate and retain hydrogen ions.

Compensation mechanisms

Should the acid–base balance be upset, initial buffering occurs plus physiological events to compensate for the imbalance. See Table 10.14.

Table 10.14 Compensation for the four acid–base states

Acid–base state	Compensation	How compensation occurs
Primary respiratory acidosis	Metabolic compensation	• Kidneys excrete acid and retain bicarbonate which takes 2–4 days • pH normalises
Primary respiratory alkalosis	Metabolic compensation	• Kidneys excrete bicarbonate through urine as bicarbonate reabsorption by the kidneys is reduced • Increased serum lactate, pyruvate and less acid excretion causing a base deficit • pH normalises
Primary metabolic acidosis	Respiratory compensation	• Hyperventilation, lowering the carbon dioxide level • This induces respiratory alkalosis by chemoreceptor stimulation in the carotid artery and aorta • pH normalises
Primary metabolic alkalosis	Respiratory compensation	• Hypoventilation, raising the carbon dioxide level • This is due to the pH depressing the respirations

Causes of acid–base imbalance

Respiratory acidosis

Due to reduced carbon dioxide excretion, an excess of carbonic acid forms in the extracellular fluid. Therefore, there is an increase in hydrogen ion concentration or a deficit in the base. There are four main causes of repiratory acidosis:

- Obstructive lung disease — secretions, loss of lung volume, atelectasis, pleural effusions.
- Factors adversely affecting the respiratory centre — head injury, oversedation, intubation into the right main bronchus.
- Respiratory muscle weakness — muscular dystrophy, neuropathies, phrenic nerve palsy.
- Hypoventilation from mechanical ventilation.

Respiratory alkalosis

This results from a reduction in pCO_2 and therefore carbonic acid and hydrogen ions. It is caused by:

- Acute or chronic hypoxaemia.
- Hyperventilation from anxiety, fever, exercise, pain or mechanical ventilation.
- Pulmonary embolus.
- Salicylate overdose.

Metabolic acidosis

This results from bicarbonate loss or increased hydrogen production. It is caused by:

- Lacticacidosis and poor tissue perfusion.
- Sepsis.
- Renal disease — renal failure, renal tubular acidosis.
- Diabetic ketoacidosis.
- Diarrhoea.
- Ingestion of acids — acetazolamide, ammonium chloride drug therapy.

Metabolic alkalosis

This results from an accumulation of bicarbonate or loss of acid in the extracellular fluid. It is caused by:

- Diuretic therapy.
- Intake of sodium bicarbonate.
- Vomiting, nasogastric tube aspiration.
- Steroid therapy.

Clinical features of acid–base balance

Acidosis

Respiratory distress (if due to an obstructive cause), shallow breathing, reduced level of consciousness, hypoventilation, hypoxia, cyanosis (if due to a respiratory centre cause), poor peripheral perfusion, grey mottled appearence, tachypnoeic, Kussmaul's respirations, lethargy and drowsiness.

Alkalosis

Tachypnoeic, dizziness, muscular weakness and twitching, tingling fingers and toes, tetany due to the shift of ionised calcium, hypokalaemia if on diuretic therapy, vomiting.

Treatment of acid–base imbalance

Respiratory acidosis

- Treat hypoxia and cyanosis with oxygen.
- Consider mechanical ventilation.
- Increase mechanical ventilation if inadequate.
- Treat the cause — head injury, oversedation, etc.
- Regular blood gases to assess effectiveness.

Respiratory alkalosis

- Treat the cause — pulmonary embolism, salicylate overdose, comfort and reassure the patient if anxious and hyperventilating.
- Reduce mechanical ventilation.

- Ask patient to breathe into a closed paper bag if old enough to understand.
- Regular blood gases to assess effectiveness.

Metabolic acidosis

- Adequate oxygen to restore pulmonary and systemic perfusion.
- Volume (plasma expander).
- Administer prescribed sodium bicarbonate to partially correct the acid–base imbalance.
- Optimise ventilation.
- Treat the cause — sepsis, ketoacidosis, diarrhoea.
- Regular blood gases to assess effectiveness.

Metabolic alkalosis

- Re-evaluate diuretic therapy.
- Treat vomiting.
- Reduce intake of sodium bicarbonate or other alkalising agents.

For an interpretation of acid–base balance see Figure 10.1 and for examples of blood gases in primary and compensatory states see Table 10.15.

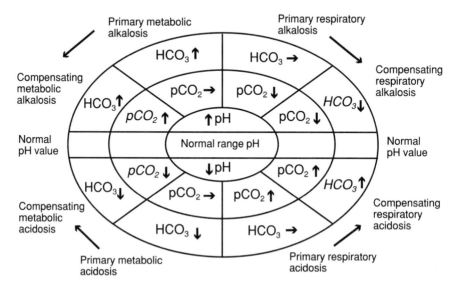

Figure 10.1 Acid–base balance. Stephen McGlaughlin, Manchester Children's Hospital. Reproduced with permission.

Table 10.15 Examples of blood gases in primary and compensated states.

Primary respiratory acidosis:		Compensated respiratory acidosis:	
pH	7.28	pH	7.34 (low to normal)
CO_2	64	CO_2	64
$NaHCO_3$	24	$NaHCO_3$	30
Primary respiratory alkalosis:		Compensated respiratory alkalosis:	
pH	7.6	pH	7.49 (high to normal)
CO_2	30	CO_2	30
$NaHCO_3$	24	$NaHCO_3$	20
Primary metabolic acidosis:		Compensated metabolic acidosis:	
pH	7.28	pH	7.34 (low to normal)
CO_2	36	CO_2	30
$NaHCO_3$	16	$NaHCO_3$	16
Primary metabolic alkalosis:		Compensated metabolic alkalosis:	
pH	7.6	pH	7.49 (high to normal)
CO_2	36	CO_2	50
$NaHCO_3$	32	$NaHCO_3$	32
		Chronically compensated respiratory acidosis:	
		pH	7.34–7.38
		CO_2	50–65
		$NaHCO_3$	36

Pulse oximetry

Pulse oximetry is a continuous non-invasive technique capable of monitoring the oxygen saturations of haemoglobin found in the arterial circulation. It is used widely in the hospital setting and in the transportation of critically ill patients.

How it works

Two light-emitting diodes (LEDs) which transmit infrared and red lights shine through the tissues to a photodetector[288]. The amount of absorbed light is related to the degree of saturated haemoglobin in the tissues. Well-oxygenated haemoglobin absorbs a relatively small amount of light and poorly oxygenated haemoglobin absorbs a larger amount of light[10]. The information is then passed to a computer/monitor. To ensure an accurate reading the appropriately sized probe must be used and placed correctly and securely around a pulsatile source — fingers, toes, ear lobe, etc. The LEDs must be opposite the photodetector.

Clinical situations which may interfere with oximetry

Poorly perfused patient

A poor signal will be emitted until the patient's perfusion improves. This is due to a reduction in the arterial blood supply, resulting in a weak pulse and therefore a poor light source. It is commonly found in peripherally shut down patients[288].

Anaemic patient

If the haemoglobin is below approximately 5 gm/dl the oximeter reading will be unreliable.

Carbon monoxide poisoning

Carbon monoxide has an approximately 250 times greater affinity for haemoglobin than oxygen, making interpretation unreliable. Arterial blood gases will give a more accurate measurement.

Methaemoglobinaemia

Haemoglobin will not transport oxygen if methaemoglobin develops following nitrate or other drug/chemical exposure. Again comparison with the arterial blood gas will be required for accuracy.

Ambient light interference

Phototherapy and surgical lights will interfere with the oximeter reading. Therefore, cover the probe with a dark material. Nail varnish should also be removed if the probe is located on a finger.

Movement of patient

Movement may mimic arterial pulsations thus leading to spurious readings.

Nitric oxide

Nitric oxide, once regarded as a toxic atmospheric substance was first recognised to have a therapeutic role in the late 1980s[289]. It was utilised in paediatric medicine primarily to treat pulmonary hypertension[290, 291] but also has several applications for use in the critically ill patient.

The role of endogenous nitric oxide

Endothelium-derived relaxing factor (EDRF) was first identified in 1980[292], but it was not until 1987 that this mystery substance released in certain situations from the endothelial lining of blood vessels was subsequently identified as nitric oxide by Palmer et al.[293] and Ignarro et al.[294]. Three major roles of nitric oxide have been identified:

- Nitric oxide causes a localised relaxation of smooth muscle which regulates the systemic and pulmonary vascular tone, coronary circulation and ischaemic related reperfusion changes[295]. Should hypoperfusion of blood vessels occur, the nitric oxide is released from the endothelium, vasodilating blood vessels, thus increasing blood flow[296] by decreasing the vascular resistance.
- Nitric oxide opposes platelet adhesion and aggregation and thus thrombus formation[297, 298] by interfering with calcium mobilisation within the platelets[299].
- Activated macrophages produce nitric oxide which plays a major role in host defence mechanisms[299, 300].

Scientists subsequently developed exogenous nitric oxide for use in a variety of clinical situations and as most clinical uses are in connection with pulmonary hypertension and severe lung disease, its application has been developed in the ventilated patient via a specially adapted circuit. Inhalation of nitric oxide directly to the alveoli will have the desired effect of relaxing the smooth muscle of the pulmonary vasculature, causing vasodilation and thus increasing blood flow to the lungs.

Clinical uses of exogenous nitric oxide

- Congenital heart disease: Nitric oxide can be used to decrease pulmonary vascular resistance in patients where a raised pulmonary vascular resistance causes a life-threatening condition, and can also increase cardiac output by reducing right ventricular afterload. As it provides selective, localised vasodilation (when the nitric oxide reaches the haem part of the red blood cell, its vasodilating properties will be stopped) it has its application in patients with primary pulmonary hypertension or pulmonary hypertension associated with left to right shunting. This is found in congenital heart lesions such as ASD, VSD, AVSD where an increased pulmonary blood flow over a period of time will cause an elevated pulmonary vascular resistance. Equally, a right to left shunt that may occur through a PDA can also elevate lung pressures. Cardiopulmonary bypass and the associated hypothermia can agitate an already increased pulmonary vascular resistance in the newborn[301].

- Acute respiratory distress syndrome (ARDS): Nitric oxide can be used to dilate the pulmonary bed thus reducing the pulmonary artery pressure.
- Persistent pulmonary hypertension of the newborn (PPHN): Elevation of the pulmonary vascular resistance will cause an extrapulmonary shunt through the PDA and patent foramen ovale[301].
- Respiratory distress syndrome and bronchopulmonary dysplasia: Hypoxia and acidosis.
- Meconium aspiration: Hypoxia and acidosis.
- Diaphragmatic hernia: Pulmonary hypertension.
- Heart and lung transplant: Complications of ischaemic and reperfusion injury perioperatively will predispose the patient to pulmonary hypertension. An increased pulmonary vascular resistance preoperatively predisposes to right ventricular failure postoperatively[302].
- Conversely, the role of nitric oxide in septic shock can be detrimental as it is thought to be responsible for the vasodilation that occurs in severe sepsis[300]. It has therefore been suggested that a substance to block the action of nitric oxide may be useful in the regulation of nitric oxide potency[303].

Levels of nitric oxide

The appropriate concentration of nitric oxide is between 1 and 100 parts per million[304] although more recent studies have suggested only 1–30 parts per million as beneficial[305]. The literature has diverse dose ranges but in the author's experience, most patients seem to improve with doses around 10–20 parts per million.

Key management issues

The key management issues for a child receiving nitric oxide therapy are shown in Table 10.16.

Table 10.16 Assessment and management of potential problems in a child receiving nitric oxide therapy

Observe for the development of pulmonary oedema and pneumonitis caused by:
- Formation of nitrogen dioxide caused by nitric oxide reacting with oxygen[296] therefore administer a dose as low as possible as the higher the dose the more rapidly nitrogen dioxide is formed.

Observe for the development of methaemoglobinaemia:
- 90% of inhaled nitric oxide is absorbed into the blood stream reacting with haemoglobin to form methaemoglobin. Methaemoglobin will not carry oxygen resulting in a very cyanosed patient so the patient needs regular blood gas analysis — 1 hour after commencing nitric oxide therapy and then twice daily. It must be remembered that a falsely high oxygen saturation may occur despite the cyanotic appearance — rely on arterial blood gases. Treatment for methaemoglobinaemia is blood transfusion, ascorbic acid or methylene blue[302]

Observe for the development of atherosclerosis due to the release of platelet derived growth factor which inhibits smooth muscle proliferation[306]

Observe for haemorrhage:
- Assess clotting times and platelet counts as nitric oxide can suppress platelet adhesion and prolong clotting time predisposing to haemorrhage
- Observe for oozing around puncture sites and wounds and perform careful suctioning

Deterioration when nitric oxide is withdrawn following prolonged usage:
- The endogenous production of nitric oxide is switched off when there is a prolonged exposure to exogenous nitric oxide therefore exogenous nitric oxide must be weaned slowly as severe hypoxaemia and cardiovascular collapse can occur if it is discontinued quickly[290, 302]. Pulmonary artery pressure and partial pressure of oxygen should be observed during the weaning process

Hand ventilating and suctioning the patient on nitric oxide:
- When hand ventilating the bagging circuit should be connected to the nitric oxide supply to prevent vasoconstriction from occurring, as the half life is between 1 and 6 seconds
- The use of closed suction catheters should be considered to prevent disconnection from the circuit if hand bagging is not required. However, remember the dead space could make the patient unstable if a complex heart lesion exists (e.g., HLHS)
- Sedating and paralysing the patient must be considered
- Minimal handling and co-ordinated cares should be employed

Environmental and patient monitoring of nitric oxide and nitrogen dioxide:
- 24 hour monitoring of the environment and patient should be used as this will negate the use of a scavenger system
- The acceptable blood concentration for nitrogen dioxide is less than 5 parts per million
- Inform the technicians and medical staff if levels become too high
- Research into the toxicity of nitric oxide therapy for employees exposed to its use is still minimal. Jones[300] raises the pertinent considerations as to whether staff with a coagulopathy or asthma or who are pregnant should look after patients receiving nitric oxide therapy, taking into account anecdotal reports of spontaneous abortion and mutagenesis

Chapter 11
Cardiovascular management

Cardiovascular management

The cardiovascular conditions associated with congenital heart disease can be divided into the following catergories.

Low cardiac output

See the section on normal cardiac output in Chapter 1.

Definition

Low cardiac output can be described as a reduction in the amount of circulating blood ejected from the ventricles subsequently affecting major organs and tissue perfusion. The determinants of cardiac output depend on the four variables of preload, afterload, contractility and heart rate. Irregularities in the aforementioned determinants will cause low cardiac output.

Factors that affect the variables

Increased preload

- Congestive heart failure.
- Vasoconstriction.
- Congestive cardiomyopathy.
- Bradycardia.
- Fluid overload.

Decreased preload

- Hypovolaemic shock.
- Dehydration.

- Restrictive cardiomyopathy.
- Capillary leak.
- Systemic vasodilation.
- Severe right ventricular failure.
- Positive pressure ventilation.
- Cardiac tamponade.

Increased afterload in the right ventricle

- Pulmonary hypertension.
- Obstructed right ventricular outflow tract.
- Pulmonary vein obstruction.
- Hypervolaemia.
- Positive pressure ventilation.
- Polycythaemia.

Increased afterload in the left ventricle

- Obstructive lesions (aortic stenosis).
- Increased systemic vascular resistance.
- Systemic hypertension.
- Vasoconstriction.
- Fluid overload.
- Cardiac tamponade.
- Hypoxia.
- Acidosis.

Decreased afterload

- Septic, cardiogenic, neurogenic and anaphylactic shock states.
- Hypovolaemia.
- Vasodilators.

Increased contractility

- Sympathetic nervous system.
- Hyperdynamic states.
- Inotropes.

Decreased contractility

- Cardiogenic shock.
- Congestive cardiac failure.

- Acidosis.
- Hypercapnia.
- Hypoxia.
- Electrolyte imbalance.
- Myocardial infarction.
- Ischaemia.
- Beta blockers.
- Inflammation.
- Congenital heart diseases (e.g., ASD, VSD, AVSD, PDA, TOF, AS)[220, 236–239].

Increased heart rate

- Sympathetic nervous system.
- Hypotension (shock).
- Fever.
- Exercise.
- Fear.
- Pain.
- Arrhythmias.

Decreased heart rate

- Parasympathetic nervous system.
- Arrhythmias.
- Raised intracranial pressure.

Clinical assessment of low cardiac output

All organs will be affected by hypoperfusion resulting in:

Cardiovascular signs and symptoms

- Arrhythmias: tachycardia initially to compensate for the onset of the low cardiac output followed by bradycardia which is a late and premorbid feature.
- Weak thready pulse.
- Reduced diastolic pressure and subsequent reduced coronary perfusion.

Respiratory signs and symptoms

- Tachypnoea progressing to a decreased rate and apnoea.
- Low oxygen saturations due to impaired oxygen transportation.

- Hypoxia.
- Hypercarbia.
- Acidosis.
- Increasing pulmonary vascular resistance.

Renal signs and symptoms

- Oliguria to anuria due to a reduction in renal perfusion.
- Increasing urea and creatinine production.

Circulating volume

- Hypovolaemia due to capillary leak or fluid overload.

Neurological signs and symptoms

- Irritability.
- Confusion.
- Agitation.
- Restlessness.
- Reduced level of consciousness, coma.

Gastrointestinal signs and symptoms

- Reduction in peristalsis resulting in nausea.
- Vomiting and paralytic ileus.
- Hepatomegaly.
- Hepatic congestion.
- Jaundice.
- Hyperglycaemia due to the stress response.
- Pancreatitis.
- Necrotising enterocolitis/ischaemic bowel.

Sepsis

- Susceptibility to translocation of bacteria from the gut.

Skin

- Cold.
- Pale.
- Mottled.

- Clammy.
- Hypothermic.
- Capillary refill prolonged.
- Lactic acidosis.
- Increasing core–peripheral temperature gradient.

Key management issues

The key management issues in a child with low cardiac output are shown in Table 11.1.

Table 11.1 Assessment and management of potential problems in a child with low cardiac output

---

Management of a decreased preload:
- Aim to optimise the preload by fluid loading to increase the filling pressures. Infuse prescribed colloids starting at 10 ml/kg to increase the central venous pressure, left atrial pressure and decrease the heart rate. Ideal pressures depend on the type of heart defect and age of the patient. The pressures may not rise should capillary leakage occur[172] and equally, over-increasing preload can affect myocardial function and predispose to multi-organ failure. Therefore, if fluid has no effect, inotropes should be considered — consider Starling's Law (see Chapter 1 on the normal heart)
- Assess effectiveness of increased preload: increased filling pressures, increased urine output, decreased core–peripheral temperature gradient, no evidence of systemic or pulmonary oedema

Management of increased afterload involves reducing the afterload by:
- Ensuring preload is maximised before reducing afterload
- Vasodilating the patient — use of either sodium nitroprusside, glyceryl trinitrate, phenoxybenzamine, enoximone, ACE inhibitors and diuretics. Avoid environmental cooling predisposing to vasoconstriction
- Assess the effectiveness of the vasodilator therapy and additionally monitor and correct the hypotension resulting from the vasodilator therapy
- Administer opiates to sedate and relax the patient, thus reducing afterload
- Administer beta blockers
- Assess effectiveness of decreased afterload: normotensive, peripherally warm, urine output of 1–2 ml/kg/hour, sinus rhythm
  Caution — reducing the afterload can also reduce contractility of the heart

Management of decreased contractility:
- Ensure preload is optimal
- Reduce the afterload to offload the ventricle
- Administer prescribed inotropes — dopamine, dobutamine, epinephrine, norepinephrine, calcium, digoxin — appropriate to the needs of the patient taking into account that inotropes vasoconstrict
- Consider the reversibility of the condition and perhaps use of the intra-aortic balloon pump or left ventricular assist device if inotropes and fluid loading fail

(contd)

Table 11.1 (contd)

- Improve oxygenation and avoid acidosis by:
  1. Correcting existing acidosis with manipulation of ventilation and sodium bicarbonate
  2. Increasing oxygen administration
  3. Increasing PEEP although this can increase intrathoracic pressure and reduce preload
  4. Ensuring endotracheal patency
  5. Administering diuretics to decrease pulmonary oedema
- Assess effectiveness of improved contractility: increased blood pressure, decreased filling pressures, improved warmth, perfusion and colour to tissues, brisk capillary refill, increased urine output and sinus rhythm
- Induced hypothermia (cooling via thermostatically controlled water blanket) to around 33°C (rectally) has been shown not only to reduce metabolic demands but also to aid myocardial contractility in the heart with low cardiac output[240]. Studies have shown myocardial contractility is improved by the positive inotropic effect on the hypothermic myocardium[219, 241]

Management of irregular heart rate or rhythm with an aim to achieve sinus rhythm to optimise the stroke volume and thus cardiac output:
- Monitor ECG continuously noting arrhythmias and report promptly
- Monitor for and correct electrolyte imbalances
- Ensure temporary pacing box is available. Connect wires to box as a precaution should arrhythmias develop
- Treat specific arrhythmias promptly (see later in chapter for details). However, if bradycardia presents consider the use of drug therapy and pacing. If tachycardic consider systemic cooling to 34–36°C to reduce metabolic demands and oxygen consumption. Treat presenting pyrexia aggressively
- Administer prescribed antiarrhythmic drugs
- Assess effectiveness of regular heart rate and rhythm: sinus rhythm, normal electrolytes and apyrexial

Management of the underlying cause of the low cardiac output, e.g., congestive heart failure, cardiac tamponade, sepsis, cardiomyopathy

Management of the respiratory distress associated with the low cardiac output:
- Sedate, paralyse and ventilate if extubated
- Correct acidosis, hypoxia and hypercapnia

Management of other multi-organ failure associated with low cardiac output:
- Brain — Observe for fitting, signs of raised intracranial pressure, hypoperfusion
- Kidneys — Observe for oliguria, anuria, deranged electrolytes
- Gut — Observe for paralytic ileus, NEC/ ischaemic bowel, hepatomegaly. Monitor liver function tests and for the presence of coagulopathy
- Immune system — Prevent translocation of bacteria from the gut and systemic inflammatory response by administering selective decontamination of the gut agents

Congestive heart failure

Aetiology

Congestive heart failure in an infant or child is normally attributed to the presence of a congenital heart defect, the age of the patient is related to the cause. Presenting at birth, congestive heart failure is usually attributed to hypoplastic left heart failure, during the first few days to TGA or TAPVD, and during the first four weeks to VSD or PDA[4]. Congestive heart failure is due to three main causes:

- Reduced contractility (cardiomyopathy, anaemia, acidosis, anomalous coronary artery and any congenital lesion with high pulmonary blood flow, congenital heart block, sepsis, fluid overload, surgery to the affected ventricle).
- Increased volume (left to right shunts causing high output heart failure).
- Increased afterload (obstructive lesions such as mitral or aortic stenosis, coarctation of the aorta, causing low output heart failure)[4, 220].

Definition

Congestive heart failure is defined as the failure of the heart to provide sufficient cardiac output for metabolic demands.

Anatomy and pathophysiology

In childhood, congestive heart failure usually involves both left and right ventricles, both being dependent on one another for adequate cardiac output.

Left ventricular failure

Myocardial contractility is decreased having a direct effect on the left ventricle's ability to eject its contents forcefully into the systemic circulation. This causes a back pressure into the left atrium, pulmonary veins and lungs resulting in congestion, pulmonary oedema and an increased pulmonary artery pressure.

Right ventricular failure

The right ventricle empties ineffectively due to reduced myocardial contractility. Back pressure therefore occurs, resulting in an increase in pulmonary artery pressure in the lungs, right atrium and systemic veins causing generalised oedema, hepatomegaly, ascites, periorbital oedema, pleural effusions and oedema in the limbs and other dependent areas.

Clinical signs and symptoms

Cardiovascular signs and symptoms

- Cardiomegaly.
- Tachycardia as a compensation mechanism.
- Weak, thready pulse.
- Hypotension.
- Raised central venous pressure if right side affected.

Respiratory signs and symptoms

- Tachypnoea.
- Dyspnoea.
- Pulmonary oedema.
- Dry, irritable cough.
- Pleural effusions.
- Cyanosis.

Renal signs and symptoms

- Oliguria.
- Renin–angiotensin–aldosterone mechanism is activated due to the reduction in renal blood flow[11]. This causes sodium and water to be reabsorbed as a compensatory mechanism.

Gastrointestinal signs and symptoms

- Failure to thrive if too breathless to feed.
- Anorexia.
- Acute weight gain due to oedema.
- Vomiting.
- Hepatomegaly.

Skin signs and symptoms

- Cold.

- Clammy.
- Mottled, pale skin.
- Sweating.
- Oedema of limbs, dependent areas, periorbital, liver and ascites formation.
- Skin breakdown due to oedema.

Other features

- Anxiousness.
- Restlessness.
- Irritability.
- Fatigue.
- Neck vein distension in older child.

Diagnosis

- Auscultation: Gallop rhythm, heart murmur associated with mitral regurgitation from left ventricular dilatation. Chest: fine crackles.
- Chest x-ray: Cardiomegaly, increased pulmonary vascular markings.
- Blood tests: Hyponatraemia.

Key management issues

Key management issues in a child with congestive heart failure are shown in Table 11.2.

Table 11.2 Assessment and management of potential problems in a child with congestive heart failure

Management of the low cardiac output with the goal of reducing oxygen demands as the infant and small child has little cardiac reserve:
- Continuous ECG monitoring and frequent assessment of cardiovascular status. Report worsening condition promptly
- Administer prescribed diuretics
- Administer prescribed digoxin to aid contractility and cardiac output
- Administer prescribed inotropes in severe low cardiac output. Consider the use of ACE inhibitors
- Administer prescribed vasodilators to reduce afterload
- Ensure the patient is normothermic to reduce metabolic and thus oxygen demands
- Ensure bedrest and minimal handling, co-ordinating care efficiently

Management of respiratory distress:
- Frequent assessment of respiratory status. Report worsening condition promptly

(contd)

Table 11.2 (contd)

- Administer prescribed oxygen, assessing effectiveness with the use of a saturation monitor and blood gases
- Sit the child up, raise the head of the cot in an infant. This should relieve respiratory distress
- Mechanical ventilation may be required if the child is in severe heart failure
- Correction of acidosis, hypoxia and hypercapnia will enhance cardiac output
- Administer prescribed diuretics
- Offer small, frequent feeds. If too breathless, consider nasogastric feeds or parenteral nutrition

Management of oedema:
- Administer prescribed diuretics to reduce systemic and pulmonary congestion
- Ensure a strict in/output balance is maintained assessing for hypovolaemia or hypervolaemia
- Restrict fluids as prescribed. Use small drinking vessels to hide the fact there is only a little fluid in it
- Administer prescribed diuretics
- Weigh daily to assess effectiveness of treatment
- Manage electrolyte balance, detecting and correcting imbalances promptly
- Meticulous skin care to prevent skin breakdown in the oedematous child
- Offer a child small, frequent, high calorie, high protein, low salt food/drinks
- Offer a baby the same, in liquid form — small amounts regularly to prevent breathlessness from the exertion of sucking. Consider topping the feed up via a nasogastric feed if the baby is too tired to finish off the feed orally. Try not to let the baby get too hungry and cry as this will use up valuable energy which would be better utilised for sucking
- Care of the child who develops pleural effusion requiring chest drains
- Care of the child who develops ascites requiring drainage

Management of the underlying cause for the low cardiac output, e.g., early surgical intervention for congenital heart disease, cor pulmonale in bronchopulmonary dysplasia, anaemia, arrhythmias

Management of the associated anxiety related to low cardiac output:
- Comfort and reassure the child and family
- Give regular updates as to the child's progress/deterioration/procedures and intervention required
- Encourage parents' and siblings' involvement in the care of their child ensuring they understand the importance of minimal handling and co-ordinating cares
- Listen to the child's/parents' worries and concerns

Postpericardiotomy syndrome

Aetiology

Postpericardiotomy syndrome is thought to be associated with localised inflammation and an autoimmune response as antiheart antibodies have been detected[10]. Between 25–27% of children will develop the syndrome after the first postoperative week but it can occur at 4–6 weeks postoperatively[242, 243]. It presents more frequently in children over two and lasts for several weeks, re-occurring in approximately 21% of patients[4, 38].

Definition

Postpericardiotomy syndrome is a febrile illness developing after a pericardiotomy which involves the pleura and pericardium.

Clinical signs and symptoms

Cardiovascular signs and symptoms

- Pericardial effusions resulting in cardiac tamponade.
- Pericarditis.
- Tachycardia.

Respiratory signs and symptoms

- Pleural effusions.
- Pleuritis.
- Chest pain radiating to the shoulder tip.
- Tachypnoea.

Inflammatory / sepsis signs and symptoms

- Fever 38–40°C.

Other signs and symptoms

- Arthralgia.
- Malaise.
- Lethargy.

Diagnosis

- Chest x-ray: Increased pulmonary vascular markings, pericardial shadow.
- ECG: ST elevation.
- Echocardiogram: Pleural and pericardial effusions.
- Blood tests: Raised ESR, CRP, white cell count with leukocytosis, presence of antiheart antibodies and a rise in antibody titres against the coxsackie B virus and cytomegalovirus in approximately 70% of patients[38].

Key management issues

The key management issues in postpericardiotomy syndrome are shown in Table 11.3.

Table 11.3 Assessment and management of potential problems in a child with postpericardiotomy syndrome

---

Management of the inflammatory response:
- Bedrest must be enforced. Providing stimulation around the bed area in the form of music, television, videos, computer games, board games, painting, visitors, etc.
- Administer prescribed anti-inflammatory drugs, e.g., aspirin, ibuprofen
- Administer prescribed steroids

Management of the pericardial effusion:
- If cardiac tamponade is developing or present, assist with pericardiocentesis. Ensure the child is prepared for the procedure, and if under local anaesthetic, reassured and comforted throughout the procedure
- Send the fluid to the laboratory for analysis

Management of the pleural effusion

Management of the pain from arthralgia and chest pain

Management of the fever

Cardiac tamponade

Aetiology

Cardiac tamponade can be caused by surgery, a stab wound, crush injury to the chest, cardiac tumour, infection, or pericardial effusion usually associated with postpericardiotomy syndrome.

Definition

Cardiac tamponade is a collection of serous fluid, blood or clots in the pericardium which compresses the heart, reducing cardiac output. It is therefore an emergency situation.

Clinical signs and symptoms

Symptoms may occur abruptly or insidiously over a few hours.

Cardiovascular signs and symptoms

- Poor peripheral perfusion with the core–peripheral temperature gradient increasing.

- Reduced urine output.
- Reduction in the amount of chest drainage expected for the condition — this is usually sudden in nature due to the clot formation.
- Bulging chest dressing in the patient with an open chest.
- Premorbid signs include increasing left atrial pressure and increasing central venous pressure, pulsus paradoxus, hypotension, bradycardia or tachycardia, electromechanical dissociation (pulseless electrical activity).

Diagnosis

This is an emergency situation so investigations may not be pertinent and diagnosis should be made from the clinical features.

- Echocardiogram: If time permits, echo will show the collection of fluid in the pericardium.
- Chest x-ray: This will show widening of the mediastinum[220].

Key management issues

The key management issues in a child with cardiac tamponade are shown in Table 11.4.

Table 11.4 Assessment and management of potential problems in a child with cardiac tamponade

Maintain cardiac output:
- Resuscitation will be required should electromechanical dissociation (pulseless electrical activity) occur
- The cardiac surgical team should be sent for urgently
- The child and bedspace should be prepared for chest exploration or needle aspiration under echocardiogram control
- Chest drains should be kept patent by gentle milking and low grade suction
- In an open chest, the patch should be checked for signs of bulging. If bulging of the patch is present, it should be fenestrated or the sutures removed to relieve the bulging
- Blood products must be available — use of the universal recipient, whole blood or packed cells
- The surgical team should be assisted in the event of a re-sternotomy or needle aspiration
- Parents must be contacted (if not present) and fully informed of the situation

Prevention of cardiac tamponade is the goal:
- Ensure patency of chest drains by gently milking at regular intervals, and by the application of low grade suction
- Observe drainage for clots and debris. Report findings to surgeons promptly
- Assess the patient for the aforementioned clinical features immediately reporting findings

Delayed sternal closure

Sternal closure perioperatively in the sick baby or child with a complex congenital heart lesion is associated with significant compromise of cardiac output[244, 245]. Complications from sternal closure are more common in the neonate with lesions such as interrupted aortic arch, TAPVD, severe coarctation of the aorta, TGA, HLHS and truncus arteriosus. Thus delayed sternal closure is frequently employed to alleviate cardiac compression to maintain output and provide a means of access should re-exploration of the chest cavity be required[246].

Complications of sternal closure

The complications associated with primary sternal closure post bypass and aortic cross clamping are shown in Table 11.5.

Table 11.5 Complications associated with sternal closure

Cardiac complications:
- Cardiac tamponade
- Haemorrhage due to post bypass coagulopathy or neonatal coagulopathy
- Myocardial, mediastinal oedema
- Persistent arrhythmia
- Access delayed should insertion of intra-aortic balloon pump or ventricular assist devices be required
- Increasing haemodynamic instability: increasing CVP, low mean BP, low urine output, cool peripheries
- Cardiac compression with a restriction in diastolic filling
- Increasing inotropic requirements

Respiratory complications:
- Increasing ventilation requirements: pulmonary hyperinflation, intrapulmonary haemorrhage, hypoxia, respiratory acidosis
- Pulmonary hypertension
- Pulmonary oedema

General complications:
- Prematurity
- Capillary leak syndrome related to the length of bypass
- Increasing fluid requirements

Advantages of delayed sternal closure

- Effective relief of mediastinal compression.
- Provision of haemodynamic stability.

- Less likely to require large doses of inotropes.
- Easier access for re-exploration of the chest cavity.
- Reduction in ventilation requirements thus increasing the functional residual capacity. This enables the mean airway pressure and oxygen requirements to be reduced and increases oxygen delivery to the tissues.

Disadvantages of delayed sternal closure

- Infection — mediastinitis and wound infection are surprisingly rare[245, 247]. Should an infection occur, the likely organism is one of the staphylococci bacteria[248] or candidae.
- Mortality is associated with the severity of the lesion and multi-organ failure, not the delayed sternal closure[245,247].
- Morbidity rates are low[245].

Technique of delayed sternal closure

At the end of the operation, the sternal wound is closed with a Goretex™ membrane and sutured to the skin edges[248]. Chest stents may be necessary in the baby with a very oedematous heart but may cause local wound complications from skin tensions[244]. A sterile dressing is placed over the latex membrane and aseptically changed only if haemorrhage or leaking occurs. Bilateral pleural drains and mediastinal drains are left *in situ*. Some centres use either iodine or antibiotic ointments and dressings[244, 247].

Management issues

The key management issues in a child with an open chest are shown in Table 11.6.

Table 11.6 Assessment and management of potential problems in a child with an open chest

Label the patient's chest with a suitable label, e.g., "my chest is open", to alert staff and parents to the fact

If the patient is stable, he or she can be allowed to wake up as a little movement will help reduce the overall oedema. However, adequate analgesia and sedation must be given to prevent discomfort and haemodynamic instability from being too restless

Enteral feeding is a priority to protect the gut

Administer prescribed selective decontamination of the gut medicine to prevent translocation of bacteria from the gut and oral flora

(contd)

Table 11.6 (contd)

Ensure echocardiograms are performed with sterile covers and sterile gel. The probe must be gently applied to the chest wall as it can compromise cardiac output

Tip the bed/cot downwards to mobilise dependent oedema

Prophylactic antibiotic cover should be for a longer period if the chest is left open

"Flat" lift the patient to prevent any strain on the open chest. Nurse in supine position only. The patient's head can be turned from side to side

Very gently milk the chest drains as vigorous milking can cause a negative pressure vacuum causing the patch to adhere to internal tissues

The patch should be inspected at regular intervals for an indication of bulging which may predispose to cardiac tamponade. The child's vital signs should be monitored closely to assess for tamponade formation

All care should be planned and co-ordinated to ensure that minimal handling is performed so that the child can benefit from long periods of rest

Elective closure of the chest

Once haemodynamic and respiratory stability have been achieved and postoperative oedema has subsided (commonly after several days) a decision can be made electively to close the sternum. This may be performed in the intensive care setting under aseptic conditions. The closure may be performed either in several stages over a period of days or in one procedure depending on the child's stability and tolerance. If the procedure is to be performed on ICU, the nurse maintains responsibility for the patient and environment before, during and after the chest closure, in close conjunction with the theatre staff. See Table 11.7.

Table 11.7 Management of the patient before elective closure of an open chest

Management of the patient	Management of the environment
• Prepare the child and parents for the impending procedure • Ensure a unit of crossed matched blood is available • Ensure 10–20ml of prescribed sodium chloride flush, 10% calcium gluconate, midazolam, fentanyl and vecuronium syringes, plus the emergency minijets are near the intensivist/anaesthetist	• Clear cubicle of locker, table, chairs • If the patient is in a cot which is not height adjustable, place an electronic lift under the cot and elevate to the surgeon's required height. Move the child to the right side of the cot or bed • Place defibrillator with appropriate internal connections in cubicle • Place screens around the bedside

(contd)

Table 11.7 (contd)

• Connect lectrocath with stopcock (distal to the patient) to a lumen on the central line • Connect a 50 ml syringe of plasma to one end of the stopcock • Connect patient to appropriate pacing box • Place inconti sheet under patient • Place diathermy pad under patient and connect to diathermy machine • Place roll under neck to elevate chest • If the patient is a baby, move him or her close to the edge of the cot, remembering that the surgeon stands on the opposite side of the cot to the heart • Connect patient up to diathermy safe ECG leads (orange) • Ensure patient has had a prescribed bolus of sedation, analgesia, paralysing agent, and antibiotic cover for the procedure	• Arrange for light source for the surgeon • The theatre staff will bring in all the appropriate equipment for the actual procedure

Management of the patient during elective closure of an open chest is shown in Table 11.8.

Table 11.8 Management during elective closure of an open chest

Management of the patient	Management of the environment
• The role of the nurse is to act as "runner" for the theatre staff • Two nurses check the number of swabs at the start of the procedure and at the end • The nurse must observe the patient's vital signs informing medical staff if stability is affected in any way	• Ensure all staff entering the patient's cubicle are wearing a theatre mask and hat • Assist in gowning of the theatre staff • Connect surgeon's light source • Connect the internal paddles to the defibrillator

Management of the patient after the elective closure of an open chest is shown in Table 11.9.

Arrhythmias

Sinus rhythm

Sinus rhythm is shown in Figure 11.1.

Table 11.9 Management after elective closure of an open chest

Management of the patient	Management of the environment
• The nurse must assess the patient at frequent intervals for signs of low cardiac output — cooling peripheries, reduction in urine output, tachycardia, low blood pressure and report promptly • Reassessment of chest drain losses	• Return bedspace to a safe working environment

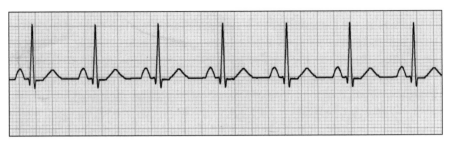

Figure 11.1 Sinus rhythm

Definition

The rate and rhythm are normal for the age of the patient. The impulse originates in the sinoatrial node and is conducted through the normal physiological pathway.

Disorders of rate

Sinus arrhythmia

- Definition: The characteristics of sinus rhythm are present but a change in heart rate occurs with respiration — on inspiration the heart rate increases and, conversely, on expiration the heart rate falls. It is more common with young children and originates in the sinus node.
- Causes: Respiration, increased vagal tone.
- Treatment: None.

Sinus bradycardia — Figure 11.2

- Definition: The characteristics of sinus rhythm are present but the heart rate is too low for the expected age. It may affect cardiac output

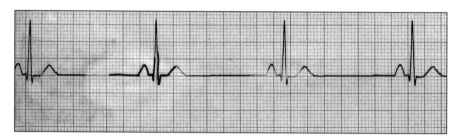

Figure 11.2 Sinus bradycardia

if prolonged or severe. If the rate falls below 100 beats per minute for an infant, 80 for a child or 60 for an adolescent it may be classed as a bradycardia.

- Causes: Prolonged bradycardia is usually a preterminal arrhythmia. Causes can include cardiac surgery around the atria, hypoxic/ischaemic damage to the heart, raised intracranial pressure, myxoedema, drugs (beta blockers, digoxin, lignocaine), increased vagal stimulation (suction, intubation, endotracheal and nasogastric tubes), increased cardiovascular fitness, sleep, neonatal sepsis.
- Treatment: The underlying cause should be treated. However, if prolonged, the following may be attempted: atropine at 20 μg/kg, epinephrine at 10 μg/kg, temporary pacing[249].

Sinus tachycardia — Figure 11.3

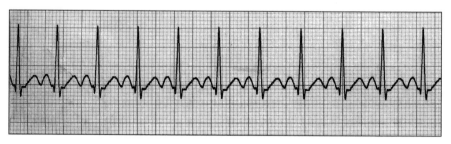

Figure 11.3 Sinus tachycardia

- Definition: The characteristics of sinus rhythm are present but the heart rate is too fast and variable for the expected age. It may affect cardiac filling and emptying and increase oxygen consumption which may be to the detriment of the critically ill child. If the rate rises above 160 beats per minute for an infant, 120 for a child or 100 for an adolescent, it may be classed as a tachycardia.

- Causes: Cardiovascular surgery, hypovolaemia, pain, excitement, exercise, fear, poor cardiac output, excessive inotropic infusion, congestive heart failure, anaemia, thyrotoxicosis, drugs (atropine, amphetamines, epinephrine, other inotropes, caffeine, nicotine), pyrexia (with each 1°C rise in temperature the heart rate increases by 10 beats per minute[10]).
- Treatment: The underlying cause should be treated, systemic cooling, digoxin.

Supraventricular tachycardia (narrow complex tachycardia) — Figure 11.4

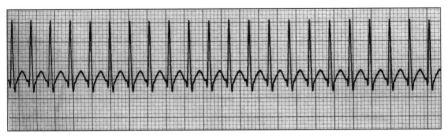

Figure 11.4 Supraventricular tachycardia

- Definition: This is a general name for a group of three types of tachycardia[4] which may compromise cardiac filling. The heart rate tends to be fixed unlike sinus tachycardia which is variable. The three types are:
  1. Nodal/AV junctional where there is loss of the P wave.
  2. AV re-enterant/paroxysmal atrial tachycardia where an accessory pathway (bundle of Kent) develops as seen in Wolff–Parkinson–White syndrome.
  3. Atrial where the single focus is in the atria[4].
- Causes: A normal heart is present in approximately 70% of cases[3], Wolff–Parkinson–White syndrome, structural accessory pathways, drugs (caffeine, nicotine), stress, cardiovascular surgery, pyrexia.
- Treatment: If cardiac output falls, treatment is urgent in the sick child. A synchronous DC shock at 0.5 j/kg to 1–2 j/kg followed by antiarrhythmic drugs, repeating the process from 2 j/kg[249].
  If cardiac output is not compromised:
  1. Carotid sinus massage — this can cause asystole.
  2. Valsalva manoeuvre — after inspiration the patient closes the glottis and tries to exhale in an attempt to reduce venous return to the heart and thus reduce cardiac output[250].
  3. Place ice on the face of infants.

4. If these manoeuvres fail then give a rapid intravenous injection of adenosine 50 µg/kg, repeated by 100 µg/kg followed by 250 µg/kg. A synchronised shock may then be required followed by other anti-arrhythmics — flecainide, digoxin, amiodarone, verapamil or propanolol (if both verapamil and propanolol are given to an infant they can cause profound hypotension).

5. In Wolff–Parkinson–White syndrome, radiofrequency ablation can be performed to interrupt the accessory pathway.

Maintenance digoxin or flecainide may be necessary in the patient prone to supraventricular tachycardias.

Ventricular tachycardia (wide complex tachycardia) — Figure 11.5

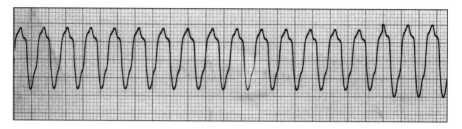

Figure 11.5 Ventricular tachycardia

- Definition: Rapidly repeating ventricular beats resulting in three or more ventricular ectopics. Complexes are wide and bizarre in appearance. P waves are usually absent. Cardiac output is severely compromised as filling, emptying and contraction are affected[220]. The patient can collapse and there is a danger of the condition developing into ventricular fibrillation.

- Causes: Drugs that prolong the QT interval (flecainide, amiodarone), antidepressants, terfenadine, digoxin toxicity, cisapride, caffeine, heart disease and long QT syndrome, cardiac tumours, congenital heart disease, acquired heart disease, myocarditis, hypoxia, hypokalaemia, acidosis, irritative (cardiac catheterisation), inflammation, infections.

- Treatment: (1) If pulse not present, treat as ventricular fibrillation, (2) if the pulse is present, give a nonsynchronous DC shock at 0.5 j/kg to 1 j/kg to 2 j/kg, antiarrhythmics, repeat from 2 j/kg, treat cause[249], (3) if pulse present and cardiac output satisfactory, give lignocaine at 0.5–1 mg/kg, synchronous shock and antiarrhythmics, treat cause[249].

Disorders of rhythm

Atrial flutter — Figure 11.6

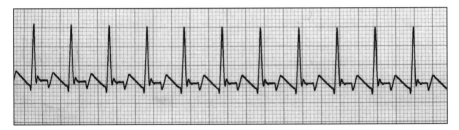

Figure 11.6 Atrial flutter

- Definition: Regular sawtooth appearance of P waves. The atrial rate is around 300 beats per minute. The ventricular rate varies but is a normal rhythm. Cardiac output can be compromised if the ventricular rate is fast.
- Causes: Congenital heart disease (mitral stenosis, Ebstein's anomaly), surgical causes (Mustard, Senning operations), drugs (digoxin toxicity), atrial enlargement.
- Treatment: Antiarrhythmics (digoxin), beta blockers (propranolol), cardioversion if not digitalised, rapid oesophageal atrial pacing.

Atrial fibrillation — Figure 11.7

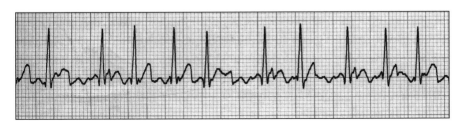

Figure 11.7 Atrial fibrillation

- Definition: Irregular, chaotic non-contracting atrial activity resulting in a rate of 350–600 beats per minute[4]. P waves are not visible and the ventricular rate is irregular. Cardiac output is affected as the stroke volume is decreased therefore peripheral pulses may differ from the apex.
- Causes: As for atrial flutter.

- Treatment: As for atrial flutter. Additionally anticoagulation before and after cardioversion to prevent thromboembolic episodes[4].

Atrial ectopics — Figure 11.8

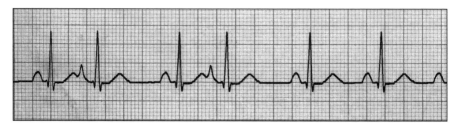

Figure 11.8 Atrial ectopics

- Definition: Abnormal P waves with the early occurrence of QRS complexes.
- Causes: Infection, inflammation, trauma, surgery, thyrotoxicosis, hypoxia, drugs (caffeine, nicotine, alcohol).
- Treatment: Not normally needed. However, digoxin can be prescribed.

Ventricular ectopics — Figure 11.9

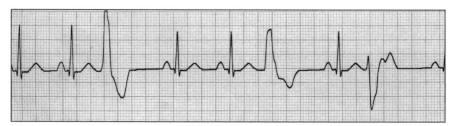

Figure 11.9 Multifocal ventricular ectopics

- Definition: Wide, bizarre, QRS complexes occurring earlier than expected. The ectopic foci originate in the ventricles and can be unifocal, occurring from a single focus, or multifocal occurring from many foci in the ventricles. In the well child, it is insignificant but if associated with heart disease, familial syncope, or runs of ectopics, it is significant as cardiac output can be affected. It may precede ventricular tachycardia occurring in groups as bi- or trigeminy where ectopics alternate with the QRS complexes or as couplets, triplets or more (ventricular tachycardia) in succession.

- Causes: Infection, inflammation, electrolyte imbalance (hypokalaemia, low magnesium), drugs (caffeine, alcohol, nicotine, digoxin toxicity, epinephrine), cardiac tumours, long QT syndrome.
- Treatment: If there is normal cardiac output, treatment is not normally required for isolated ectopics. However, if cardiac output is affected, lignocaine at 0.5 mg/kg, beta blockers and antiarrhythmics are given. Any underlying cause is treated.

Disorders of conduction

First degree heart block — Figure 11.10

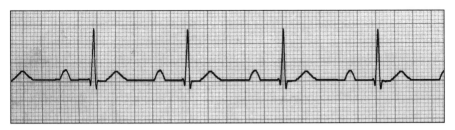

Figure 11.10 First degree heart block

- Definition: Prolonged PR interval for the age of the patient. There is a normal QRS complex but this can progress to second degree heart block. It is due to prolonged conduction through the AV node.
- Causes: It can occur in otherwise healthy patients, cardiomyopathies, surgery, congenital heart disease (e.g., ASD, AVSD), digoxin toxicity, electrolyte imbalance.
- Treatment: None except if due to digoxin toxicity or electrolyte imbalance.

Second degree heart block — Figure 11.11

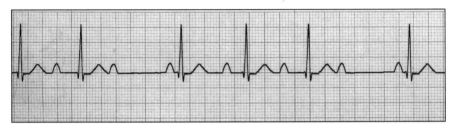

Figure 11.11 Second degree heart block

- Definition: Intermittent disruption of conduction down the bundle of His from the atria to the ventricles, resulting in a faster atrial rate than ventricular. There are two types:
  1. Mobitz I (Wenckebach) — Variable PR interval until it is so prolonged that a QRS is omitted.
  2. Mobitz II - There is a fixed PR interval with extra-atrial contractions that are not always accompanied by a QRS complex. It can progress to third degree heart block.
- Causes: Congenital heart disease, surgery, drugs (digoxin toxicity), cardiomyopathy.
- Treatment: Treat the underlying cause, pacing, atropine.

Third degree heart block — Figure 11.12

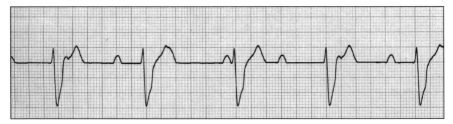

Figure 11.12 Third degree heart block

- Definition: Disruption of conduction down the bundle of His from the AV node. The atria and ventricles beat independently of each other. Atrial impulses are not conducted to the ventricles resulting in an atrial rate of 90–120 and a very slow ventricular rate of 30–50 beats per minute. Cardiac asystole can occur if the ventricular rate is very slow resulting in up to 10 seconds of cardiac output and syncope. This obviously can be very dangerous.
- Causes: Congenitally from maternal systemic lupus erythromatosus, congenital heart disease, cardiac surgery along the septum, myocarditis.
- Treatment: Isoprenaline infusion until temporary pacing can be established. Most patients will require insertion of a permanent pacemaker.

Cardiac arrest

Upon finding a patient with inadequate cardiac output or in cardiac arrest, help should be summoned immediately and cardiopulmonary resuscitation commenced. A senior doctor or resuscitation leader should control the situation, assessing the effectiveness of the intervention at regular intervals.

Asystole — Figure 11.13

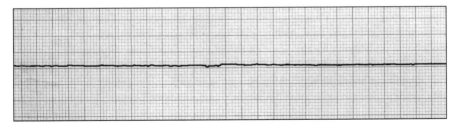

Figure 11.13 Asystole

- Definition: Cardiac standstill with no output. The patient appears collapsed. The ECG has the characteristics of a straight line, with or without P waves.
- Cause: Normally results from an acidic, hypoxic, ischaemic episode which causes a bradycardia prior to the asystole[249].
- Treatment: Ventilate, epinephrine IV at 10 µg/kg, cardiopulmonary resuscitation (CPR) 60 cycles/3 minutes. Colloid and sodium bicarbonate are given, then the epinephrine repeated at 100 µg/kg, CPR for 3 minutes and repeat from epinephrine 100 µg/kg[249].

Ventricular fibrillation — Figure 11.14

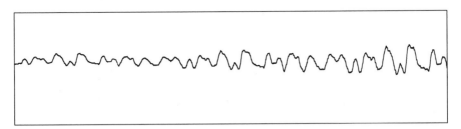

Figure 11.14 Ventricular fibrillation

- Definition: No cardiac output. Collapsed patient. There are no recognisable complexes on the ECG, just bizarre, "quivering" patterns.
- Cause: This arrhythmia is rare in paediatrics unless hypothermic, or overdose of tricyclic antidepressants[249], hypoxia, hyperkalaemia.

- Treatment: A precordial thump is administered if the cardiac arrest is witnessed. An asynchronous DC shock at 2 j/kg, repeated at 2 j/kg then 4 j/kg. Ventilate the patient, give epinephrine at 10 µg/kg, shock at 4 j/kg repeated a further two times, epinephrine at 100 µg/kg, 20 CPR cycles/1 minute. Treat the cause, give colloid and sodium bicarbonate then repeat from shocking three times at 4 j/kg[249].

Electromechanical dissociation (pulseless electrical activity)

- Definition: No cardiac output despite the presence of normal PQRS complexes on the monitor.
- Causes: Shock, hypovolaemia, cardiac tamponade, tension pneumothorax, drug overdose, electrolyte imbalance. This can occur in a child with a pacemaker who has arrested but still shows ECG complexes if connected to a monitor.
- Treatment: Ventilate, give epinephrine 10 µg/kg, fluids at 20 ml/kg, treat cause, epinephrine at 100 µg/kg, 3 minutes/60 cycles of CPR and repeat from epinephrine 100 µg/kg[249].

Key management issues for cardiac arrest

For most children, cardiac arrest will have resulted from a respiratory arrest which allows for a more successful outcome than initial cardiac arrest which occurs in children with heart disease[251]. Following cardiac arrest, the child should be assessed frequently for further episodes and the complications associated with no or reduced cardiac output. The sustained effects will depend on the length of time the child was without cardiac output and the cause of the arrest. Whatever the cause, the child should be assessed and managed systematically commencing with an "ABC" approach (Table 11.10).

Table 11.10 Key management issues in cardiac arrest

System   Management and intervention during and following cardiac arrest

Respiratory
- Maintenance of airway — establish a secure airway
- Administer oxygen, air or oxygen/air if ductus arteriosus dependent
- Administer appropriate ventilation for effective oxygen delivery and carbon dioxide elimination
- Observe for presence of respiratory distress
- Blood gas analysis
- Oxygen saturations
- Regularly assess effectiveness of interventions

(contd)

Table 11.10 (contd)

Circulation
- Establish secure vascular access
- Give prescribed fluid resuscitation therapy including colloids, crystalloids, buffering agents to neutralise acidosis, inotropes

Cardiovascular
- Heart rate, rhythm and regularity — if inadequate, provide cardiac compressions and defibrillation or cardioversion depending on the rhythm/rate
- Pulse strength
- Assess intracardiac pressure if postoperative patient
- Assess peripheral perfusion — colour, temperature, capillary refill
- Assess systemic perfusion — urine output, neurological perfusion
- Assess patency of the ductus arteriosus in a duct dependent baby
- Assess potential for cardiac tamponade in a postoperative patient

Investigations
- Chest x-ray
- Echocardiogram
- ECG
- Urea and electrolytes
- Full blood count
- Clotting
- Blood gases
- Lactate

Multi-organ failure
- Over the next few hours/days assessment of all systems will be required to establish the degree of hypoxic/ischaemic damage to vital organs

Brain
- Minimise brain damage from the effects of hypoperfusion — maintaining effective oxygenation, circulation and electrolytes, reduce intracranial pressure by sedating, paralysing and hyperventilating the child, prevent acidosis, hypercapnia, administer cerebral diuretics, control fits and reduce cerebral oxygen demands by cooling the patient. In the infant perform a cranial ultrasound scan to assess the damage. If stable, perfom a CT or MRI scan of head

Kidneys
- Minimise renal damage from the effects of hypoperfusion — maintain effective oxygenation and circulation, maintain effective urine output by administration of diuretics but consider peritoneal dialysis should anuria persist. Care should be taken if administering nephrotoxic drugs in the presence of renal failure

Liver
- Minimise liver damage from the effects of hypoperfusion — maintain effective oxygenation and circulation, correct coagulopathies by administration of fresh frozen plasma, cryoprecipitate, assess liver function tests regularly

Gastrointestinal
- Minimise gut damage from the effects of hypoperfusion by administering prescribed selective decontamination of the gut drugs, administering enteral feeding,

(contd)

Table 11.10 (contd)

especially breast milk which may have antibodies to protect the gut, assessing gastrointestinal losses and types of losses (e.g., bloody stools, nasogastric aspirate) and girth measurements

Metabolic/sepsis
- Consider the use of antibiotics, monitoring for sepsis over the next few days
- Monitor lactate levels

Parental care
- The parents should be notified immediately should respiratory or cardiac arrest occur. If the parents are not present during resuscitation, a member of staff should be available to stay with them and to communicate the child's progress from the resuscitation team.The time passes very quickly for the staff busy resuscitating a child, but agonisingly slowly for parents waiting for news. Updates need to be given every 5 minutes or so. Should no progress have been made after 10 minutes, the probability of poor outcome must be conveyed to prepare the parents for the event of their child's death. An honest, caring attitude is paramount. The child's name should always be used. Provision of privacy from other parents, free use of the telephone, tissues, drinks and religious and cultural needs have to be addressed
- Debate as to whether or not parents should be present during resuscitation commonly arises. It is a controversial issue in which opposing views prevail. The professional often feels parents should not be present as it is perceived as too stressful

Parental perspectives
- Parents may want to be with their child at this time[252–254]. Equally, knowing that everything possible had been done for their child in the event of death would have more impact should the parents witness the attempted resuscitation[255]. Feelings of guilt and helplessness may present in the relative who has not participated in the care of their child at this time[256]
- Certain advantages have been identified for relatives being present:
  1. Avoidance of denial of the death of their child
  2. Can be with the dying child to give comfort
  3. Can see everything possible has been done for their child
  4. Parental involvement is possible[255]

Staff perspectives
- Many nursing and medical staff have valid concerns regarding the presence of parents during resuscitation — there is little time to prepare the parents for what they are about to witness and the effects could be detrimental to the parents for years afterwards[257], especially if the chest has to be reopened. However, if a senior member of staff is present he or she can prepare the parents before entering and stay with them during the event giving honest explanations whatever the outcome
- It is a stressful and difficult time for staff[258]. Nevertheless, if staff are trained effectively they can perform confidently, dispelling some elements of stress associated with resuscitation[259]. Staff may be concerned about any legal implications as to whether the parents would interfere with the attempts at the resuscitation and the decision to stop or carry on with the resuscitation. Whatever the circumstances, each situation is unique so parental presence will have to be considered individually in a sensitive and caring manner by an experienced member of staff

Cardiovascular interventions

Cardioversion and defibrillation

Cardioversion and defibrillation are rarely performed in babies and children due to the main cause of cardiac arrest being respiratory arrest leading to bradycardia and asystole. Conversely, in adults, ventricular fibrillation is the prime cause of arrest, necessitating defibrillation.

Cardioversion

- Description: Delivery of an electrical current synchronised with the patient's own abnormal heart rate to depolarise the cells, thus allowing the sinus node to initiate the heart's rhythm once again[260].
- Uses: Rapid rates (SVT, VT, atrial tachyarrhythmias).
- Procedure: The patient is sedated with a light anaesthetic if not already ventilated. Metal jewellery is removed. The defibrillator is turned on and the patient is connected to the ECG monitor by means of the ECG leads. Appropriate sized paddles are chosen and jelly pads placed on the area of the right upper lobe and over the apex of the heart. The "sync" button is pressed which allows the defibrillator to recognise the components of the PQRST complex thereby automatically discharging the shock at the appropriate time. The defibrillator is charged and the paddles placed on the chest wall. Staff are asked to stand back, the discharge button is pressed and the effects of the intervention are assessed.

Defibrillation

- Description: Delivery of an electrical current either internally or externally through the chest wall to the fibrillating heart. This depolarises the myocardium allowing subsequent organised repolarisation and a resumption of regular contractions.
- Uses: Terminal abnormal rhythm (ventricular fibrillation, pulseless ventricular tachycardia and to restart the heart in asystole).
- Procedure: CPR is commenced until the defibrillator is ready. Metal jewellery is removed. ECG leads are attached, the defibrillator is turned on and the jelly pads applied to the right upper lobe area and apex of the heart. Appropriate-sized paddles are chosen, charged to 2 j/kg and placed on the jelly pads. Staff are told to stand back and the current is discharged. The resulting rhythm is assessed and other pertinent treatment performed.

Problems associated with cardioversion and defibrillation

- Arrhythmias: R on T phenomenon causing ventricular fibrillation, atrial fibrillation, SVT, VT, VF.
- Burns to the paddle area if inadequate gel/pads or excess gel on the skin. There must be a firm contact between the paddles and the chest wall to minimise the severity of the burns. Burns can occur to the myocardial wall if too many joules are used.
- Staff may receive a shock if in contact with the bed or patient or via fluid on the floor acting as an electrical arc.

Pacing

Pacing may be necessary to treat the heart rate or rhythm disturbance which is compromising cardiac output. It is normally indicated for the following reasons:

- Arrhythmias caused by cardiomyopathy, hypoxia, electrolyte imbalances, hypothermia, sick sinus syndrome, myocardial infarction, hypersensitive carotid sinus syndrome.
- Failure to respond to inotropes, oxygen and antiarrhythmics.
- Cardiac surgery — damage to the conduction tissue resulting in heart block.

Types of pacing

Temporary pacing

- Oesophageal: An electrode is passed up the nose and fed down into the oesophagus until it is behind the left atrium. Discomfort is felt if the voltage is very high.
- Transthoracic: A needle is passed through the anterior chest wall and an epicardial pacing wire is attached through the needle to the epicardium.
- Transcutaneous: Two adhesive pads are placed on the chest wall. This can cause all muscle groups to contract causing a degree of discomfort for the patient.
- Epicardial: During open heart surgery, pacing wires are inserted through the epicardial surface. Wires on the surface of the right side of the chest are atrial wires and on the left are ventricular wires. Insertion of two wires will allow pacing of either atria or ventricles.

- Transvenous: A wire is passed via a major vein into the right atria or ventricle. However, risks are associated with this procedure, i.e. pneumothorax, heart perforation, air emboli, haemorrhage, infection and arrhythmias.
- Permanent pacing: This is required two to three weeks after temporary pacing is initiated. The pacemaker is implanted subcutaneously. If the patient is a small neonate, an open surgical approach may have to be used.

Concepts associated with pacing

Three basic concepts must be understood:

- Capturing: This is whether the pacemaker is pacing the desired chamber(s).
- Sensing: This is whether the pacemaker is sensing the patient's own (intrinsic) contractions of the heart chambers. This is necessary so that the pacemaker avoids competing with the patient's own rhythm. The pacemaker only "kicks in" when it cannot detect (sense) the patient's own effort.
- Threshold: This is the least amount of stimulus required to stimulate the myocardium or the least amount of voltage for the patient's own beats to be sensed.

Modes of pacing

The North American Society of Pacing and British Pacing and Electrophysiology groups have standardised a code to describe the modes of pacing available (Table 11.11). There are five positions but for the purpose of this book, only positions I to III will be discussed.

Table 11.11 Pacing modes

Code position	I	II	III
Code letter	V	V	T
	A	A	I
	D	D	D
	O	O	O

Code position

I: Which chamber is paced — either the ventricle (V), atrium (A), dual chamber (D) or neither (O).

II: Which chamber is sensing — this is the patient's own effort. Letters V, A, D, O may not be set as position I; for example, in VDD mode, (V) ventricle is paced, and the pacemaker senses both the atrium and ventricle (D).

III: The response of the pacemaker to the sensed beat — for example, in VVI mode, the ventricle (V) is paced, the ventricle is sensed (V) but the pacemaker withholds pacemaker output in the presence of a sensed beat (I). That is, if the pacemaker is set for a rate of 100 bpm, it will discharge if the rate falls below 100, but only sense if the rate is above 100.

The (T) position is rarely used but locates the sensed intrinsic (patient's own) events.

The (D) position is when the pacemaker reacts to the sensed beat by inhibiting its response by tracking the sensed event. For example, in DDD mode, the pacemaker senses the atrial beat, inhibits atrial output and triggers the ventricular output after a predetermined interval.

In fixed pacing, the pacemaker will give a preset heart rate but does not synchronise with the patient. Therefore, there is the chance of R on T wave phenomena.

Choosing the correct pacing mode

The following is an example of how to determine the correct mode of pacing.

The initial assessment must be to establish whether there is atrioventricular conduction:

- A--------- V: If the atrial rate is slow during AV conduction — pace the atria, e.g., AAI mode
- A × V: (1) If there is no AV conduction and the atrial rate is good — sense the atria and pace the ventricle, e.g., DDD.
- If there is no AV conduction and the atrial rate is slow — pace both the atria and ventricle, e.g., sick sinus syndrome.

If the pacing is to combat a tachyarrhythmia such as SVT, two methods can be used:

- Set the pacemaker atrial rate higher than the patient's own rate and reduce slowly (AAI mode).
- Overdrive the atria up to 2:1 block, e.g., set the pacemaker at 360 atrial beats per minute compared with the patient's own 180 beats per minute.

Key management issues

The key management issues for a child requiring pacing are shown in Table 11.12.

Table 11.12 Assessment and management of potential problems in a child requring pacing

Assess and record:
- Patient's own heart rate and blood pressure. The heart rate and tracing on the monitor may be the pacemaker's electrical stimuli. If hypotension is present or blood pressure is unrecordable, the patient may be in electromechanical dissociation (pulseless electrical activity) requiring resuscitation
- Mode of pacing
- Output threshold — this is the lowest voltage required to capture or initiate the pacing. It will have to be increased over a period of two weeks as there will be fibrosis around the wire tip. After two weeks or so a permanent pacemaker will be necessary if the patient's rhythm/rate has not returned to normal
- Pacing spike on the ECG recording
- Battery life

Failure of the pacemaker to capture:
- The patient may require CPR if cardiac output is compromised
- Increase the threshold voltage
- Check for a loose connection between the wires and pacemaker. Secure connections
- Check for a wire fracture
- Check for battery failure
- Consider pacing box failure and change the box

Failure to sense or undersensing of patient's own rate:
- Same as for failure of pacemaker to capture (above)
- Check for inadequate QRS signal — increase the threshold sensitivity
- Reposition the patient

The pacemaker is oversensing:
- Turn down the sensitivity
- Remove electromagnetic interference

(contd)

Table 11.12 (contd)

Removal of pacing wires:
- Performed 4+ days postoperatively
- Perform a 12 lead ECG prior to removal noting for any remaining arrhythmias
- Monitor the patient for pericardial effusion and cardiac tamponade after wire removal

If the pacemaker is permanent, education for the child and parents:
- A full explanation is required and with most makes of pacemaker, an accompanying booklet is provided by the manufacturing company
- The patient cannot have an MRI scan or go through an airport metal sensing machine as it will set off the alarm and a body search may be required, mobile phones can be used but only by using the right ear for reception
- Follow-up will be required for life

Haemodynamic monitoring

Invasive blood pressure monitoring

Indications for use

An invasive catheter for continuous monitoring of the blood pressure is most valuable in the intensive care setting where patients may be unstable with labile blood pressures. The main indications for invasive arterial blood pressure monitoring include:

- Cardiovascular surgery.
- Neurosurgery or head injury.
- Septic shock states.
- Drug therapy — inotropes, vasodilators, antihypertensive therapies.
- Frequent arterial blood gas sampling.

Sites of cannulation

The radial, femoral, dorsalis pedis and umbilical arteries are the most utilised sites for arterial cannulation. The brachial artery can be used but has inherent risks as it is an end artery.

Key management issues

The key management issues for a child with an arterial line are shown in Table 11.13.

Table 11.13 Assessment and management of potential problems in a child with an arterial line

---

Risk of disconnection resulting in catastrophic haemorrhage:
* Ensure all connections are luer lock, tight and the line is held in place securely with appropriate strapping
* Ensure the line can be viewed at all times and that the inquisitive child's hands do not tamper with the connections
* Ensure alarm parameters are set appropriately and are audible
* On removal of the arterial line, pressure must be applied for a minimum of five minutes, remembering that the child with a coagulopathy will require longer pressure[14]. A haematoma may occur at the puncture site

Risk of air emboli/thrombosis from frequent blood gas sampling and the presence of a coagulopathy in the critically ill child[14]:
* Ensure tubing, transducer, infusion and syringes are free from air
* Always aspirate before injecting to prevent air or old blood in the tubing or at the tip of the catheter being injected into the patient's artery
* A constant, slow infusion can prevent thromboembolic episodes[261]

Inaccurate blood pressure monitoring:
* Ensure the line is calibrated at the start of each shift
* Ensure the height of the transducer correlates with the patient's right atrium. Use a spirit level for accuracy
* Maintain patency of the line with infusion of saline if a big vessel or heparinised saline if a small vessel is cannulated

Interruption of blood supply to the distal limb — this may be caused by too big a cannula related to the size of the artery, a thromboembolic episode, arterial spasm or the injection of a solution other than saline or heparinised saline:
* Use the appropriate sized cannula for the artery
* Gentle aspiration and flushing of the cannula may prevent a thromboembolic episode or spasm of the artery
* Frequent observation of the distal limb for absent pulse, blanching, change in colour from normal colouration, to blue to white (ominous sign) and cool skin need reporting promptly
* Do not inject fluids other than prescribed saline or heparinised saline as gangrene may occur — umbilical arterial lines being the exception

Risk of sepsis:
* The site should be inspected at regular intervals for signs of infection — redness, tenderness, hotness, oedema — and reported promptly. Blood cultures from the line can be taken should septicaemia/bacteraemia be suspected. Appropriate sepsis treatment should be commenced on discovery of an infection
* An aseptic insertion technique and blood sampling technique should be employed
* Dressings should be performed after assessment of the site. Swabs of the site can be taken at dressing takedown
* Flush solutions and tubing should be changed as per hospital policy

Arterial wave form interpretation — Figure 11.15

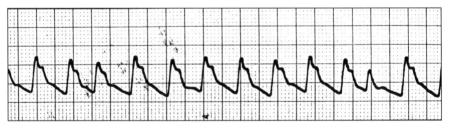

Figure 11.15 Normal arterial wave formation

- A sharp upstroke to . . .
- A peak indicative of systole.
- A gradual downstroke to . . .
- The dicrotic notch indicative of the aortic valve closing.
- A gentle curve at the bottom indicating the end of diastole.
- The area under the curve up to the dicrotic notch relates to stroke volume.

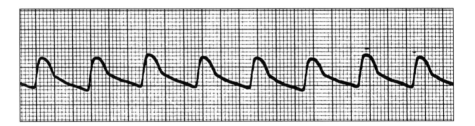

Figure 11.16 Dampened arterial wave formation

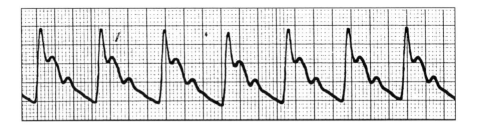

Figure 11.17 Over-shoot on an arterial wave formation

Arterial waveform issues

Potential waveform problems are shown in Table 11.14.

Table 11.14 Potential waveform problems

Dampened trace (Figure 11.16) (loss of dicrotic notch) caused by:
* Occlusion of the cannula tip due to debris. Do not flush forcefully, aspirate gently
* Cannula tip up against the wall of the artery — reposition the cannula
* Air in the transducer set up/line — aspirate air. Re-zero the transducer
* Blood in the line — turn the rate of the flush up. Check all connections are tight and stopcock position correct
* Patient hypotensive — compare the arterial blood pressure against a cuff pressure to establish whether the trace is dampened or the patient is hypotensive
* Fluid infusing through system at a high rate

Overshoot (Figure 11.17) resulting in a falsely high blood pressure, although the mean is accurate. Caused by:
* Long, soft tubing causing a degree of resonance frequency — ensure short, stiff tubing is used
* Air bubbles — remove
* Ensure the transducer height is at the level of the patient's right atrium and recalibrate

No reading caused by:
* Stopcock occluded — reposition
* Catheter occluded — unblock

Incorrect reading caused by:
* Transducer level not at height of right atrium
* Air in the system
* Leak in the system
* Faulty monitor or transducer

Low dicrotic notch caused by:
* Slow emptying of the ventricle and low circulating volume — give fluids

Pulsus paradoxus caused by:
* A systolic decrease of 3–10 mmHg which is present upon respiration indicating hypovolaemia — fluid challenge to increase the stroke volume

Pulsus alterans — alternate high and low waveforms — indicative of left ventricular failure

Central venous pressure (CVP) monitoring

A central venous catheter is placed to assess vascular tone and venous volume[262] and for monitoring right ventricular filling pressures (preload).

Indications for use of central venous access

* Assess effectiveness of volume resuscitation.
* Management of central venous pressure.
* Administration of drugs which are irritant to peripheral veins.

- Administration of total parenteral nutrition.
- Venous access in the peripherally shut down patient.
- To give large volumes of fluid.
- Safe and continuous administration of inotropes.
- Long-term venous access.

Sites of cannulation

The femoral, internal and external jugular, subclavian, antecubital fossa and umbilical veins can all be used.

Normal values

- Normal child, non-ventilated: 2–4 mmHg.
- Normal child, ventilated: 6–8 mmHg.
- Some degree of RV failure (e.g., TOF): 12–14 mmHg.
- Fontan type procedure: 14–20 mmHg.

Key management issues

The key management issues specific to a child undergoing CVP monitoring are shown in Table 11.15.

Table 11.15 Assessment and management of potential problems in a child undergoing CVP monitoring

---

Low CVP caused by:
- Low preload, hypovolaemia, insufficient venous return — fluid load

High CVP caused by:
- High preload, hypervolaemia — administer prescribed diuretics
- Right ventricular failure — maintain a high CVP to help right ventricular emptying
- High intrathoracic pressure from positive pressure ventilation during inspiration — take the CVP measurement upon expiration
- Right sided heart surgery — tetralogy of Fallot, Fontan type procedure

Arrhythmias caused by:
- Tip of the catheter migrating — perform a check x-ray after insertion to establish the position

Risk of sepsis — as for arterial blood pressure monitoring. Use of bacterial filters to minimise microbial contamination

Risk of thromboembolic complications — as for arterial blood pressure monitoring

Risk of air emboli — air enters the systemic and cerebral circulation in children with intra-cardiac mixing, that is, a right to left shunt. Therefore no air must enter the venous line in children with a right to left shunt. Aspirate before flushing. Additionally, filters to remove air and debris should be used

(contd)

Table 11.15 (contd)

Venous stasis and discoloration of the distal limb – check the pulses of the distal limb to ensure it is only a venous problem, not arterial. Monitor for signs of congestion. Elevate the affected limb

Risk of haemorrhage — as for arterial blood pressure monitoring

Specific complications pertaining to the site of insertion:
- Femoral vein — renal vein thrombosis, portal vein thrombosis, venous stasis of the leg
- Subclavian vein — pneumothorax, haemothorax, brachial plexus injury, chylothorax, haemorrhage. Check x-ray after insertion
- Internal jugular — insertion must be avoided in babies with TGA as cannulation of the ascending aorta is possible
- Umbilical vein — portal vein thrombosis and hepatic necrosis[263]

Pulmonary artery pressure monitoring

Indications for use

- To assess the pressure of the pulmonary vasculature. This is of particular use in babies with TAPVD, AVSD, VSD and other lesions predisposing to pulmonary hypertension.
- To assess left ventricular function by management of the pulmonary artery wedge pressure. However, this is not commonly performed in paediatric cardiac management due to the size of available catheters. Therefore this function will not be discussed further.
- For intravenous access — prostacyclin is a potent pulmonary vasodilator and can be infused safely through the catheter directly into the area where it is required.

Sites of insertion

- Directly through the chest wall into the pulmonary artery.
- Indirectly, fed up through the femoral vein.

Normal values

Normal mean pulmonary artery pressure is one third of the mean arterial blood pressure.

Key management issues

The key management issues in a child undergoing pulmonary artery pressure monitoring are shown in Table 11.16.

Table 11.16 Assessment and management of potential problems in a child undergoing pulmonary artery pressure monitoring

As for arterial blood pressure monitoring

Pulmonary artery rupture is more common in patients with pulmonary hypertension who are anticoagulated — observe for haemoptysis

Removal of direct line — this should only be performed by a surgeon 5–7 days postoperatively. The child should have a unit of blood available as there is a risk of haemorrhage

Indirect lines, e.g., via the femoral vessels, can be removed by nursing staff

Left atrial pressure monitoring

Indications for use

- Often used in paediatrics due to the inaccessibility of pulmonary artery wedge monitoring.
- For accurate assessment of left ventricular filling pressures (LV preload).
- For inotrope infusions if central venous access is limited.

Site of insertion

- Directly through the chest wall into the left atrium.
- Indirectly fed through the femoral vein to the right atrium and across the septum into the left atrium.

Normal values

The normal value of left atrial pressure is 6–10 mmHg. The mean value is usually slightly higher than the CVP recording.

Key management issues

The key management issues in a child undergoing left atrial pressure line monitoring are shown in Table 11.17.

Table 11.17 Assessment and management of potential problems in a child undergoing left atrial pressure line monitoring

As for arterial blood pressure monitoring

Low left atrial pressure caused by:
- Reduced pulmonary venous return from the lungs especially in a pulmonary hypertensive crisis

High left atrial pressure caused by:
- Cardiac tamponade
- Fluid overload

Removal of direct line should be performed by a surgeon as there is a risk of haemorrhage and cardiac tamponade. Therefore a unit of blood should be available and the mediastinal drain left *in situ* until the line has been removed. Quarter hourly observations for haemorrhage should be performed. Indirect lines can be removed by the nursing staff

Intra-aortic balloon pumping

Intra-aortic balloon pumping (IABP) is a temporary cardiac assist device which has been used in adults since 1968[264]. The device was first used in paediatrics in 1981 with disappointing results[265] but has subsequently been developed and advanced for use in babies as small as 3 kg. See Figures 11.18 and 11.19

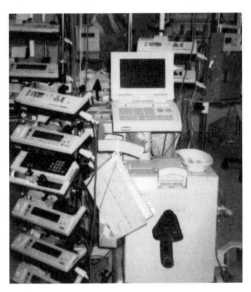

Figure 11.18 Arrow showing an intra-aortic balloon pump surrounded by the numerous pieces of equipment a child will require whilst being balloon pumped (it is important not to forget the child amongst all the equipment!)

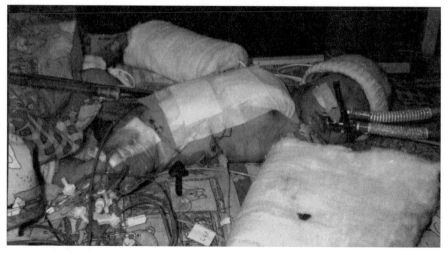

Figure 11.19 Arrow showing direct entry of intra-aortic balloon through the chest wall

Physiological principles of IABP

Counterpulsation (inflation and deflation of the balloon during diastole and systole, respectively) within the aorta displaces the blood volume, thus increasing the diastolic blood pressure[266]. This augmentation of perfusion during diastole increases coronary perfusion in the failing heart. It is achieved by sending blood back to the aortic root and hence the coronary arteries[10]. Additionally, afterload is reduced by deflation of the balloon before ventricular ejection.

The overall cardiac effects will reduce myocardial demands, increase myocardial oxygen supply and increase cardiac output in the patient with poor left ventricular function. The systemic effects include increased perfusion to the brain, kidneys, lungs, gut and other tissues.

Indications for use

Balloon pumping can be used in various scenarios, however, it should not be used if there is little chance of recovery. Therefore, anticipating its use will increase the success and survival rates as it assists, not replaces the left ventricle[267].

Indications for IABP

- Low cardiac output with increasing inotropic requirement[172].
- Weaning from cardiopulmonary bypass.

- As a bridge to transplant (rare in the UK within paediatrics).
- Septic shock.
- Cardiogenic shock.
- Myocarditis.
- Congenital heart disease (postoperatively in anomalous coronary artery, AVSD, aortic and mitral valve replacement, Fontan procedure, tetralogy of Fallot, TGA[267]).

Contraindications to IABP

- Patent ductus arteriosus.
- Aortic insufficiency.
- Aortic aneurysm.
- Congenital heart diseases (interrupted aortic arch, coarctation of the aorta, hypoplastic left heart syndrome, hypoplastic aortic arch).

Mechanics of IABP

An appropriately sized balloon is selected depending on the size and weight of the neonate or child. It is inserted aseptically either directly through the chest wall or indirectly in a femoral artery into the thoracic descending aorta. The ideal position being between the left subclavian artery and the renal arteries[267].

The balloon is connected into a pump which inflates and deflates the balloon with an inert gas (helium), synchronised with the cardiac cycle. Helium is used as it is a very light gas and so increases the speed of balloon inflation and deflation. A check x-ray is taken to ensure the correct position has been attained. Heparinisation is required to prolong the clotting to twice its normal value. Activated clotting times (ACT) should be monitored 1–2 hourly until the ACT is 120–180 seconds. Clotting profiles should be performed 6 hourly.

Timing of the IABP

Timing is vital to optimise the best cardiac augmentation for the patient. The pump needs to be triggered to inflate and deflate the balloon when the appropriate time with the cardiac cycle is reached. Inflation of the balloon is timed to occur at the dicrotic notch, that is closure of the aortic valve, on the arterial pressure tracing or when the R wave occurs on the ECG recording. As the balloon inflates, diastolic pressure is augmented, increasing coronary artery blood flow and myocardial oxygen supply.

The greater elasticity of the young aorta gives variable augmentation. However, increased myocardial oxygen supply can be achieved even in the neonate. The balloon must be deflated before the aortic valve opens thus allowing forward flow of the blood. Deflation decreases the aortic end diastolic pressure and the next peak systolic pressure which will reflect the reduction in afterload.

Problems exist with timing in paediatrics as the heart rate is faster at this age. In adults the pump times automatically but in paediatrics or patients with a heart rate of greater than 120 beats per minute, manual timing is preferred. This is due to the R wave interval being shorter, leaving less time for the pump to react between the electrical events of the heart and the mechanical events shown on the screen. It is preferable therefore to use the arterial waveform in paediatrics. However, two arterial lines will be required — one for the IABP and one for arterial sampling.

Whichever trigger is used, when the pump is set to manual timing, an increase or decrease in heart rate by 10 beats per minute or arrhythmias warrant frequent re-evaluation of the timing and fine tuning to ensure correct inflation and deflation timing. If the child is paced, newer machines have pacing modes which recognise the pacing spike on ECG.

Timing is set to inflate the balloon at an inflation ratio of 1:1, 1:2 or 1:3. The choice of ratio depends on the amount of support needed — the higher the support, the higher the ratio. If the pump cannot inflate quickly enough, e.g., with a fast tachycardia of 200 beats per minute, the balloon inflation can be set for 1:2 ratio, that is every second beat, the balloon will inflate thus ensuring a more effective augmentation.

Helium fills

The balloon is filled with helium, a light gas, which allows for fast inflation and deflation[267]. Rapid heart rates will cause the helium to diffuse and evaporate more quickly, necessitating filling of the balloon at least every 45 minutes. Should augmentation reduce, preloading of the balloon with helium may be required[267].

Assessing the effectiveness of the IABP

Within paediatrics, balloon pumping has less chance of marked diastolic augmentation due to the pliable aorta. The aorta in adults becomes calcified over the years, thus allowing the balloon to inflate against a more rigid aorta, augmenting diastole more effectively. However, assessing the effectiveness of balloon pumping can reveal the advantages of:

- Increased diastolic pressure.
- Increased mean arterial pressure.
- Increased urine output.
- Increased tissue perfusion with a reduction in the core–peripheral temperature gradient.

and disadvantages of:

- An increasing heart rate.
- Lowered systemic vascular resistance.
- Lowered mean arterial pressure.

Should the patient's condition not improve or indeed worsen, consideration must be given to mechanical faults such as a kinked balloon, helium leak, too small a balloon, migration of the balloon or inaccurate timing.

Weaning of the IABP

Initially, inotropic support and other drug support should be significantly weaned and the child assessed for stability. Augmentation is then weaned to 50%, the cardiac output assessed and the timing ratio frequency lowered from 1:1 to 1:2 to 1:3. During the weaning period, the child should be further assessed for a deterioration in cardiac output[268].

Once satisfied that the child is stable, the balloon can be surgically removed as it must not lie immobile in the aorta due to the potential formation of thrombi and emboli. This is crucial in cardiac arrest situations when the balloon pump is set to pressure trigger, allowing augmentation of diastolic pressures during cardiac compression. This provides augmentation of coronary and cerebral perfusion. Alternatively, the balloon can be put into internal trigger with half augmentation to allow movement without impeding ventricular outflow on cardiac compression.

Key management issues

Nurses should be familiar both with the principles of intra-aortic balloon pumping and with operating the pump itself as they are accountable for their actions. The child is often very sick and it usually takes two nurses to care for him or her — one to operate and interact with the balloon pump, which is unlikely to be in automatic mode, and one to provide the other necessary nursing care. The key issues are shown in Table 11.18.

Table 11.18 Assessment and management of potential problems in a child undergoing intra-aortic balloon pumping

Assessment for alterations in cardiac output:
- Monitor heart rate and regularity, systolic, mean and diastolic blood pressure, left atrial pressure, central venous pressure
- Ensure correct timing of balloon pump to maximise its effectiveness
- Assess urine output, which is indicative of kidney perfusion
- Assess core–peripheral temperature gradient and general tissue perfusion
- Monitor for increasing balloon pump requirements to maintain falling cardiac output

Management of the balloon pump timing for optimal performance:
- Assess when the balloon inflates and deflates in relation to the cardiac cycle
- Time the balloon to inflate at the dicrotic notch, that is, aortic valve closure
- Time the balloon to deflate before the aortic valve opens, that is, before systole
- Correct any inaccurate timing
- Ensure electrolytes are in balance to avoid the development of dysrrhythmias
- Maintain the trigger — if ECG, do not take leads off; if arterial, maintain patency of the line
- Should the heart rate change within 10 beats per minute, check the accuracy of the timing as it may require fine tuning
- Record the heart rate at which the timing was set
- If the heart rate is over 190 beats per minute and augmentation is poor, consider changing the inflation ratio to 1:2

Assess for a reduction in renal perfusion due to renal artery occlusion:
- Monitor urine output hourly reporting amounts less than 1 ml/kg/hour
- Monitor changes in biochemistry particularly a rising urea, creatinine and potassium
- Monitor for generalised oedema. Weigh if possible

Assess for a reduction in gut perfusion due to the balloon occluding the mesenteries:
- Is enteral feeding potentiating a hypoxic gut?
- Monitor girth 2–4 hourly
- Monitor for clinical features of a distended abdomen, shiny and grey in appearance, bloody stools, abdominal pain/tenderness, increasing nasogastric losses, reduced or absent bowel sounds and report promptly
- Check x-ray daily to assess the balloon position and potential migration

Monitor for the development of limb ischaemia and poor tissue perfusion:
- Palpate right and left popliteal and pedal pulses hourly
- Palpate left radial pulse hourly to ensure that the balloon tip is below the left subclavian artery and not in the left subclavian artery or ascending aorta
- Assess the colour, temperature, perfusion and capillary refill of limbs hourly and report immediately if any changes documented
- Avoid leg flexion if the balloon is sited in the femoral artery

Prevention, detection and management of thromboembolic formation:
- Administer prescribed anticoagulants
- Monitor effectiveness by assessing ACT hourly until stability of anticoagulation achieved. Aim for an ACT of 120–180 seconds
- Perform full clotting screens 6 hourly. Aim for a partial prothrombin time twice normal

(contd)

Table 11.18 (contd)

- Never allow the balloon to lie idle for periods longer than 20–30 minutes as clots will develop on the surface of the balloon which when activated again will embolise into major organs causing severe problems for the already critically ill child
- Monitor and assess the patient for the development of thromboembolic episodes

Detection and management of haemorrhage:
- Units of blood must always be available whilst the patient is on a balloon pump should the aorta rupture or anticoagulation cause a bleed
- Monitor surgical sites, nasogastric losses, endotracheal losses, stools, urine and other areas for signs of bleeding and report promptly

Management of thrombocytopenia due to the mechanical action of counterpulsation which destroys the platelets:
- Monitor platelet levels daily
- Administer prescribed platelets should the level be low and bleeding occur

Management of infection due to invasive procedure:
- Administer prophylactic antibiotics
- Screen for infection at regular intervals and on suspicion of the development of clinical features associated with infection — raised white cell count, raised C-reactive protein, positive blood cultures, thrombocytopenia, pyrexia, tachycardia, cooling peripheries, hypotension and redness, tenderness, oozing around operative sites

Management of mechanical problems:
- Loss of triggering — check the ECG lead placement and arterial line patency
- Balloon leak — assess for loss of augmentation and potential gas emboli
- Balloon malposition — check x-ray daily to ascertain position, left radial pulse

---

Chapter 12
Haematological and
neurological management

Haematological management

Haematological management encompasses the following issues.

Neonatal coagulation

As a significant proportion of newly diagnosed patients with congenital heart disease are in the neonatal period, it is important to consider that due to a deficiency of clotting factors II, VII, IX, X, neonates are at risk from haemorrhagic disease of the newborn[38]. This disease normally occurs within 48–72 hours post birth so it is imperative that vitamin K is administered shortly after birth as it is necessary for the production of clotting factors.

Key management issues

The key management issues for a neonate with a coagulopathy are shown in Table 12.1.

Disseminated intravascular coagulation

The seriously ill neonate, infant or child having undergone a prolonged period of hypoperfusion and thus tissue injury due to hypoxia, can activate a coagulation mechanism which causes diffuse clotting and profound haemorrhage[10, 38, 333]. This may further develop down the systemic inflammatory response pathway potentiating multi-system organ failure. This mechanism is known as disseminated intravascular coagulation

Table 12.1 Assessment and management of potential problems in a neonate with a coagulopathy

Establish if/when the neonate has had vitamin K and whether it was oral or intravenous

Perform a baseline clotting to assess for the presence of a coagulopathy:
- Prothrombin time — This measures the activity of the extrinsic and common pathways of the clotting cascade and will assess for abnormalities of factors V, VII, X[38, 332]
- Activated partial prothrombin time — This measures the activity of the intrinsic and common pathways of the clotting cascade and will assess for abnormalities of all factors except VII, XIII[38, 332]
- Reptilase time — Although this measures the same factors as the prothrombin time, it is unresponsive to heparin. Therefore, if there is an abnormal prothrombin time but the reptilase time is normal, the coagulopathy is likely to be due to heparin[38, 332]

Perform a baseline full blood count to analyse the haemoglobin, haematocrit, platelets, white cell and differential

Correct presenting coagulopathy with prescribed FFP, cryoprecipitate, platelets and vitamin K (see later in this section for the appropriate choice of replacement)

(DIC) which is a secondary acquired coagulopathy describing a systemic imbalance of coagulation and results in a prolonged activation of both the clotting mechanism and fibrinolytic system[10, 332, 333]. DIC presents with a prolonged prothrombin time, activated partial prothrombin time and reptilase time, indicative of the consumption of intrinsic coagulation factors, and a low fibrinogen and platelet count.

Features indicative of plasmin generation (haemorrhage), include purpura, petechiae and haemorrhage into major organs (the head, liver, kidneys, lungs, skeletal system, and gastrointestinal tract). Additionally features pertaining to thrombin generation (thrombosis) occur in major organs and present as a cerebral vascular accident, pulmonary embolus, right ventricular thrombosis or peripheral thrombosis causing gangrene.

Other signs of DIC include pyrexia, acidosis, proteinuria, hypoxia, joint pain, thrombocytopenia, cytokinin and kinin generation manifested in the form of shock, and oedema formation[334].

Key management issues

Disseminated intravascular coagulopathy is potentially fatal and the main aim is to treat its effects on the body and support coagulation. See Table 12.2.

Table 12.2 Assessment and management of potential problems in a child with DIC

Management of the underlying condition — sepsis, low cardiac output, acidosis

Assessment and management of the plasmin generation (haemorrhage):
- Assess and observe major organs for haemorrhage:
  1. Brain — headaches, fitting, loss of consciousness, confusion, irritability
  2. Kidneys — haematuria, anuria, oliguria, increasing urea and creatinine
  3. Lungs — pulmonary haemorrhage
  4. Gastrointestinal — gum bleeding, coffee ground aspirate, malaena, fresh blood
  5. Liver — hepatomegaly, raised liver function tests
  6. Skeletal — joint pain
  7. Skin — petechiae, bruising, oozing of blood from orifices, wounds or puncture sites. Avoid IM injections, adhesive dressings, razor blades[333]
- Assess puncture sites, wounds, orifices for bleeding which will start to ooze[333]
- Regular clotting profiles, D-Dimer assay (D-Dimer is formed when plasmin digests fibrin[333]) and a full blood count to evaluate the disease process
- Administration of blood products to manage the coagulopathy
  1. Fresh frozen plasma to replace the consumed clotting factors
  2. Platelets to replace the consumed platelets
  3. Cryoprecipitate to raise the fibrinogen levels
  4. Vitamin K for the production of clotting factors
  5. Blood transfusion if anaemic

Assessment and management of the thrombin generation (thrombosis):
- Administer prescribed heparin to prevent the formation of microemboli, although its use in purpura fulminans is doubtful[333, 335]
- Assess and observe major organs for thrombosis formation:
  1. Brain — cerebral vascular accident, fitting, loss of consciousness
  2. Kidneys — vessel thrombosis, oliguria to anuria[333], raised creatinine and urea
  3. Lungs — pulmonary embolus with increasing respiratory support
  4. Peripheries/skin — purpura fulminans with gangrene

Postoperative bleeding

Mediastinal and pleural bleeding plus bleeding from puncture sites must be assessed closely and prolonged bleeding treated aggressively[172]. The aim of management is to prevent the bleeding from getting worse which will directly affect haemodynamics, the circulating volume, tissue perfusion, haematocrit, oxygen carrying capacity and coagulation.

Blood loss is assessed by volume/kg/hour. Acceptable losses are usually 3ml/kg/hour for 3 hours or 5 ml/kg/hour for the first hour. Blood loss amounting to 5–10 ml/kg/hour must be reported to the medical staff and appropriate treatment given. Once approaching 10 ml/kg/hour the decision to reopen the chest is normally made.

Risk factors predisposing to bleeding

- The chronically cyanosed patient who will have changes to the bone marrow and hence associated thrombocytopenia.
- Re-operation due to the previous formation of fibrous tissue and adhesions which are very vascular.
- Prolonged cardiopulmonary bypass causing abnormal platelet aggregation, activation[172] and depletion of 30–60% of clotting factors[336].
- Pre-existing coagulopathy (e.g., congenital, haemorrhagic disease of the newborn, DIC, idiopathic, drug-induced e.g., warfarin, aspirin, heparin).

Key management issues

The key management issues for a patient who is bleeding are shown in Table 12.3.

Table 12.3 Assessment and management of potential problems in a patient who is bleeding

---

Assessment of blood loss:
- Measure amount at quarter hourly intervals until there is evidence that the bleeding is slowing down. Calculate loss/kg/hour
- Observe blood pressure, heart rate, central venous pressure, left atrial pressure, urine output and peripheral perfusion. If low, this may be indicative of hypovolaemia which must be reported promptly and the appropriate replacement given

Establish the cause:
- Perform clotting profiles and full blood counts at regular intervals
- Lack of coagulation factors – prolonged prothrombin and activated partial prothrombin times. Administer prescribed fresh frozen plasma and vitamin K
- Thrombocytopenia – administer prescribed platelets
- Hypofibrinaemia – administer prescribed cryoprecipitate
- Anaemia (haematocrit less than 0.35) – administer prescribed packed cells (blood)
- Inadequate filling pressures (left atrial or central venous pressures). Administer blood or plasma depending on the patient's haematocrit — less than 0.35 give blood, above 0.35 give plasma
- Effects of heparin — administer prescribed protamine 1 mg/kg/hour over 10 minutes

Maintain chest drain patency — see later in this chapter

Prevention of hypertension by adequate analgesia, sedation and vasodilation

Consider normothermia if the patient does not need to be cooled to reduce metabolic demands and oxygen consumption. Hypothermia causes suppression of the coagulation mechanism [172]

Consider increasing the positive end expiratory pressure as it can compress mediastinal blood vessels by reducing the venous return. However, this could be dangerous if the patient is haemodynamically unstable as it may reduce cardiac output and cause hypotension in the presence of hypovolaemia [172]

Colloid transfusion

Key management issues

The management issues for a patient undergoing colloid transfusion are shown in Table 12.4

Table 12.4 Assessment and management of potential problems in a patient undergoing colloid transfusion

Each unit of colloid must be checked by two members of staff as per hospital policy

Neonatal blood should be CMV negative and leukocyte depleted. Di George patients must have irradiated blood products. Other infectious risks include hepatitis, CMV, AIDS and malaria

- Blood must be filtered and administered through the appropriate blood giving set (170–200 mesh filter). This removes the microaggregates and leukocytes which develop in processed blood
- Platelets must be administered via a platelet giving set, having only been removed from the agitator immediately prior to use
- FFP must be filtered through a blood giving set (170–200 mesh filter)
- Cryoprecipitate must be defrosted and administered through a blood giving set (170–200 mesh filter)

The patient must be monitored for signs of transfusion reaction:
- Vital signs must be taken before commencement of the transfusion to serve as a base-line and then every 15 minutes for the first hour of the transfusion. Thereafter, every hour of the remaining transfusion should be adequate
- A haemolytic reaction due to incompatible blood would cause pyrexia, shivering, vomiting, flank pain, headache, haematuria, purpuric rash and shock. The nurse should stop the transfusion immediately, call for medical assistance and keep the transfusion bag to recheck the donor against the recipient
- A circulatory overload may occur if the transfusion is administered too quickly or too much is given. The patient would present with dyspnoea, pulmonary oedema and cough. The nurse should ensure that the transfusion is given by a syringe or infusion pump to prevent accidental over-transfusion although care must be taken when programming the pump. The amount of prescribed colloid should not be excessive for the patient's weight and haemoglobin — see later in this section. Whilst administering it, the blood pressure and central venous and left atrial pressures, if present, must be observed
- A risk of allergic reaction increases with repeated transfusions even over several years due to the patient forming antibodies. Wheezing, flushing, urticaria and anaphylactic shock can occur. The nurse should stop the transfusion, call for medical assistance and maintain the patient's airway if compromised. Prescribed antihistamines, epinephrine and steroids may be given

When large amounts of blood are transfused, serum ionised calcium must be monitored as it will become depleted due to the citrate anticoagulant binding with the calcium. 1 ml of IV calcium gluconate 10% can be given with every 100 ml of blood transfused. Serum potassium must additionally be monitored should large transfusions be given as processed blood contains large amounts of potassium

Consider the use of furosemide half way through the transfusion

Fresh blood products

See Table 12.5 for fresh blood products and their uses.

Table 12.5 Fresh blood products and their uses

Type	Products and uses
Blood	**Packed cells** • Used to increase the haematocrit by 70% • Have no clotting factors • Weight (kg) x 3 x desired rise in haemoglobin = ml of packed cells required or 15 ml/kg • Cross match **Whole blood** • Rarely used as the extra volume of blood that has to be given only contains a few clotting factors which is not advantageous to cardiac patients • Weight (kg) x 6 x desired rise in haemoglobin = ml of whole blood required or 20 ml/kg • Cross match **Saline adenine glucose and mannitol (SAGM) blood** • This is a solution added to red cells used to replace the plasma removed from the whole blood • Weight (kg) x 6 x desired rise in haemoglobin = ml SAGM required or 20 ml/kg • Cross match
Plasma	**Fresh frozen plasma** • Contains all clotting factors • Used for patients with a coagulopathy or if bleeding is profuse (above 5 ml/kg/hour) and haematocrit above 0.35 • Group and save wherever possible. Otherwise AB negative is the universal donor in emergencies • 10–15 ml/kg will raise the coagulation factor by 20%
Cryoprecipitate	• Only indicated if the fibrinogen level is low • Group and save • One bag/6 kg body weight will raise the fibrinogen level by 1 g/l
Platelets	• Administered in the presence of low platelets (less than 30,000/microlitre) and bleeding • One unit/5 kg body weight raises the platelet count by $50 \times 10^9/l$ • Group and save • Short duration of effectiveness. If planning a surgical intervention in the presence of thrombocytopenia, platelets should be administered one hour before • Must be agitated constantly, until transfused

Helen Hill, PICU and Jenny Minards, Haematology Dept. Royal Liverpool Children's NHS Trust, (adapted with permission)

Chest drain management

Numerous chest drain systems are available but all ultimately have the same function of removing air or fluid from the pleural space or mediastinum.

The drain maintains a negative pressure which must be lower than that of the pleural space. A pressure gradient must therefore be created enabling movement of the air or fluid from an area of high pressure to one of lower pressure, that is from the pleural or mediastinal space to the chest drain bottle. To achieve this, the distal end of the chest drain is placed beneath 2 cm of water creating a water seal thus enabling the desired movement of air or fluid[10].

Key management issues

The key management issues for a patient with a chest drain are shown in Table 12.6.

Table 12.6 Assessment and management of potential problems in a child with a chest drain

Maintain patency of the chest drain:
- The patient should be assessed for signs of respiratory distress
- The chest drain must be attached to low grade suction system of 5 kPa
- All connections must be secure. The chest drain at the bottle end is beneath the water level. Two clamps and a roller should be close to hand should disconnection occur
- The chest drain at the bottle end must be beneath a predetermined water level
- Gentle milking of the drains at quarter hourly intervals immediately postoperatively or until the drainage is less than 3 ml/kg/hour. Note that vigorous milking can generate pressures of up to –300 cm/water in the mediastinum and thus increase bleeding and discomfort for the patient [172]. The characteristics of the drainage should be assessed
- Drains should have the slack taken off them and not be allowed to dangle straight off the bed. They should be taped to the chest wall
- Ensure that the bottles are kept lower than the level of the chest when moving the patient to prevent a siphoning effect
- In the presence of a pleural drain a chest x-ray is performed to assess the lung expansion
- Chest drains should not be clamped for prolonged periods

Assess for complications of drain insertion:
- Blocked or decreasing mediastinal drainage — if early in the postoperative period, this could be one of the initial causes of cardiac tamponade. Therefore, milk gently and call for surgical advice. However, it could be a sign that the patient is getting better!
- Disconnected pleural drains — a pneumothorax may occur if the patient is not receiving positive pressure ventilation. Connect up the drain immediately and observe the patient's oxygen saturation, and vital signs. Ask for immediate medical assessment. A chest x-ray is indicated
- Infection — maintain strict aseptic technique upon handling or changing the drains. Send a sample of fluid for culture and sensitivity should infection be suspected

(contd)

Table 12.6 (contd)

- Pain — adequate intravenous opiate analgesia, paracetamol and oral non-steroidal anti-inflammatory analgesia or codeine phosphate must be given as pain from the drains can cause chest wall splinting, subsequent shallow breathing and a chest infection with a need for increased respiratory support
- Turbulent bubbling — usually represents a leak in the system so check all connections. However, it can occur in patients whose chest is open or in the presence of a bronchopleural fistula
- Increase in drainage — may represent chylothorax, pleural effusions, haemorrhage from the removal of direct left atrial or pulmonary artery catheters

Chest drain removal:
- The losses should amount to less than 3 ml/kg/day before removal is indicated [38]
- The patient must have adequate sedation and analgesia
- Remove the suction
- Ideally, the patient should be asked to inspire deeply to maintain a positive intrapleural pressure but this is hard to achieve in paediatrics for obvious reasons
- The drain is removed swiftly
- A purse string suture is secured
- A clean dressing is applied
- A chest x-ray is performed to assess for the formation of pneumothorax or pneumo-mediastinum during removal

Neurological management

A thorough examination should be made on admission to provide a baseline with which to gauge potential neurological deterioration. This may occur postoperatively, following acute hypoxic periods in the chronically cyanosed, or after thrombolytic episodes.

Cerebral vascular accident (CVA)

Congenital heart disease is responsible for up to 30% of childhood cerebral vascular accidents (CVA) and is normally associated with a thromboembolic event from either an intracardiac source, the passage of venous emboli into the cerebral circulation or venous stasis[307].

Causes of CVA

- Chronic hypoxia and polycythaemia: In developed countries the risk of CVA from chronic hypoxia and polycythaemia has reduced significantly due to earlier surgical intervention[308].
- Particulate emboli: This can be from several sources, the most common being intraoperatively whilst on cardiopulmonary bypass. The use of membrane oxygenators reduces the risk of particulate emboli as

opposed to bubble oxygenators[309]. The causes of particulate emboli are:
1. The patient's own platelets and leukocytes due to a massive stress response.
2. Particles in the oxygenator which occur during the manufacturing process.
3. Debris from blood transfusion or intravenous infusions[220].
4. Septic emboli from bacterial endocarditis.
- Air emboli: Air may enter the systemic circulation in a variety of ways. For example, during IV therapy in patients with a right to left shunt; when coughing, which causes a rise in intrathoracic pressure in patients with a left to right shunt; air left in the heart during open heart surgery; bubble oxygenators.
- Postoperative emboli can result from the operative insertion of synthetic materials or stasis of blood flow from a Blalock–Taussig shunt with a low blood pressure and elevated central venous pressures[307].

Signs and symptoms

- Fitting.
- Impaired level of consciousness.
- Hemiplegia.
- Language or visual impairment.

Key management issues

The key management issues for a patient with a CVA are shown in Table 12.7.

Table 12.7 Assessment and management of potential problems in a child with a CVA

Preventative measures can be taken to minimise the risk of developing a CVA:
- Use of membrane oxygenators during cardiopulmonary bypass
- Identification of the child at increased risk — polycythaemia, hypoxia, right to left shunts, bacterial endocarditis, the child who has had a prosthetic valve replacement and increased right atrial pressure
- Use of intravenous filters to remove air and debris
- Prophylactic anticoagulation in the high risk child

Management after a CVA has occurred:
- Assess and observe the patient for further deterioration. Perform neurological observations — this may not be possible in the paralysed and sedated child. Reflexes and posturing must be documented
- The safety of the child must be maintained whilst fitting

(contd)

Table 12.7 (contd)

- Oxygenation and cerebral perfusion is maintained by:
  1. Paralysing and heavily sedating the child
  2. Hyperventilating the child to reduce pCO_2, to increase cerebral perfusion — caution is needed in babies with hypoplastic left heart syndrome
  3. Diuretics are administered to reduce cerebral oedema
  4. Fluids are restricted
  5. The head of the bed is elevated by 30°
  6. The head is kept in a midline position
- A CT scan is performed as soon as the child is stable to assess the extent of the bleed/clot
- Rehabilitative measures should be employed sooner rather than later. The physiotherapist can teach staff and parents about correct posturing
- Once the child has regained consciousness, staff must inform the child of the problem and what is being done to help him or her recover from the CVA. Some children will have experienced extensive brain damage from which they may not recover completely

Intraventricular haemorrhage

Intraventricular haemorrhage (IVH) is usually associated with prematurity but can occur in approximately 11% of neonates having sustained haemodynamic instability and hypoperfusion of the brain[310]. Coagulopathy in conjunction with cardiopulmonary bypass may additionally increase the risk[307].

Neonates presenting with haemodynamic instability, coagulopathy or who are of low birth weight (less than 1500 g) must all be scanned for potential IVH by cranial ultrasound[307]. Children with congenital heart lesions who are particularly at risk from developing IVH include those with hypoplastic left heart syndrome[311], and coarctation of the aorta with its associated hypertension[312].

Grades of IVH[313]

- 0 No bleed.
- 1 Germinal layer.
- 2 Intraventricular haemorrhage.
- 3 Intraventricular haemorrhage with distension of the ventricular system.
- 4 Intraventricular haemorrhage with parenchymal bleeding, that is intracerebral.

Signs and symptoms

- Apnoea.
- Fitting.
- Tense bulging fontanelle, with separated sutures.
- Anaemia.
- Low packed cell volume.
- Pale.
- Acidosis.
- Later, increasing head circumference with the development of hydrocephalus in severe cases.

Types 1, 2 and 3 may not be symptomatic, however type 4 can render the baby very ill, with the prospect of severe handicap if he or she survives.

Key management issues

The key management issues for a patient with IVH are shown in Table 12.8.

Table 12.8 Assessment and management of potential problems in a baby with IVH

Management of the apnoea and acidosis:
- The baby should be ventilated, sedated and paralysed
- The acidosis should be corrected with intravenous sodium bicarbonate or equivalent (THAM)

Management of the anaemia:
- The baby must be transfused as the haemoglobin level may have fallen to around 7–9 g/l. This should help in the correction of acidosis

Management of fitting: See later in this section

Preventative measures include:
- Minimal handling, co-ordinating cares
- Prevention of raised intracranial pressure (suctioning, coughing and hypoxia)
- Loud noises — avoid banging bins/doors, tapping on incubators

---

Cerebral abscess

Cerebral abscess presenting in the presence of a congenital heart defect occurs due to the mobilisation of septic emboli in the child with a right to left shunt or chronic hypoxia and polycythaemia (however, this does not normally present in developed countries where surgical intervention takes place before the chronic effects of cyanosis occur).

Signs and symptoms

- Vomiting.
- Lethargy.
- Pyrexia.
- Headache.
- Fitting.
- Visual disturbances.
- Hemiplegia.

Diagnosis

The diagnosis is confirmed by CT scan.

Key management issues

The patient is managed with antibiotic therapy, with or without surgical drainage.

Fitting

The most common neurological feature post cardiac surgery is fitting[314]. One study found that 26% of babies fitted following deep hypothermic circulatory arrest and yet only 11% of the babies fitting were detected by staff[314].

Causes of fitting

- Deep hypothermic circulatory arrest/post pump.
- Electrolyte imbalances.
- Temperature changes.
- CVA (thromboembolic episodes).
- Sepsis (brain abscess, generalised sepsis).
- Hypoxia.

Key management issues

The key management issues for a patient who is fitting are shown in Table 12.9.

Table 12.9 Assessment and management of potential problems in a child who is fitting

---

Assess and observe the child for fits:
• This may be difficult to establish in the paralysed/sedated child

Management of the child who is fitting:
• Place child on his or her side
• Describe what is observed, in the order that it occurs and for how long
• Observe
    1. Eyes – deviating upwards, to the opposite side?
    2. Muscle contraction — tonic (muscles contracted/rigid for a time), clonic (muscles contract and relax rhythmically)
    3. Consciousness altered, is patient lucid?
    4. Colour changes — cyanosed, red, pale?
    5. Vital signs change — BP, heart rate, SaO$_2$, respiration
• Establish the cause if possible and treat
• Comfort and reassure the child and parents as fitting can be very distressing for the parents

Drug management:
• Administer prescribed anticonvulsants. Usually to stop the fit a benzodiazepine such as diazepam is prescribed, followed by regular phenobarbitone, adding phenytoin once phenobarbitone levels are therapeutic

---

Pain

What is pain? McCaffery[315] describes pain as "Whatever the experiencing person says it is, existing whenever he says it does". However, in a non-verbal intensive care patient or in a patient too young to verbalise, the nurse has to be the patient's advocate, assessing pain objectively and effectively, communicating findings to other members of the health care team and formulating an appropriate treatment plan[316].

Unfortunately, as nurses do not know what patients are experiencing, they can only imagine, usually using their own prior experience of pain. Pain can therefore be described as an elusive concept as it is difficult to define, difficult to measure and the level of suffering caused by the pain varies from individual to individual.

This section is certainly not an exhaustive guide to pain assessment and management as there are numerous texts for that purpose, rather an introduction to a few aspects that cardiac staff should consider when nursing a child in pain.

Assessment of pain related to age and cognitive development

The assessment of pain in children has come a long way over the past 20 years, although it will always be a subjective phenomenon. One area where little progress has been made is in the ventilated, sedated/paralysed patient. As most children having cardiac surgery will undergo a period of ventilation and sedation/paralysis, it is a disturbing concept to know staff are not in a position to assess with accuracy their patient's level of pain. Parents are often very perceptive as to whether or not their child is comfortable so they may be invaluable in helping to assess their child's level of pain[317].

The child's perception of pain varies according to his or her age and level of cognitive development.

Pain in the baby or infant

The infant in pain will exhibit pain behaviour which may be assessed by staff aware of the measurable parameters an infant will display.

Behavioural cues

- Body movement: Is the baby settled or restless (fussing, squirming, fisting) or is body tension present (rigidity, trembling, drawing knees up, withdrawing from surroundings)?
- Facial expression: Is the baby's face relaxed, neutral, peaceful or grimacing (frowning, brow bulge, facial twitch) or is there a severe grimace (eye squeeze, wide open mouth, taut tongue) [22, 318–321]?
- Crying: Is the baby crying? Crying gently (moaning) or screaming (long duration with tears)?

Physiological cues

- Mild pain: Heart rate, blood pressure, respiratory rate and oxygen saturations show approximately 10% difference from the baseline.
- Severe pain: Heart rate, blood pressure, respiratory rate and oxygen saturations show approximately 20% difference from the baseline. Bradycardia is common and there is palmar sweating.
- Other physiological changes include increased secretions of cortisol, glucose, endorphins, and cool, pale, mottled, dusky and sweaty skin[321–323].

There are no studies available discussing how infants' understanding of pain relates to their illness or injury as, clearly, they are unable to verbalise[11]. From the age of 8 months, separation anxiety (the baby from his or her parents) makes procedural pain worse[11].

Pain in the toddler

Toddlers' reaction to pain is complicated by variables such as their limited understanding and capability of verbalising their pain, the strange environment and procedures, loss of control and autonomy, their emotional reaction being greater than in infants, and separation anxiety being more marked[11, 324]. Additional behavioural cues include biting, kicking, running away, restlessness, irritability, altered position (fetal) and guarding[317]. These reactions are in response not only to pain but also to the perceived pain associated with the procedure or the event about to take place[11].

Toddlers are only able to communicate their pain in a limited fashion, vaguely pointing to an area where the pain is thought to be. For this reason, abstract pain assessment tools are not useable in this age group but a concept such as facial pain scales can be used around 3 years of age. The "Oucher" facial pain tool is the most recognised one and consists of a series of faces starting with a smiling face and progressing to a sad, very upset, crying face. The child points to the face that resembles how he or she feels when in pain[325].

Pre-school age children

Pre-schoolers' pain is seen as a physical experience, one in which they hold someone responsible for the pain. They may also attribute pain as a form of punishment for something they have done[326]. Their limited understanding makes it difficult for them to understand why their heart "has to be fixed". Words such as "small scratch", "take out", "remove" and so on may be totally misunderstood.

Behavioural reactions to pain

Behavioural reactions usually fall into three categories[11].

- Aggression: Push the person away.
- Verbal expression: "I hate you", "Go away", "I'll be good if…".
- Dependency: "Help me", clinginess.

An example of a pain assessment tool useful in this age group is the Eland Colour Tool whereby the child is given different coloured crayons and is instructed to pick a colour which depicts the worst pain imaginable, choosing different colours to represent no pain at all. The child then colours in a body chart with the colour they find appropriate for their intensity of pain, around the area where the pain is.

School age children

School age children know their body parts, relating them to the pain they are experiencing which can lead to the fear of mutilation and death[326]. Later abilities include the concepts of "if" this happens, "then" ____, for example, "if" your appendix is taken out, "then" you will feel much better.

Behaviourally, these children exhibit signs of anxiety. Therefore factual explanations may help reduce their anxiety and hopefully some of their pain. They are not very often aggressive but will clench their fists and grit their teeth in response to pain. They will begin to understand abstract phenomena, for example, numeric pain assessment tools which start at 0, being representative of no pain, to 10, the worse pain imaginable. Professionals can utilise behavioural check-lists, to assess patients' pain[327].

Adolescents

Adolescents fear mutilation, loss of privacy, loss of dignity and loss of control. They are likely to remain very controlled throughout a painful procedure fearing loss of control and may even deny having pain in an attempt to maintain control even further. Self-reporting tools are excellent for this age group, for example, the visual analogue numerical tool, and pain questionnaires[328].

Ventilated, sedated/paralysed patients

For the ventilated, sedated/paralysed child on intensive care, pain assessment will have to be based on an assessment tool similar to that for a neonate utilising behavioural and physiological cues. A modified Children's Hospital of Eastern Ontario Pain Scale (CHEOPS)[328] can be useful in this patient population, in addition to other scales mentioned previously, but to date there is no one tool that assesses this group of patients with any accuracy.

It must be remembered however, that due to the sedation and possible paralysing agent, the child may only exhibit some of the cues associated with pain. Equally, physiological cues may be responsible for other variables, namely inotropic use, inadequate sedation, haemorrhage, respiratory distress and so on.

Management of pain

Ideally, pain management should be preventative, being assessed and evaluated frequently. However, this is not always possible so once the pain intensity has been assessed, the most appropriate combined interventions should be given to the patient. Pain management can be divided into pharmacological and non-pharmacological management.

Pharmacological management of pain

Numerous preparations are available for pain management from paracetamol to morphine, administered in a myriad of ways.

Opiate preparations

Opiate preparations are chosen especially in the postoperative period following cardiac surgery. Contrary to many people's beliefs, a thoracotomy is much more painful than a sternotomy, yet it is only in recent years that patients undergoing a thoracotomy have been administered opiate analgesia and paravertebral blocks.

The choice of preparation is usually the consultant's preference although the pain service can provide much advice. Other variables must also be taken into consideration such as the use of fentanyl in neonates with hyper-reactive pulmonary vasculature who benefit from a preparation which dulls the stress response of the vasculature, minimising episodes of pulmonary hypertension and imbalances between the pulmonary and systemic vascular resistance.

The administration of opiates is usually intravenously in this patient population and is of most benefit when a bolus is given, followed by a continuous infusion. Intermittent, isolated boluses are not conducive to the prevention or titration of pain for maximum comfort[11].

Non-steroidal anti-inflammatory drugs (NSAIDs)

NSAIDs, for example diclofenac and ibuprofen, can help bridge the gap between weaning the opiate and starting paracetamol. NSAIDs are particularly useful in bony, muscular pain where there is usually much inflammation. However, they have to be used with caution in critically ill patients as they are a gastric irritant. They must be given with milk feeds so as to avoid a gastric bleed. Additionally, they must be used with caution in patients who are anticoagulated because of the risk of bleeding.

Paracetamol

Paracetamol is excellent for mild pain or mild to moderate pain in conjunction with an NSAID or even an opiate if the pain is still not relieved. Again it must be given regularly, not ad hoc, so as to maximise its effects.

Route of administration

- Orally/nasogastrically: This is acceptable unless the pain is severe or there is a history of gastrointestinal bleed or gastrointestinal surgery and the patient is nil by mouth.
- Rectally: This is acceptable unless the child is embarrassed by the procedure or there is evidence of necrotising enterocolitis.
- Topically: Local anaesthetic creams to anaesthetise the skin prior to venepuncture are most important. This is easily forgotten on the intensive care unit but also depends on how urgent the need for venous access is.
- Intravenously: This is the usual route postoperatively with a continual infusion being the one of choice.
- Intramuscularly: This route is usually "banned" from paediatrics as it is very painful and alternative routes can be used. Additionally, in the critically ill child, altered tissue perfusion can cause unpredictable drug absorption[10]. A child on anticoagulants must not have IM injections as a large haematoma will develop.
- Regional: Paravertebral blocks in thoracotomy patients as small as 3 kg have been used successfully with superb results[329].
- Entonox: This is being used with growing popularity in patients having chest drains removed who are above 4–5 years of age. At this age children are capable of following instructions on how to use the equipment.
- Patient controlled analgesia: A continuous opiate infusion can be given with an additional bolus administered by the patient should breakthrough pain occur. There is no danger of overdosing as there is a lock-out period and dose limits are set for the individual patient according to his or her weight[10].

Non-pharmacological management of pain

The child must be adequately prepared for surgery, painful procedures and events to ensure co-operation and to minimise pain. Parents should be present for painful procedures to comfort and reassure their child.

- Guided imagery: Children are asked to think of something, a place, etc. which gives them great pleasure and is non-threatening. They then must describe the place in detail, concentrating only on the pleasurable experience when the painful procedure is being done[11].
- Diversional therapy: Play in all its forms can be used – music, computers, creative play (drama, painting, crayoning, Play-doh), Lego, videos, television and so on. Equally, play can be used as a tool for the child to act out his or her fears and worries or as a teaching aid for procedures and events[10].
- Relaxation therapy: This can be used in young infants by cuddling, stroking and gentle rocking, whilst talking to them softly. Older children can be placed in a comfortable position and encouraged to breathe deeply, tensing and subsequently relaxing areas of the body.
- TENS: Transcutaneous electrical nerve stimulation is where electrical waves are delivered via electrodes to the skin, stimulating endorphin release[329].
- Touch: Normal, non-threatening touch is very important, especially in critically ill children or children who are chronically ill and requiring numerous painful procedures.
- Hypnosis: Hypnosis has been used for several years in patients who fear dental pain and in children with cancer[330, 331]. It could perhaps also be used in children undergoing painful cardiac procedures such as chest drain removal or insertion, needle aspirations and so on.
- Minimising parental separation: This is important for all age groups, even for independent adolescents who must be given the option of whether or not they want their parents present.

Chapter 13
Renal, fluid and electrolyte management and gastrointestinal management

Fluid management in the postoperative cardiac patient

Crystalloid fluid

The aim of crystalloid fluid management post open heart surgery is to restrict input. This is necessary because of the haemodilution which occurs whilst on cardiopulmonary bypass[337] and the stress of surgery causing increased secretion of anti-diuretic hormone and the associated water and sodium retention[10, 337]. For details of fluid management after open heart surgery see Table 13.1.

Table 13.1 Fluid management post open heart surgery

Day of surgery	1 ml/kg/hour	24 ml/kg/day
Day 1 postoperative	2 ml/kg/hour	48 ml/kg/day
Day 2 postoperative	3 ml/kg/hour	72 ml/kg/day
Day 3 postoperative	4 ml/kg/hour	96 ml/kg/day

Ten per cent dextrose is used as maintenance fluid for neonates due to the increased metabolic demand and to maintain blood glucose. The neonate must be assessed for the development of hyperglycaemia. Infants and children usually only require 5% dextrose.

Fluid management following closed heart surgery is not as restrictive as the patient has not had to endure the effects of cardiopulmonary bypass and the associated stress response. The patient usually starts on double the regime of open heart surgery patients, that is, 2 ml/kg/hour, increasing to 4 ml/kg/hour on day 1.

Colloid management

Although the open heart surgery patient is usually totally body fluid over-loaded, he or she is often intravascularly depleted[38]. The desired filling pressures have to be communicated to the nursing staff so appropriate colloid replacement can be given. Additionally, once the patient starts to warm postoperatively, vasodilation may predispose to extra boluses of colloid, usually requiring 5–10 ml/kg. For further colloid management see the section on haematological management.

Electrolyte management

Potassium

Normal values

Normal values for potassium are 3.5–5 mmol/l.

Functions

- Major intracellular electrolyte.
- Increases myocardial contractility.
- Increases skeletal and smooth muscle contractility.
- Helps in the regulation of acid–base balance.
- Increases neuromuscular transmission.

Hypokalaemia

Causes of hypokalaemia include:

- Diuretics.
- Vomiting.
- Inadequate intake.
- Steroid therapy.
- Alkalosis.
- Prolonged cardiopulmonary bypass.
- Insulin which causes the movement of potassium from intravascular to intracellular compartments.

Clinical features:

- Atrial and ventricular ectopics, weak pulses, tachycardia.
- Muscle weakness.
- Flaccid paralysis.
- Fatigue.
- Anorexia.
- Vomiting, reduced peristalsis.
- Hypotension.

Treatment:

- Treat the cause.
- IV replacement therapy.
- Normal requirements 2–4 mmol/kg/day.
- Potassium less than 2.5 mmol/l administer 20 mmol potassium in 40 ml sodium chloride at a maximum rate of 0.5 ml/kg/hour via a central line only. The line must not be flushed. Check potassium levels 1–2 hourly.
- Potassium 2.5–3.5 mmol/l, administer 10 mmol potassium in 100 ml maintenance fluid to run at 1–3 ml/kg/hour.
- Potassium 3.5–5 mmol/l, administer 5 mmol potassium in 100 ml maintenance fluid to run at 1–3 ml/kg/hour.
- Oral supplements can be given if tolerating enteral feeds.
- Administer potassium sparing diuretics.

Hyperkalaemia

Causes of hyperkalaemia include:

- Low cardiac output.
- Renal failure — oliguria/anuria.
- Acidosis.
- Haemolysis/tissue necrosis.
- Cardioplegia.
- Massive blood transfusions.
- Potassium infusions.
- Potassium sparing diuretics.

Clinical features:

- Arrhythmias, asystole, prolonged P–R interval, ST depression, tall T waves, widening QRS, flat P waves.

- Muscle weakness.
- Twitching.

Treatment:

- Frequent potassium monitoring.
- IV sodium bicarbonate if acidotic (1 mmol/kg) to move potassium from intravascular to intracellular compartments.
- Calcium resonium orally (1 g/kg in four divided doses/day).
- Insulin and glucose (0.1 units/kg Actrapid).
- Diuretics.
- Stop potassium additives.
- Maximise cardiac ouput.
- Dialysis/haemofiltration.

Sodium

Normal values

Normal values for sodium are 135–145 mmol/l.

Functions

- Controls water excretion and retention intra- and extracellularly.
- Increases neuromuscular transmission.
- Extracellular osmolarity regulator.
- Maintains acid–base balance.

Hyponatraemia

Causes of hyponatraemia include:

- Inadequate intake.
- Gastrointestinal losses.
- Sweating.
- Fever.
- Diuretics.

Clinical features:

- Weakness.
- Dizziness.
- Muscle twitching.
- Cramps.

- Nausea.
- Diarrhoea.
- Oliguria.
- Hypotension.

Treatment:

- Fluid restriction.
- Diuretics.
- IV or oral supplementation, maintenance dose 1–2 mmol/kg/day.

Hypernatraemia

Causes of hypernatraemia include:

- Increased intake of sodium.
- Diarrhoea.
- Dehydration.
- Sweating.
- Sodium bicarbonate during cardiac arrest.
- Sodium chloride via monitoring lines (LA, PA, CVP, arterial).
- Decreased output during renal disease.

Clinical features:

- Increased cardiac contractility.
- Very thirsty.
- Nausea and vomiting.
- Fitting.
- Irritability.
- Oliguria.
- Flushed appearance.
- Dehydration.

Treatment:

- Reduce sodium intake.
- Liberalise fluids.

Magnesium

Normal values

Normal values for magnesium are 0.78–1.02 mmol/l.

Functions

- Maintains intra- and extracellular potassium equilibrium — a low magnesium level allows movement of potassium to the extracellular fluid causing hypokalaemia.
- Increases myocardial contractility.
- Increases neuromuscular transmission.

Hypomagnesaemia

Causes of hypomagnesaemia include:

- Diuretic therapy.
- Hypocalcaemia.
- Diarrhoea.
- Dietary deficiency.
- Renal failure.

Clinical features:

- Decreased myocardial contractility, low cardiac output.
- Arrhythmias — ventricular ectopics, ventricular fibrillation.
- Bronchoconstriction.
- Pulmonary hypertension.
- Fitting.
- Parasthesiae.

Treatment:

- IV 50% magnesium sulphate 0.2 ml/kg diluted over 1 hour.
- Treat cause.

Calcium

Normal values

Normal values for calcium are total: 2.1–2.6 mmol/l, ionised: 1.13–1.32 mmol/l. Calcium can be measured as the total or ionised, that is the amount freely available for use by the cells. The total calcium may be within normal limits with a low ionised calcium therefore the ionised level is the figure to treat as it is the most active, available form.

Functions

- Myocardial contraction.
- Positive inotropic effect, thus increased cardiac output.
- Skeletal muscle contraction.
- Blood clotting.
- Cellular permeability.
- Maintains teeth and bone integrity.

Hypocalcaemia

Causes of hypocalcaemia include:

- Di George syndrome.
- Inadequate calcium intake.
- Vitamin D deficiency.
- Phosphate deficiency.
- Cardiopulmonary bypass — ionised levels are diluted when on bypass and are additionally lowered when large volumes of plasma are given, when the patient is shocked or hypoxic (especially in the neonate)[38].
- Large blood transfusions.
- Alkalosis or acidosis.
- Abnormal albumin levels as it affects the protein binding capacity.

Clinical features:

- Tingling of fingers and toes.
- Carpopedal spasm.
- Tetany.
- Fitting.
- Laryngospasm.
- Reduced cardiac output.
- Prolonged repolarisation of the myocardium.
- Bleeding.
- Fractures.

Treatment:

- Calcium replacement therapy — IV via a central vein 0.5 ml/kg of calcium gluconate 10% as a short infusion. Severe deficiency administer 0.2 ml/kg/hour.
- Oral supplementation.
- Increase vitamin D and phosphate intake.

Urine output

The urine output of cardiac patients is of prime importance and indicates how well the kidneys are being perfused, thus how effective cardiac output is and how effective glomerular filtration is.

Urine output according to age

- Neonates and infants: 2 ml/kg/hour.
- Young children: 1–2 ml/kg/hour.
- Older children: 0.5–1 ml/kg/hour.

Should urine output fail to reach the desired amount, several steps can be undertaken as described by Elliott and Delius[337]:

- Assess the patient's filling pressures and vital signs.
- Fluid challenge the patient with 10–20 ml/kg/hour of colloid if hypovolaemic.
- Maximise cardiac output with inotropes.
- Administer IV furosemide at 1 mg/kg.

Should the above steps fail, discuss with the nephrologist the possibility of implementing renal replacement therapy sooner rather than later.

The examination of urine postoperatively may indicate the presence of haemolysis with blood stained/rusty coloured urine. This occurs during cardiopulmonary bypass and especially if bypass was prolonged. However, it could be the result of transfusion incompatibility so a direct and indirect Coomb's test should be carried out[337].

Acute renal failure

Classification

- Prerenal: This is due to hypoperfusion of the kidneys from hypoxia, hypotension and low cardiac output, or hypovolaemia and is the most likely cause of renal failure in intensive care patients. Following open heart surgery approximately 8% of patients will have some degree of prerenal failure[338].
- Intrinsic: This is associated with kidney disease such as haemolytic uraemic syndrome, systemic lupus erythematosus, polycystic kidney disease. Should a neonate present with a cardiac lesion and acute renal

failure, the appropriate tests must be performed to rule out any congenital abnormality of the renal tract. This is especially important in neonates diagnosed with Vater's, Edward's or Turner's syndromes[220].

- Postrenal: This classification of renal failure is caused by an obstructive disease of the kidneys.

Pathophysiology of prerenal failure

Prerenal failure results from hypoperfusion of the kidneys which causes a reduction in renal blood flow. Initially, the kidneys respond by vasoconstricting the efferent arterioles to maintain glomerular capillary pressure and reabsorption of sodium and water. However, if the hypoperfusion is severe and prolonged, the glomerular filtration rate will fall dramatically[10].

Clinical features

Blood parameters

- Rising creatinine above 80 μmol/l.
- Rising urea above 7 mmol/l.
- Hyperkalaemia.
- Hyponatraemia.

Urine parameters

- Urine output less than parameters stated previously.
- Creatinine above 30 μmol/l.
- Urea above 14 mmol/l.
- Sodium less than 10 mmol/l.
- Osmolarity greater than 2.

Other features

- Fitting from hyponatraemia.
- Metabolic acidosis.
- Oedema

Key management issues

The key management issues for a patient with acute renal failure are shown in Table 13.2.

Table 13.2 Assessment and management of potential problems in a child with acute renal failure.

Prevention, if possible, of hypoperfusion:
- Maximise cardiac output by optimising preload, reducing afterload and improving contractility with the use of inotropes (dopamine above 5 µg/kg/min can cause renal arteriole vasoconstriction so avoid). Control arrhythmias
- Aggressively manage hypoxia and metabolic acidosis
- Treat hypovolaemia by assessing filling pressures and vital signs
- Fluid challenge if filling pressures low with 10–20 ml/kg of colloid

Manage fluid balance:
- Accurately record input and output of crystalloid and colloid fluid balance
- Administer prescribed furosemide 1–2 mg/kg IV qds or a continuous infusion. Additionally, aminophylline administered as a short infusion prior to the furosemide, can potentiate an effective diuresis. Should these methods fail, renal replacement therapy should be initiated promptly
- If oliguric, fluids should be restricted
- Insertion of urinary catheter to accurately assess urine output

Management of electrolytes:
- Assess and manage imbalances, particularly hyperkalaemia

Management of the hypervolaemia due to sodium and water retention
- Assess the degree of overload — increased filling pressures, systemic venous oedema, tachycardia, hypertension, bulging fontanelle in infants
- Administer prescribed diuretics and monitor effectiveness by calculating urine output in ml/kg/hour
- Restrict fluid intake
- Maintain tissue integrity which is prone to break down due to oedema, by use of pressure relieving devices, a diet rich in protein, ensuring tubes and monitoring equipment not pressing into skin, keeping skin dry and clean

Management of anaemia due to bone marrow suppression

Avoid a high intake of sodium or potassium, either enterally or intravenously

Careful administration of nephrotoxic drugs:
- Aminoglycoside and cefotaxime antibiotics are commonly used for cardiac prophylaxis so must have levels taken regularly (if appropriate) and the doses adjusted to compensate for the renal failure
- Digoxin is nephrotoxic so levels must be taken and the dose altered accordingly to compensate for the kidneys' inability to excrete effectively during acute renal failure

Peritoneal dialysis

Peritoneal dialysis is a form of renal replacement therapy which can be used in both acute and chronic renal failure, when oliguria persists and urea and electrolytes become severely deranged. A sterile catheter is placed into the peritoneum and fluid runs in and out, having contact with the peritoneal membrane which is a highly vascular and semi-permeable area.

Uses of peritoneal dialysis (PD)

- Urea and electrolyte imbalances.
- Hypervolaemia.
- Metabolic acidosis.
- Multi-organ failure.
- Poisoning.

Advantages of PD therapy

- Causes less haemodynamic instability than haemodialysis. Haemofiltration once established, however, can be more unstable than PD.
- Relatively easy access as opposed to vascular access.
- Inexpensive.

Disadvantages of PD therapy

- It is less effective in removing solutes and water quickly[172].
- Can cause respiratory compromise.
- The omentum can wrap around the catheter tip, thus blocking the catheter, particularly in the neonate.
- Can cause hyperglycaemia, particularly if the dialysate is high in glucose.
- Sepsis.
- Can cause problems with thermoregulation especially in neonates and infants as it acts as an effective heat exchanger.

Contraindications to PD therapy

- Abdominal surgery within 7 days (if the wound is still draining).
- Peritonitis.
- Necrotising enterocolitis.
- Congenital gastrointestinal anomaly — gastroschisis, diaphragmatic hernia or exomphalos[10, 337].
- Severe pulmonary disease.

How PD works

The peritoneum is a large semi-permeable membrane which allows the passage of solutes across the membrane by osmosis and diffusion[337]. By inserting a catheter into the peritoneum, diffusion of water and electrolytes occurs between the peritoneal capillaries and the dialysate[10]. It then removes water and electrolytes from the blood by the process of osmosis, the amount depending on the electrolyte concentration of the dialysate.

The dialysate

The dialysate is made up of various electrolytes, the one having the greatest effect on osmotic pull being dextrose. Three strengths of dextrose are available, the highest concentration pulling off the largest amount of fluid – 1.36%, 3.86%, and 6.36% (which is rarely used as it causes hypovolaemia). Additionally 3.86% and 6.36% can cause hyperglycaemia requiring the administration of insulin. Blood sugars therefore need careful monitoring. Heparin, usually 500 units/l of dialysate is required to maintain tube patency. Potassium may also be added if hypokalaemia becomes a problem. If the patient is very sick and has lacticacidosis, a lactate free dialysate can be obtained.

- The dialysate must be warmed to body temperature before instillation.
- 25–50 ml/kg of dialysate is instilled. The dialysate is more effective in smaller patients as the surface area is proportional to the size of the patient.
- Samples of PD fluid should be sent to the laboratory for culture and sensitivity on a twice weekly basis or if infection is suspected and the drainage is cloudy. Antibiotics can be added to the dialysate bags using a strict aseptic technique.
- Frequent urea and electrolyte samples must be taken.

The cycle

- 5 to 10 minutes instillation time.
- 35 minutes dwell time — this can be varied depending on the amount of fluid to be pulled off.
- 15 minutes drainage time — by the end of the 15 minutes, should the output not reach the same as the amount instilled, extra time must be

allowed rather than starting another cycle and risking the patient becoming fluid overloaded and the abdomen distended.

Fluid balance status

A strict input and output incorporating both colloid and crystalloid balances must be undertaken to assess accurately the patient's needs.

Key management issues

The key management issues for a patient undergoing peritoneal dialysis are shown in Table 13.3.

Table 13.3 Assessment and management of potential problems in a child undergoing PD

Peritonitis (occurs in approximately 33% of patients undergoing PD therapy[10]):
- Monitor for changes in appearance of the drainage, particularly if cloudy
- Assess the patient for a tender, painful, distended abdomen, pyrexia, vomiting, paralytic ileus and report promptly if observed
- Send a sample for culture and sensitivity analysis
- Administer prescribed antibiotics
- Manage the pain, pyrexia and vomiting

Hypoproteinaemia:
- Proteins, particularly albumin, are lost into the dialysate solution. This occurs more often in paediatric patients[337]
- Ensure enteral intake is protein rich

Fluid and electrolyte imbalance:
- Monitor for hyperglycaemia, hypernatraemia and hyperkalaemia which can be due to too high a dextrose concentration in the dialysate
- Hypocalcaemia can present once the dialysis has been effective in lowering the potassium

Haemodynamic instability:
- The blood pressure can fall in critically ill patients when the PD is draining, therefore drain out more slowly and use a less strong concentration of dialysate. There is little advantage in having to treat the dialysis-induced hypovolaemia with plasma, when it will invariably move from the intravascular compartments to the tissues making the patient even more oedematous

Respiratory compromise:
- During the dwell period, respiratory splinting can occur, especially in small babies. Therefore, it may be advisable to instil small amounts for short periods only

(contd)

Table 13.3 Assessment and management of potential problems in a child undergoing PD

Leakage of the catheter to the:
- Outside — leakage can occur around the insertion site. The site should be covered in sterile gauze which is weighed to assess the degree of leakage. Consider smaller instillations
- Chest drains — cardiac surgeons often insert a PD catheter whilst in theatre, passing from the thoracic cavity to the abdominal cavity. Therefore, there is the possibility of leakage into the chest drains which can be established by testing the chest drainage for the presence of glucose. It does not normally cause problems and dialysis can usually continue

Failure of the catheter to drain due to:
- Lines kinked or clamped
- Leakage into chest drains or outside insertion point
- Catheter blocked — this is usually due to the presence of fibrin strands and requires the catheter to be flushed in the first instance with saline. If this fails, heparinised saline or urokinase may be considered
- Omentum can wrap around the catheter, blocking its tip. This may necessitate replacement of the catheter[339]
- Child being constipated can impede the fill and drain
- Consider changing the child's position to help drain any catheter which is slow to empty

Haemofiltration

Haemofiltration is another renal replacement therapy which has inherent advantages and disadvantages. However, it is rarely used in the child with a cardiac defect mainly due to the vascular access required, especially if the child will require further cardiac catheterisations and heart surgery in the future. Therefore, it is not discussed further in this book.

Gastrointestinal management

Gastrointestinal management encompasses the following issues.

Nutrition

The infant, child or adolescent with a condition that exists along a continuum of critical to chronic illness, poses a challenge for those involved in nutritional management. A well child has a higher metabolic rate than an adult. The ultimate goal of nutrition in sick children is to provide sufficient calories and thus energy, which allows for tissue growth and development in a non-anabolic state.

The nurse must continuously assess the child's nutritional state. Working with the dietitian and other members of the multidisciplinary team will help in achieving this goal. Assessment should include weighing the child, measuring height and head circumference and calculating the body surface area. Plotting results on a centile chart provides an accurate record of the child's progress over a period of time, although the child with congenital heart disease may have periods of oedema and thus false weight gain. Obtaining a dietary history from the child and parents allows the nurse and team to assess the balance of carbohydrates, proteins, fats, vitamins and minerals which provide the calories and nutrition for growth and development. The dietitian usually has close links with the child who has a congenital heart defect as gaining weight may be a problem if persistent heart failure occurs.

Nutrition in critical illness

The child with sepsis or fever may have an increased metabolic rate requiring more calories to prevent a hypermetabolic, catabolic state (tissue breakdown or destruction). Ideally, indirect calorimetry should be performed to estimate rate and energy expenditure in critically ill children, although this is difficult in ventilated children with uncuffed endotracheal tubes. A diet rich in protein is required as provision of a diet too high in carbohydrates can increase carbon dioxide production[272]. Electrolyte balance is vital in critical illness as a potassium, sodium, calcium, magnesium or glucose imbalance can threaten vital organ function, muscle physiology or nerve conduction[10, 272].

When in intensive care, nutritional intake is delivered preferably via a nasogastric tube or gastrostomy. Drug therapy and the period of critical illness can obviously have an impact on the body's ability to absorb enterally but the advantages of enteral feeding outweigh parenteral feeding in most circumstances (Table 13.4)

Nutrition in heart failure

The baby with heart failure from a congenital heart defect needs calories for growth and development. However, if the heart failure is uncontrolled, breathlessness can prevent a baby from sucking effectively. Sucking in itself is a very energy consuming activity so the breathless baby tries hard to ingest milk but becomes tired quickly therefore requiring even more calories to account for the energy expended. This downward spiral of events predisposes the baby to failure to thrive.

Measures can be employed to assist these hungry babies to grow. Initially giving small feeds regularly — two hourly — may be of help. Should the baby still be too tired or take an hour or so to feed, then a cup and spoon can be used to take the energy out of the sucking. Some parents often see an improvement when the baby is weaned for that very reason. Continuous 24-hour feeding, as opposed to overnight feeding with daily supplements or plain oral feeding has been shown to benefit this group of patients in increasing their weight and improving their nutritional status and intake[340]. Should this method be employed, it is important to allow the baby to have some oral intake for comfort reasons and so that he or she does not forget what eating is like! Alternatively, some babies try feeding normally and when too tired are "topped up" with a nasogastric feed. The baby should not be pushed too hard when attempting oral feeding and if the heart failure is severe, parenteral feeding may required to prevent the respiratory embarrassment associated with sucking. This method of inducing weight gain is not ideal as parenteral nutrition has known disadvantages (Table 13.4)

Breast feeding

The mother wanting to breast feed her baby should be encouraged to do so. If fluid balance assessment is important or the baby is too ill to suckle, the mother can be encouraged to express her milk as the emotional benefits of doing this are most important. The mother with a baby facing major heart surgery needs to bond with her child and feel some control in his or her management. Knowing "breast is best" allows her to regain the knowledge that she is providing and caring for her sick infant, something which the nursing staff cannot do.

Whether breast or bottle fed, the dietitian will assess the calorie intake, increasing it with preparations such as Duocal or Polycal, thus maximising calorie intake in as concentrated a form as possible. Equally, the child managing to eat will be assessed for likes and dislikes, a diet tailor-made to the child's requirements being provided. Should the child refuse food then high protein, high calorie drinks should be encouraged to provide the essential nutrients required.

Enteral versus parenteral feeding

The advantages and disadvantages of enteral and parenteral feeding are shown in Table 13.4.

Table 13.4 Advantages and disadvantages of enteral and parenteral feeding

	Advantages	Disadvantages
Enteral feeding	• Easy access • Relatively inexpensive • Provision of calories, carbohydrates, fats, vitamins and minerals in a most acceptable form for the body to digest • Helps in the prevention of stress ulcers • Maintains the gut mucosal barrier, thus preventing the translocation of bacteria from the gut which can result in a systemic inflammatory response and multi-organ failure[341, 342] • Improves wound healing • Prevents immune dysfunction • Improved morbidity and mortality rates[343, 344]	• Risk of aspiration • Discomfort on placement of the tube • Nasal obstruction from the tube could increase respiratory distress in small babies, however an orogastric tube may then be placed
Parenteral feeding	• A means of calorie and nutritional provision should enteral feeding be impossible, for example after gastrointestinal surgery, severe cardiac failure, necrotising enterocolitis	• Provision of a long or central line with its associated complications: 1. Infection 2. Accessibility 3. Haemorrhage 4. Pneumothorax 5. Air emboli 6. Blood vessel thrombosis 7. Catheter sepsis 8. Arrhythmias • Metabolic problems: 1. Hypoglycaemia 2. Hyperglycaemia 3. Electrolyte imbalances 4. Liver damage if prolonged use 5. Cholestatic jaundice • The need for daily serum electrolytes to tailor-make the feed may not be sufficient in a critically ill patient with rapidly changing electrolytes • The expense of the preparation and use of equipment • The discomfort and restriction associated with the catheter

Necrotising enterocolitis (NEC)

Aetiology

Although the aetiology is unknown, this disease is normally associated with the preterm infant but equally can present in a critically ill neonate who has undergone a period of hypoxia, hypotension and sepsis, for example, a baby with a duct dependent cardiac lesion in which the duct has closed[345]. If enteral feeding is then commenced, it provides a substrate for micro-organisms that occur in the ischaemic gut[313]. Although other factors have been linked with the development of NEC, studies are not conclusive in their findings. However, it appears that multi-organ failure often accompanies NEC and there can be a history of increasing respiratory support in the preceding 24 hours before NEC is diagnosed[346], thus suggesting implications for the treatment of the disease. The neonate's immature immune system has also be studied as a potential factor in its development[347, 348].

Definition

Necrotising enterocolitis (NEC) is the development of necrotic patches in the bowel, commonly in the ileum and colon.

Signs and symptoms

Cardiovascular signs and symptoms

- Cardiovascular collapse as characterised by bradycardia, hypotension, profound shock and cool peripheries.

Respiratory signs and symptoms

- Increasing respiratory support in the 24 hours prior to diagnosis.
- Tachypnoea.
- Apnoea.

Gastrointestinal signs and symptoms

- Nasogastric aspirations increased.
- Vomiting — bile stained.
- Mild to severe abdominal distension, grey and shiny in appearance.
- Abdominal tenderness.

- Rectal bleeding/blood stained stool.
- Absent bowel sounds,
- Increased passage of stools, particularly seedy in nature[349].

Renal signs and symptoms

- Metabolic acidosis.
- Oliguria.

Other signs and symptoms

- Irritability.
- Lethargy.
- Listlessness.
- Mottled skin.
- Pallor.
- Hypothermia.

Diagnosis

- Abdominal x-ray: Dilated loops of bowel, free intraperitoneal gas, fluid levels present[313].

Key management issues

Early recognition is vital as early intervention has a significantly lower morbidity and mortality rate than in late diagnosis. Depending on the clinical condition of the baby, conservative management may be tried, however if the condition worsens or the baby is unresponsive to conservative treatment, surgical intervention is required. See Table 13.5.

Table 13.5 Assessment and management of potential problems in a baby with NEC

Management of septic shock:
- Administer prescribed IV antibiotics for gram negative and gram positive organisms for 7–10 days
- Administer prescribed plasma to correct hypovolaemia and thus hypotension
- Administer prescribed inotropes should the cardiac output need support
- Assess cardiac output at regular intervals including urine output, core–peripheral temperature gradient
- Monitor clotting profile to detect for disseminated intravascular coagulation

(contd)

Table 13.5 (contd)

Management of increasing respiratory distress:
- Assess for degree of respiratory distress
- Ventilate if increasing acidosis, hypoxia, carbon dioxide retention or apnoea. Optimise ventilatory support by sedating and paralysing the baby if very sick

Management of gastrointestinal problems:
- Stop enteral feeding. Assist in the siting of a central line for parenteral nutrition. If the baby is improving enteral feeding can be started slowly in 7–10 days. Slow introduction of enteral feeding is required[313]. Breast milk is preferable as it contains maternal antibodies (IgA) which may help in the prevention of NEC
- Place the nasogastric tube on continuous low grade suction, replacing losses with prescribed saline or equivalent[345]
- Remove rectal thermometer if present
- Perform regular girth measurements
- Observe for bowel movements. Note for the presence of blood
- Take regular blood sugars to monitor for hypoglycaemia

Management of anaemia:
- Anaemia will present if the baby is septic. Transfuse as required

Management of bowel perforation:
- Daily abdominal x-rays, or more often if indicated, should be taken to detect free fluid. If found, the general surgeons should be notified immediately
- Any worsening of the baby's condition is an indication for surgical intervention although surgery in the baby with a perforated gut carries a risk of mortality of approximately 25%[313]
- Care of the baby who has undergone a laparotomy, bowel resection and formation of an ileostomy or colostomy is not covered here

Management of pain and discomfort:
- Assess for pain
- Administer analgesia and assess effectiveness
- Do not lay the baby in the prone position as the abdomen cannot be monitored, plus it will be too uncomfortable for the baby

Long-term care and follow-up

Complications of NEC include short bowel syndrome, secondary to bowel resection, requiring long-term parenteral nutrition and its aforementioned problems with the addition of failure to thrive.

Chapter 14
The dying child

Not all childhood congenital heart disease can be cured, however, it is still tragic for the family and staff when a death, expected or unexpected, occurs. There are many excellent texts on death and dying so this subject will be covered briefly.

The expected death

The family who have lived with a chronically ill cardiac child will, no doubt, have undergone the fear of death on several occasions. Being admitted to hospital and especially to an intensive care unit, heightens awareness of the severity of the problems and whether or not their child is going to survive. This question crosses their minds even when the surgery for the heart defect is planned as all procedures are potentially life-threatening. Examples of congenital heart lesions with the greatest risk are hypoplastic left heart syndrome, obstructed TAPVD, IAA with ductal dependence, but other lesions can be equally hazardous, e.g., in TGA when the coronary arteries kink, performing a Fontan procedure with high pulmonary artery pressures and so on. Each child's condition and the risks pertaining to it must be considered on an individual basis and the child and family spoken to appropriately.

Should the child for whom treatment has been discontinued ask questions about dying, staff must answer honestly and compassionately. The child, understandably, may express fear.

Should it become inevitable that the child is not going to survive, the family will start to experience anticipatory grief[350], similar to the stages described by Kubler-Ross[351] — shock and denial, anger, bargaining, depression, then eventual acceptance. This anticipatory grief is a way in which parents can prepare for the loss of their child before the event occurs[352]. The phase can occur during episodes of critical illness when the child's condition is very unstable and the future uncertain[10] and may occur several days before the event. Denial, one of the phases identified, can help the parents in the initial period of shock as it acts as a coping mechanism when things appear too overwhelming[10]. It may manifest itself with the parents refusing to withdraw treatment. Staff should treat this sensitively although they should convey messages to the parents that their child's condition is severe, for example, "He doesn't look as well today", or "The blood pressure isn't responding to the epinephrine as quickly today"[10]. Parents must not feel that the staff have "given up" on their child[10] thus avoidance of confrontation is paramount. Other emotions experienced by parents are anger, loss of control, guilt, failure and sadness, all of which occur during the period of anticipatory grief and after the child has died[353].

The effect on the siblings depends on their age — young children may appear unaffected, continuing to play with their toys, whereas older children may bottle up emotions if parents shield them from the reality of the situation. The best approach is to be honest with the siblings, involve them in decision making and be an open listener.

Withholding or withdrawing treatment

Although the medical staff have the final say in whether to prolong life or withdraw/withhold treatment, it should be a decision made in conjunction with the multidisciplinary team and, of course, the parents. It is obviously not an easy decision to make as emotional, cultural, religious, ethical and legal considerations have to be taken into account[10]. Once decided, however, it must be documented in the patient's notes by the child's doctor to avoid ambiguity and confusion.

The death

The parents and family need to know what to anticipate during an "expected" death. The nurse will have to ascertain their perceived conceptions and any fears and anxieties which the family may be experiencing about their child dying. Their worries must be dealt with in a caring, sensitive manner. Additionally they must have opportunity to discuss what will happen to their child at the time of death, whether any extra pain relief is to be given, what their child will look like (colour, changes in appearance) and so on. Equally, any wishes pertaining to what they want for their child must be met to ease this very difficult time. As parents probably will not have been in this situation before, they may need guidance from the staff[353] as to where they want their child to die (in a cubicle, in ICU, on the ward, at home), do they want to be holding their child if small or get into bed with the child if older, do they want siblings, the extended family and friends to come and say goodbye and do they want to be left alone after withdrawal has taken place?

Other physical and emotional needs have to be met such as privacy for the family, free use of telephones, and access to drinks, food and sleeping facilities in close proximity to their child (ideally in the cubicle with their child). Should the child deteriorate over a few days, periods of rest for the parents are a must and assurance must be given that staff will contact the family should the need arise. The family should be encouraged to participate in the care of their child at every possible opportunity.

When the child dies, the family should be informed by the most appropriate person — someone known to them if at all possible. The news should be conveyed gently, simply and always using the child's name. A request for post mortem may be asked for now or later depending on the parents' response.

After the death

The child's dignity and privacy must be maintained at all times following death. Emotional reactions inevitably vary from family to family, whether it is an expected or sudden death. Whatever the response, the nurse must support the family in a caring, compassionate manner. Staff who shed a tear are often respected by the family who realise that the team do genuinely care. However, should staff end up needing emotional support from the family, they must leave the area as the family's needs must come first[10].

The family must be able to stay with their child as long as they feel necessary, holding, touching and saying goodbye[353]. Photographs can be taken, a lock of hair, hand and footprints and a memory booklet are given to the parents if they wish. A bereavement booklet with information about help groups and the Alder Hey/Great Ormond Street help line for anyone affected by the death of a child should be available. Information about registering the child's death and so on is helpful.

Staff must inform the health visitor liaison nurse about the child's death. He or she will contact the school nurse, midwife and community nurses as appropriate. The child's GP and social worker must be contacted. Any prebooked outpatient appointments must be cancelled and completion of the required hospital documentation undertaken.

When, and only when, the family are ready to say goodbye, should their child be taken to the mortuary. The family can go if they wish and carry the child if not too heavy. Unfortunately, the mortuary trolley has to be used for children who are too big to carry, which is distressing for both the family and staff. Families should be informed that they can visit their child in the chapel at any time, having first rung staff to inform them of their intention. Some families will want to take the child home which again is fine as long as a post mortem is not required and the death certificate has been issued. The nurse must check that the family can get home safely, especially if very upset. An appointment is usually sent to the parents to see the consultant within six to eight weeks or sooner if required, although a longer gap will give the parents time to think of unanswered questions. Staff often like to attend the funeral although this is up to the individual; parents often appreciate the gesture. Some staff will keep in contact with the family, visiting them periodically, again this is up to the individual member of staff[353].

Sudden death

See the section on cardiac arrest.

Sudden death is often perceived as more stressful than an anticipated death. However, studies have shown there is little difference between the two in terms of the responses of the family members[354]. Conversely, parental reaction to sudden death can result in more guilt, numbness, shock and anger[355]. Additionally, the advantages of anticipatory death in being able to prepare oneself are removed when a child dies suddenly[11].

Chapter 15
Drug management

Calculation of drug doses into micrograms (µg) or nanograms (ng)/kg/minute

- Drug in milligrams (mg) or µg × 1000.
- Divided by the volume it is in.
- Divided by 60 (minutes).
- Divided by weight of patient.
- Multiplied by the rate of the infusion.
- Equals µg or ng/kg/minute.

Calculation of rate in ml/hour

- Weight (kg) × dose (µg/kg/minute) × 60 (minutes) divided by the concentration (µg/ml).

Inotropic therapy

Digoxin

Dose (oral)

Age	Total digitalising dose (TDD) (divided by 4 doses in 24 hours)	Maintenance dose start 12 hours after TDD (divided by 2 doses in 24 hours)
Premature	15–20 µg/kg	5 µg/kg
Newborn	40 µg/kg	8 µg/kg
1 month–12yrs	40 µg/kg	8 µg/kg
12yrs +	1–1.5 mg	62.5–500 µg

Dose (IV)

- 75% of the oral dose by short infusion.

Actions

- A cardiac glycoside's main action is to increase the force of contraction of the myocardium (positive inotropic effect). Additionally it reduces conductivity in the atrioventricular node.

Indications

- Heart failure, supraventricular arrhythmias (SVT, atrial fibrillation), low cardiac output, post-ventriculotomy.

Contraindications

- Second and third degree heart block, Wolff–Parkinson–White syndrome, use with caution in hypertrophic cardiomyopathy.

Side effects

- Nausea, vomiting, anorexia, diarrhoea, abdominal pain, heart block, arrhythmias, headache, drowsiness, confusion, visual disturbances.

Nursing considerations

- Monitor the heart rate, respiratory rate, potassium, calcium, magnesium, urea and creatinine.
- Monitor levels for digoxin toxicity. Therapeutic range being 1.28–2.56 nmol/l. Take levels 6 hours after last dose.
  1. Reduce dose in renal failure
  2. Increased risk of high levels when using digoxin with amiodarone, erythromycin and in hypokalaemia.

Dobutamine

Dose

- 2–10 µg/kg/minute IV infusion via a central line. Can be increased to 40 µg/kg/minute.
- Suggested concentrations: 40/80/160/320 mg dobutamine in 45 ml of 5% dextrose.

Actions

- Beta 1 adrenergic stimulator causing an increase in myocardial contraction and thus stroke volume, increase in heart rate, accelerated conduction through the sinoatrial node and atrioventricular node.
- Beta 2 adrenergic stimulator relaxing the smooth muscle of the bronchus, inhibiting the release of histamine, stimulating renin release and peripheral vasodilation as the pulmonary vascular resistance lowers.

Indications

- Cardiac surgery, myocardial failure, moderate cardiogenic and septic shock and hypotension, low cardiac output.

Contraindications

- Severe hypotension, idiopathic hypertrophic subaortic stenosis.

Side effects

- Tachyarrhythmias, hypotension, nausea, vomiting, headache.

Nursing considerations

- Continuously monitor the heart rate, blood pressure and other haemodynamic parameters.
- Dobutamine is inactivated by alkaline solutions — sodium bicarbonate, furosemide, enoximone.

Dopamine

Dose

- 1–5 µg/kg/minute renal dose.
- 5–20 µg/kg/minute cardiac dose.
- IV infusion via a central line.
- Suggested concentration: 40/80/160/320 mg in 45 ml of 5% dextrose.

Actions

- 1–5 µg, dopaminergic effects — increases perfusion to the kidneys (increasing urine output), brain, splanchnic and coronary blood supplies.

- 5–20 μg, beta 1 and 2 adrenergic effects, although more tachyarrhythmic than dobutamine.
- 20+ μg, alpha adrenergic effect — increases the systemic and pulmonary vascular resistances causing marked peripheral vasoconstriction, thus raising the blood pressure.

Indications

- Renal failure at low dose, low cardiac output, cardiogenic shock, cardiac surgery.

Contraindications

- Tachyarrhythmia, phaeochromocytoma.

Side effects

- Hypo/hypertension, tachycardia, peripheral vasoconstriction, nausea and vomiting.

Nursing considerations

- Continuously monitor the heart rate, blood pressure and other haemodynamic parameters.
- Correct hypovolaemia before use.
- Inactivated by alkalising agents as dobutamine.

Epinephrine (adrenaline)

Dose

- 0.1–1 μg/kg/minute IV infusion via a central line. Higher concentrations may be required.
- Suggested concentrations: $0.3 \times$ body weight (kg) = mg epinephrine (1:1000 = 1 mg) up to 50 ml with 5% dextrose therefore 1 ml/hour = 0.1 μg/kg/minute.

Actions

- 0.01–0.15 μg beta 1 adrenergic effects.
- 0.2–5 μg alpha adrenergic effects.
- Beta 2 adrenergic effects.

Indications

- Low cardiac output, cardiac surgery, bronchospasm.

Cautions

- Diabetes mellitus, hypertension, hyperthyroidism.

Side effects

- Tremor, tachycardia thus increasing oxygen and metabolic demands which may be to the detriment of the patient.
- Reduced renal perfusion, increased gluconeogenesis inhibiting insulin release and causing hyperglycaemia.
- Hypertension, peripheral vasoconstriction, nausea, vomiting, sweating, bronchodilation, pulmonary oedema, cerebral haemorrhage.

Nursing considerations

- Continuously monitor heart rate, blood pressure and other haemodynamic parameters, peripheral perfusion.
- Increased doses may necessitate the introduction of vasodilator therapy.

Isoprenaline

Dose

- 20–200 ng/kg/minute IV infusion via central line. Increase to 1000 ng/kg/minute as necessary.
- Suggested concentrations: $0.3 \times$ weight (kg) = mg isoprenaline up to 50 ml with 5% dextrose, therefore 1 ml/hour = 0.1 µg/kg/minute.

Actions

- Beta 1 adrenergic effects.
- Beta 2 adrenergic effects.
- Peripheral vasodilation.

Indications

- Heart block, severe bradycardia, bronchoconstriction.

Cautions

- Diabetes mellitus, hyperthyroidism, ischaemic heart disease.

Side effects

- Arrhythmias, tachycardia, hypotension, sweating, headache.

Nursing considerations

- Continuously monitor heart rate, blood pressure and other haemodynamic parameters.

Enoximone

Dose

- 5–20 μg/kg/minute IV infusion via central or peripheral cannula.
- Concentration: Must be diluted in equal parts of the drug: diluent = 100 mg (20 ml) made up to 40 ml with 0.9% sodium chloride or water for injection.

Actions

- Positive inotropic effects.
- Vasodilator.
- Phosphodiesterase inhibitor which causes an increase of cyclic AMP in the vascular smooth muscle and myocardium. This results in arteriolar dilatation and increases myocardial contraction.

Indications

- Congestive heart failure where cardiac output is reduced and filling pressures are high.

Caution

- Hypertrophic cardiomyopathy, stenotic or obstructive valvular disease, risk of propylene glycol toxicity in patients with renal impairment or on long-term treatment.

Side effects

- Hypotension, headache, nausea, ectopics, urinary retention.

Nursing considerations

- Continuously monitor heart rate, blood pressure and other haemodynamic properties.
- Long half-life (12 hours).
- Very alkaline solution (pH 12), therefore only mix with water or sodium chloride in equal proportions.
- Incompatible with all drugs.

Vasodilator therapy

Glyceryl trinitrate/nitroglycerin

Dose

- 200–1000 ng/kg/minute IV infusion via central line. Can be increased to 5 µg/kg/minute.
- Suggested concentration: 3 × weight (kg) = mg nitroglycerin up to 50 ml with 5% dextrose to a maximum concentration of 50 mg in 50 ml.

Actions

- Systemic and pulmonary vasodilator reducing preload and dilating coronary vessels.

Indications

- Pulmonary hypertension, afterload reduction with systemic hypertension.

Contraindications

- Hypovolaemia, mitral stenosis, cerebral haemorrhage, hypotension.

Side effects

- Postural hypotension, headache, flushing, tachycardia, methaemoglobinaemia and therefore impaired oxygen transportation.

Nursing considerations

- Continuously monitor haemodynamic parameters.

- Monitor methaemoglobin.
- Administer via polyethylene tubing — incompatible with PVC.

Sodium nitroprusside

Dose

- 500 ng/kg/minute IV infusion via central line.
- Suggested concentration: 3 × weight (kg) = mg nitroprusside up to 50 ml with 5% dextrose, therefore 1 ml/hour = 1 μg/kg/minute.

Actions

- Calcium channel blocker.
- Relaxes smooth muscle.
- Afterload reducing agent.
- Peripheral vasodilator.

Indications

- Hypertension, with or without peripheral vasoconstriction, to improve myocardial function.

Contraindications

- Severe hepatic impairment.

Side effects

- Palpitations, retrosternal pain, hypotension, headache, abdominal pain, cyanide toxicity — nausea, disorientation, fatigue, hepatic dysfunction, metabolic acidosis.

Nursing considerations

- Continuously monitor haemodynamic parameters.
- Optimise preload/correct hypovolaemia before therapy.
- Monitor thiocyanate levels if prolonged usage intended.
- Protect from light, use aluminium foil.

Vasopressor therapy

Phenylephrine

Dose

- 10–20 µg/kg/dose IV every 15 minutes if required.
- 0.1–0.5 µg/kg/minute via IV infusion.

Actions

- Alpha adrenergic agent which increases systemic vascular resistance and therefore systemic perfusion.

Indications

- Low systemic vascular resistance and acute hypotension.

Side effects

- Hypertension, arrhythmias, bradycardia, tachycardia.

Nursing considerations

- Continuously monitor haemodynamic parameters.

Alpha adrenergic blocking therapy

Phenoxybenzamine

Dose

- 0.5–2.0 mg/kg in one or two divided doses IV infusion over 1–2 hours.

Actions

- Blocks the alpha adrenergic effects, thereby reducing systemic vascular resistance. Afterload reduction thus occurs, causing vasodilation of the peripheries.

Indications

- Heart failure, hypertension, vasoconstriction.

Side effects

- Profound hypotension, dizziness, tachycardia, gastrointestinal disturbances.

Nursing considerations

- Continuous haemodynamic monitoring.
- Ensure adequately preloaded (not hypovolaemic).
- Ensure plasma is readily available.

Angiotensin converting enzyme (ACE) inhibitor

Captopril

Dose

- Infants 500 µg or 100 µg/kg as a test dose orally and slowly increased to 3 mg/kg/dose, in three divided doses.

Actions

- Angiotensin converting enzyme inhibitor.
- Inhibits the conversion of angiotensin I to angiotensin II resulting in an increase in sodium excretion and renin release.

Indications

- Hypertension, heart failure in combination with digoxin and diuretics.

Contraindications

- Aortic stenosis and outflow tract obstructions.

Side effects

- Profound hypotension, tachycardia, acidosis, renal impairment, hyponatraemia, sinusitis, rhinitis, nausea, vomiting, diarrhoea, taste disturbance, thrombocytopenia, leucopenia, neutropenia, headache, dizziness, parasthesia, hyperkalaemia.

Nursing considerations

- Continuously monitor haemodynamic parameters whilst initial test dose and maintenance dose established.
- Patients taking diuretic therapy and ACE inhibitor are likely to become more hypotensive especially if volume depleted.
- Patients should not take potassium sparing diuretics (amiloride) as hyperkalaemia can occur.

Diuretic therapy

Furosemide

Dose

- Oral 1–5 mg/kg/dose in one to four divided doses.
- IV bolus 0.1–1 mg/kg/dose.
- IV infusion 0.1–4 mg/kg/hour continuous.

Actions

- Potent, quick acting diuretic.
- Inhibits reabsorption of water from the ascending loop of Henle in the renal tubule (loop diuretic).

Indications

- Pulmonary oedema, left ventricular failure, congestive heart failure, oedema, oliguria.

Cautions

- Diabetes mellitus, liver failure.

Side effects

- Hypokalaemia, hyponatraemia, hypomagnesaemia, hypocalcaemia, deafness if rapid IV injection, alkalosis, rash, nausea.

Nursing considerations

- Monitor renal function — urea and electrolytes, urine output.

- Alkaline solution therefore incompatible with dextrose. Dilute with sodium chloride.
- Risk of nephrotoxicity with non-steroidal anti-inflammatory analgesia.
- Risk of ototoxicity with aminoglycosides.
- Monitor effectiveness of diuresis — urine output and weight.

Amiloride

Dose

- 400 µg/kg/day in two divided doses or give with furosemide using approximately 10% of the furosemide dose as amiloride.

Actions

- Potassium sparing weak diuretic.
- Causes retention of potassium which usually avoids the need for potassium supplements.

Indications

- Oedema, potassium conservation.

Contraindications

- Hyperkalaemia.

Side effects

- Postural hypotension, hyperkalaemia, hyponatraemia, dry mouth, gastrointestinal disturbance.

Nursing considerations

- Monitor potassium levels.
- Monitor effectiveness of diuresis — urine output and weight.

Antiarrhythmic therapy

Adenosine

Dose

- 50 µg/kg extremely rapid IV injection as half-life 10 seconds. Repeat to a maximum of 500 µg/kg.

Actions

- Rapid reversal from SVT to sinus rhythm by slowing down the conduction through the atrioventricular node.
- Interrupts the re-enterant pathways.

Indications

- SVT.

Cautions

- Atrial fibrillation or flutter.

Contraindications

- 2nd or 3rd degree heart block, asthma.

Side effects

- Severe bradycardia (20–50 bpm) which is usually short-lived due to the rapid half-life of the drug, chest pain, bronchospasm, choking sensation, dizziness.

Nursing considerations

- Monitor haemodynamic parameters.
- Comfort the patient as it can be a frightening experience.

Amiodarone

Dose

- Oral 15 mg/kg/day in three divided doses for 1 week, then 10 mg/kg/day in two divided doses for 1 week, then 5mg/kg/day thereafter.
- Loading dose IV infusion 5 mg/kg over 20 to 120 minutes.
- Maintenance infusion 10 μg/kg/minute.

Actions

- Lengthens the refractory period of the atrial and ventricular muscles.
- Negative inotropic alpha and beta blocker.
- Reduces the systemic vascular resistance.

Indications

- Wolff–Parkinson–White syndrome, SVT, ventricular tachycardia, atrial fibrillation and flutter, ventricular fibrillation if other anti-arrhythmics unsuccessful.

Cautions

- Liver, kidney and thyroid disease.

Contraindications

- Sinus bradycardia, severe hypotension, cardiac arrest.

Side effects

- Eye problems — optic neuritis, corneal microdeposits, peripheral neuropathy, myopathy, phototoxicity, pneumonitis, hypo/hyper-thyroidism, nausea, vomiting, headache, fatigue, hypersensitivity.

Nursing considerations

- Monitor haemodynamic parameters.
- Monitor thyroid, liver and kidney function.
- Monitor trough levels — therapeutic range = 0.6–2.5 mg/l.
- Has a very long half-life — 2–3 weeks — so if oral administration, it may take several weeks to reach a desired therapeutic level.
- Enhances the effect of warfarin and increases digoxin levels (halve digoxin maintenance dose).
- Increased risk of bradycardia and AV block with beta blockers.
- Toxicity with loop diuretics if hypokalaemia occurs.

Atropine

Dose

- 20 µg/kg IV (minimum 100 µg) to a maximum dose of 3 mg.
- 40 µg/kg via ETT.

Actions

- Anticholinergic effect which blocks acetylcholine at SAN and AVN, increases heart rate and AV conduction.

Indications

- Bradycardia, asystole.

Side effects

- Tachycardia, dry mouth and bronchial secretions, confusion.

Flecainide

Dose

- 2 mg/kg to maximum of 150 mg IV bolus or short infusion.
- 100–250 μg/kg/hour continuous infusion.
- Oral 2–3 mg/kg/day in two divided doses.

Actions

- Sodium channel blocker slowing the AV conduction through the AVN and bundle of His.

Indications

- Atrial and ventricular ectopics, Wolff–Parkinson–White syndrome arrhythmias, atrial fibrillation, ventricular tachycardia.

Contraindications

- Heart failure, myocardial depression.

Side effects

- Dizziness, visual disturbances, rarely nausea, vomiting, photosensivity, increased liver enzymes, peripheral neuropathy, pneumonitis.

Nursing considerations

- Monitor ECG.
- Monitor levels — therapeutic level 200–800 ng/ml. Take oral trough after 2–4 days or IV, any time during a continuous infusion.
- Increased levels with amiodarone and hypokalaemia.
- Reduce levels in renal and liver failure.

- Digoxin levels are increased by 15%.
- Give dose at different time to milk feeds.

Lignocaine

Dose

- 0.5–1 mg/kg/loading dose IV as an antiarrhythmic.
- 10–50 µg/kg/minute maintenance dose, IV continuous infusion.
- 1 mg/kg IV single dose for cardiopulmonary resuscitation, ventricular tachycardia or fibrillation.

Actions

- Sodium channel blocker and membrane stabiliser.
- Depresses ventricular depolarisation.

Indications

- Ventricular arrhythmias.

Contraindications

- Heart block.

Side effects

- Hypotension, shock, bradycardia, fitting, respiratory depression, drowsiness, confusion, anxiety, parasthesia.

Nursing considerations

- Monitor haemodynamic parameters and mental status.
- Half-life of 10–15 minutes.

Propranolol

Dose

- 10–50 µg/kg IV over 10 minutes for arrhythmias up to three or four times daily.
- 100–200 µg/kg/dose IV for spelling in tetralogy of Fallot.
- 3–4 mg/kg/day orally in three to four divided doses.

Actions

- Beta blocker — beta adrenergic blocker.
- Antiarrhythmic by attenuating effects of sympathetic nervous system and conductivity within the heart.
- Cyanotic spelling in tetralogy of Fallot — thought to reduce infundibular spasm causing the spelling, although this is under debate at present.

Indications

- Hypertension, arrhythmias, cyanotic spelling.

Contraindications

- Asthma.

Side effects

- Severe hypotension if IV, bradycardia, heart block, bronchospasm, nausea and vomiting.

Nursing consideration

- Monitor haemodynamic parameters.
- Use a short infusion, monitoring heart rate and rhythm.

Ductus arteriosus patency

Prostaglandin E_1/prosin VR/alprostadil

Dose

- 5–100 ng/kg/minute IV infusion centrally or peripherally.
- Suggested concentration: 500 µg in 500 ml of 5% dextrose.

Actions

- Maintains ductal patency until corrective or palliative surgery for congenital heart disease can be undertaken.

Indications

- Duct dependent lesions, e.g., TGA, coarctation of the aorta, HLHS, tricuspid atresia.

Side effects

- Hypotension, apnoea, bradycardia, tachycardia, cardiac arrest, pyrexia, flushing, fitting, hypokalaemia.

Nursing considerations

- Continuous monitoring of haemodynamic and respiratory parameters.
- Correct hypovolaemia before starting therapy.
- Observe for signs of ductal closure should the IV infusion infiltrate the tissue — reducing oxygen saturations, reducing to absent peripheral pulses, mottled/grey appearance, decreased urine output, acidosis, cardiovascular collapse.

Antiplatelet therapy

Aspirin

Dose

- 5 mg/kg/day.
- Or less than 10 kg = 37.5 mg daily.
- Greater than 10 kg = 75 mg daily.

Actions

- Reduces platelet aggregation thereby inhibiting thrombus formation in the arterial circulation.
- Clotting is by platelet action in the faster flowing vessels (arteries).

Indications

- Post cardiac surgery, valve and conduit surgery, and to maintain shunt patency (i.e., 4 mm shunts and below, which will be prone to turbulence from the sutures resulting in platelet aggregation).

Contraindications

- Asthma, gastrointestinal ulceration, haemophilia.

Side effects

- Bronchospasm, gastrointestinal and other organ haemorrhage, Reye's syndrome.

Nursing considerations

- Administer after food.

Anticoagulation therapy

Heparin

Dose

- Loading dose 50–100 units/kg IV infusion.
- Maintenance dose starts at 10 units/kg/hour and is increased until APTT is twice normal.
- 10 units/kg/hr, e.g., 500 u × weight in 50 ml diluent @ 1 ml/hour.
- 20 units/kg/hr, e.g., 1000 u × weight in 50 ml diluent @ 1 ml/hour.

Action

- Prevents thrombus formation on the venous side of the circulation.

Indications

- Prophylaxis against thromboembolic events, after valve, conduit and shunt surgery (cavopulmonary anastomosis and Fontan procedures), cardiomyopathy, atrial fibrillation.

Cautions

- Renal and liver impairment, surgery.

Contraindications

- Haemophilia, thrombocytopenia, cerebral haemorrhage, hypertension, hypersensitivity.

Side effects

- Haemorrhage, thrombocytopenia after 5 days, hypersensitivity.

Nursing considerations

- Monitor clotting profile.
- If thrombocytopenic after 5 days stop infusion and ask advice of a haematologist.

Warfarin

Dose

- Oral loading — see own hospital policy. Usually based on Toronto Sick Children's Sliding Scale.
- Maintenance dose 1–5 mg/kg once a day.

Actions

- Antagonises the effects of vitamin K.
- See heparin.

Indications, cautions, contraindications

- See heparin.

Side effects

- Haemorrhage, rash, hypersensitivity, skin necrosis, alopecia, hepatic dysfunction.

Nursing considerations

- Monitor levels — INR (prothrombin time reported as the INR) to be 2–3, APTT twice normal.
- Takes 48–72 hours to work fully therefore cover with heparin infusion for 5–6 days.
- Chloral hydrate enhances the effect of warfarin.
- Patient and parent education.

Antidotes to anticoagulation

Protamine

Dose

- 1 mg IV via short infusion for each 100 units of heparin given at the last dose.

Action

- Reverses the effects of heparin.

Indications

- Profuse haemorrhage following cardiopulmonary bypass, heparin overdose.

Side effects

- Hypotension, bradycardia, dyspnoea, flushing, "anticoagulant" effect if overdosed.

Nursing considerations

- Continuous monitoring of haemodynamic and respiratory parameters.
- Hypocoagulable effects may occur after initial heparin reversal due to protamine metabolism or a heparin rebound effect.

Vitamin K1/phytomenadione

Dose

- IV 300 μg/kg short infusion.

Actions

- Reverses the effects of warfarin.
- Necessary for the production of clotting factors.

Indications

- Warfarin overdosage, haemorrhagic disease of the newborn.

Contraindications

- Hypersensitivity.

Side effects

- Anaphylaxis, peripheral vascular collapse if too fast IV injection, chest constriction, flushing, cyanosis, sweating.

Nursing considerations

- Stop warfarin.

- Monitor for anaphylaxis.
- Monitor degree of haemorrhage.
- Consider use of fresh frozen plasma.
- Measure the prothrombin time.

Antibiotic therapy (prophylaxis in cardiac surgery)

Teicoplanin

Dose

- Cardiac prophylaxis:
    1. Neonate 16 mg/kg/day for one dose IV infusion then 8 mg/kg once day IV infusion.
    2. Infant + 10 mg/kg twice day for three doses, IV bolus, maximum dose 400 mg. After three doses, stop if extubated, otherwise reduce for 5 days to 6 mg/kg twice day IV bolus.

Actions

- Glycopeptide antibiotic active against aerobic and anaerobic gram positive bacteria.

Indications

- Prophylaxis in endocarditis and cardiac surgery.

Side effects

- Nausea, vomiting, diarrhoea, leucopenia, thrombocytopenia, bronchospasm, rash, anaphylaxis.

Nursing considerations

- Full blood count to monitor for blood complications.
- Reduce dose in renal failure.

Netilmicin

Dose

- Cardiac prophylaxis 3 mg/kg/dose twice a day IV bolus.
- Continue for three doses and stop if extubated or if intubated, for 5 days.

Actions

- Aminoglycoside antibiotic active against some gram positive and a large number of gram negative bacteria.

Indications

- Prophylaxis in endocarditis and cardiac surgery.

Cautions

- Renal impairment.

Side effects

- Ototoxic, nephrotoxic, colitis, nausea, vomiting, rash.

Nursing considerations

- Monitor levels — therapeutic levels: trough less than 3 µg/ml, peak 4–12 µg/ml. Levels should be taken at third dose or before each dose in renal failure.
- Avoid use with other ototoxic drugs, e.g., furosemide or ensure both are administered at different times,

Antibiotic therapy (second line therapy)

Cefotaxime

Dose

- 50 mg/kg dose IV bolus twice or four times daily depending on severity of infection.

Actions

- Third generation cephalosporin which is a broad spectrum antibiotic active against gram negative bacteria and some gram positive bacteria.

Indications

- Meningitis, gram negative and positive infections, second line antibiotic post cardiac prophylaxis after blood cultures.

Contraindications

- Hypersensitivity.

Side effects

- Nausea, vomiting, colitis, hypersensitivity, thrombocytopenia, leuco-penia, agranulocytosis, aplastic anaemia, interstitial nephritis.

Gentamicin

Dose

- Neonates under 1.5 kg, 3 mg/kg 18 hourly as IV bolus.
- Neonates over 1.5 kg, 6 mg/kg IV in two divided doses.
- Infants + 7.5 mg/kg in three divided doses as IV bolus.

Actions

- Same as netilmicin.

Indications

- Septicaemia, endocarditis, second line antibiotic post cardiac prophy-laxis after blood cultures.

Contraindications and side effects

- Same as netilmicin.

Nursing considerations

- Drug level monitoring — therapeutic levels peak 5–10 µg/ml, trough less than 2 µg/ml.
- Take before every third dose and one hour after third dose.

Antimicrobial therapy

Selective decontamination of the digestive tract (SDD therapy)

Note

- Comprises 3 oral antimicrobials, plus a paste for the mouth which combines all three antimicrobials.

Dose

	Neonate to 5 yr	5–12 yr	12 yr +
• Colistin	25 mg qds	50 mg qds	100 mg qds
• Amphotericin	100 mg qds	250 mg qds	500 mg qds
• Tobramycin	20 mg qds	40 mg qds	80 mg qds
• SDD paste	Pea sized blob to buccal mucosa qds.		

Action

- Selective decontamination of the digestive tract.
- Prevents translocation of bacteria from the gut to other areas especially the lungs (highest cause of nosocomial pneumonia in ICU patients), thereby preventing systemic inflammatory response syndrome and multi-organ failure.

Indications

- Cardiac surgery, prolonged hypoxic episodes, cardiovascular collapse, prolonged chest opening, cardiac failure.
- Organisms detected on surveillance swabs (rectal and throat swabs performed on admission and thereafter twice weekly).

Side effects

- Risk of side effects low as not absorbed by gut when administered enterally:
  1. Colistin: Parasthesia of mouth and peripheries, muscle weakness, apnoea, nephrotoxicity.
  2. Tobramycin: Same as gentamicin.
  3. Amphotericin: Nausea, vomiting, diarrhoea, headache, hypokalaemia, hypomagnesaemia, hearing loss, diplopia, fits, peripheral neuropathy.

Alkalising agent

Sodium bicarbonate

Dose

- Weight × base deficit × 0.3 divided by 2 = ml of 8.4% bicarbonate = mmols which will half correct the deficit.

Indications

- Acidosis, hyperkalaemia.

Cautions

- Alkalosis, hypernatraemia, hypokalaemia.

Side effects

- Exacerbation of the hypokalaemia, from the sodium, hypertension, fluid retention, pulmonary oedema.

Nursing considerations

- Monitor blood gases, electrolytes and fluid balance.
- Inactivates adrenaline, dopamine and dobutamine therefore use a separate IV line.
- Treat the underlying cause.
- If serum sodium levels high, consider THAM.
- Dilute to 1:10 for peripheral administration or 1:5 for central administration. Only give neat in an emergency situation.

References

A number of texts have been sourced in this chapter[4, 10, 172, 356, 357].

References

1. Feit LR (1998) Genetics in congenital heart disease: strategies. Adv Ped 45: 267–92
2. Waterston T, Helms P, Wardplatt M (1997) Paediatrics. Understanding of child health. Oxford: Oxford Core Texts.
3. Jordan SC, Scott O (1989) Heart disease in paediatrics (3rd ed). London: Butterworths.
4. Park MK (1997) The pediatric cardiology handbook (2nd ed). St Louis: Mosby.
5. Goldmuntz E (1999) Recent advances in understanding the genetic etiology of congenital heart disease. Curr Opin Ped 11(5): 437–43.
6. Grech V, Gaff M (1999) Syndromes and malformations associated with congenital heart disease in a population based study. International Journal Cardiology 68(2): 151–6.
7. Goldmuntz E, Emanuel BS (1997) Genetic disorders of cardiac morphogenesis. The Di George and velocardiofacial syndrome. Circ Res 80(4): 437–43.
8. Benson DW, Basson CT, MacRae CA (1996) New understanding in the genetics of congenital heart disease. Curr Opin Ped 8(5): 505–11.
9. Castaneda AR, Jonas RA, Mayer JE, Hanley FL (1994) Cardiac surgery of the neonate and infant. Philadelphia: WB Saunders.
10. Hazinski MF (1992) Nursing care of the critically ill child (2nd ed). St Louis: Mosby Year Book.
11. Whaley LF, Wong DL (1995) Nursing care of infants and children. St Louis: CV Mosby.
12. Tortora GJ (1995) Principles of anatomy and physiology. Australia: Wiley and Sons.
13. Urban P (1986) Integrating haemodynamic parameters with clinical decision making. Critical Care Nurse 6(2): 48–61.
14. Jowett N (1997) Cardiovascular monitoring. London: Whurr Publishers.
15. Berman W (1991) Handbook of pediatric ECG interpretation. St Louis: Mosby Year Book.
16. Hampton JR (1991) The ECG made easy. Edinburgh: Churchill Livingstone.
17. Perloff JK (1994) Clinical recognition of congenital heart disease (4th ed). Philadelphia: WB Saunders.
18. Tabery S, Daniels O (1997) How classical are the clinical features of the ostium secundum ASD? Cardiology in the Young 7: 294–301.
19. Salih M, Demirel LC, Kurtay G (1998) Prenatal diagnosis of ostium secundum ASD by M-mode fetal echocardiography. Gynecol Obstet Invest 45(1): 68–70.
20. Ross D, English CT, McKay R (1992) Principles of cardiac diagnosis and treatment. A surgeon's guide (2nd ed). London: Springer-Verlag.

21. Zufelt K, Rosenberg HC, Li MD et al. (1998) The ECG and secondum ASD: A re-examination in the era of echocardiogram. Canadian Journal Cardiology 14(2): 227–32.

22. Frankel A, Kuhl HP, Rulands I et al. (1997) Quantitative analysis of the morphology of secundum type atrial septal defects and their dynamic change using transoesophageal 30 echocardiology. Circulation 96–99 (Supp II): 323–7.

23. Gundry SR, Shattuck OU, Razzouk AJ et al. (1998) Facile minimally invasive cardiac surgery via mini sternotomy. Ann Thoracic Surgery 65(4): 1100–4.

24. Hausdorf G, Schneider M, Franbach B et al. (1996) Transcath closure of secundum atrial septal defect with atrial septal defect occlusion system (ASDOS). Heart 75(1): 83–8.

25. Bjornstad PG, Masura J, Thaulow E et al. (1997) Interventional closure of ASD with the Amplatzer device – First clinical experience. Cardiology in the Young 7: 277–83.

26. Nugent EW, Plaut WH, Edwards JE et al. (1994) ASDs. In Hurst (ed) The heart (8th ed). New York: McGraw Hill Inc.

27. Chang CH, Lin PJ, Chu JJ et al. (1998) Surgical closure of atrial septal defect. Minimally invasive cardiac surgery or median sternotomy? Surgical Endoscopy 12(6): 820–4.

28. Grech V (1998) Epidemiology and diagnosis of ventricular septal defect in Malta. Cardiology in the Young 8: 329–36.

29. Ewing CK, Loffredo CA, Beatty TH (1997) Paternal risk factors for isolated membranous VSD. American Journal Medical Genetics 71(1): 42–6.

30. Gatzoulis MA, Li J, Ho S (1997) The echocardiographic anatomy of a ventricular septal defect. Cardiology in the Young 7: 471–84.

31. Abu-Harb M, Hey E, Wren C (1994) Death in infancy from unrecognised congenital heart disease. Arch Dis Child 71: 3–7.

32. Alpert BS, Cook DH, Varghese PJ (1979) Spontaneous closure of small VSDs: 10 year follow-up. Pediatrics 63: 204–6.

33. Carotti A, Marino B, Bevilacqua M et al. (1997) Primary repair of isolated VSD in infancy guided by echocardiogram. American Journal of Cardiology 79(s11): 1498–501.

34. Meijboom K, Szatmari A, Uteris E et al. (1994) Long term follow-up after surgical closure of VSD in infancy and childhood. Journal American College of Cardiology 24: 1358–64.

35. Pacileo G, Pisacane C, Giovanna R et al. (1998) Left ventricular mechanics after closure of the VSD: Influence of the size of the defect and age at surgical repair. Cardiology in the Young 8: 320–8.

36. Van den Heuvel F, Timmers T, Hess J (1995) Morphological, haemodynamic and clinical variables as predictors for the management of isolated VSD. British Heart Journal 73(1): 49–52.

37. Anderson RH, Wilcox BR (1992) The surgical anatomy of VSD. Journal of Cardiac Surgery 7: 17–35.

38. Rogers MC (ed) (1992) Textbook of pediatric intensive care. Baltimore: Williams and Wilkins.

39. Redmond JM, Silove ED, De Giovanni JV et al. (1996) Complete AVSD – Influence of associated cardiac anomalies on surgical management and outcome. European Journal Cardiothoracic Surgery 10(11): 991–5.

40. Clapp S, Perry BL, Farooki ZQ (1990) Downs syndrome, complex atrioventricular septal defect and pulmonary vascular obstructive disease. Journal of Thoracic Cardiovascular Surgery 100: 115.

41. Michielon G, Stellin G, Rizzoli G et al. (1997) Repair of complete AV canal defects in patients younger than four months. Circulation 96(9 Supple II): 316–24.

42. Tweddell JS, Litwin SB, Berger S et al. (1998) 20 years experience with repair of complete AVSD. Ann Thorac Surgery 62(2): 419–24.

43. Campbell RM, Adatia I, Gow EM et al. (1998) Total cavopulmonary anastomosis (Fontan) in children with Down's syndrome. Ann Thorac Surgery 66(2): 523–4.

44. Kirklin JW, Barratt-Boyes BG (eds) (1986) Cardiac surgery: Morphology, diagnostic criteria, natural history, techniques and results. New York: John Wiley and Sons.

45. Weintraub RG (1990) Two patch repair of complete AVSD in the first year of life. Journal Thoracic Cardiovascular Surgery 99: 320.

46. Mavroudis C, Bauler CL (1997) Two patch technique for complete atrioventricular septal canal. Semin Thorac Cardiovascular Surgery 9(1): 35–43.

47. Levine DR, Simpser M (1982) Alveolar hypoventilation and cor pulmonale associated with chronic airway obstruction in infants with Down's. Clinical Paediatrics 21: 25–9.

48. Wilson SK, Hutchins GN, Neill A (1979) Hypertensive pulmonary vascular disease in Down's syndrome. Journal of Paediatrics 95: 722–6.

49. Green T, Thompson T, Johnson D (1981) Furosemide use in premature infants and the appearance of patent ductus arteriosus. American Journal Diseases in Children 135: 239.

50. Heymann MA (1994) Patent ductus arteriosus. In Adams FH, Emmanouilides AC, Riemenschneider TA (eds) Moss' heart disease in infants, children and adolescents, including the fetus and young adult. Baltimore: Williams and Wilkins.

51. Elliot RB, Starling MB, Neutze JM (1975) Medical manipulation of the ductus arteriosus. Lancet 1 (7899): 140–2.

52. Freed MD, Heymann MA, Lewis AB et al. (1981) Prostaglandin E_1 in infants with ductus arteriosus dependent congenital heart disease. Circulation 64(5): 899–905.

53. Rao PJ (1995) Coarctation of the aorta. Semin Nephrol 15(2): 87–105.

54. Shinebourne EA, Tam ASV, Elseed AM et al. (1976) Coarctation in infancy and Childhood. British Heart Journal 38: 375.

55. Hoffman JIE (1990) Congenital heart disease. Pediatric Clinics of North America 37: 25.

56. Pfammatter JP, Ziemer G, Kaulitz R et al. (1996) Isolated coarctation in neonates and infants: Results of resection and end to end anastomosis. Ann Thorac Surgery 62(3): 778–82.

57. Gersony WM (1994) Coarctation of the aorta. In Adams FH, Emmanouilides GC, Riemeischreider TA (eds) Moss' heart disease in infants, children and adolescents including the fetus and young adult. Baltimore: Williams and Wilkins.

58. Gersony WM (1989) Coarctation of the aorta and ventricular septal defect in infancy: Left ventricular volume and management issues. Journal American College of Cardiology 14: 1553.

59. Ho SY, Anderson RH (1979) Coarctation of the aorta. In Godman MJ, Marquis RM (eds) Paediatric cardiology (volume II). Edinburgh: Churchill Livingstone.

60. Rudolph AM, Heyman MA, Spitznas U (1972) Haemodynamic considerations in the development of narrowing of the aorta. American Journal of Cardiology 30: 514.

61. Hasegawa T, Yoshioka Y, Sasaki T et al. (1997) Necrotising enterocolitis in a term infant with coarctation of the aorta complex. Pediatric Surgery Int 12(1): 57–8.

62. Schamberger MC, Lababidi ZA (1998) Successful balloon angioplasty of a coarctation in an infant. Pediatric Cardiology 19(5): 418–19.

63. Jonas RA (1991) Coarctation – Do we need to resect ductal tissue? Ann Thoracic Surgery 54: 604.

64. Golman S, Hernandez J, Pappas G (1986) Results of surgical technique of coarctation of the aorta in the critically ill neonate. Journal of Thoracic Cardiovascular Surgery 91: 732.

65. Connolly JE (1998) Hume memorial lecture. Prevention of spinal cord complications in aortic surgery. American Journal of Surgery 176(2): 92–101.

66. Sealey WC (1979) Complications following repair of coarctation. In Cordell AR, Ellison RG (eds) Complications of intrathoracic surgery. Boston: Little and Brown.

67. van Son JAM, van Aste WNJC, van Lier HJJ et al. (1990) A comparison of coarctation resection flap angiography using ultrasonography monitored post occlusive reactive hyperemia. Journal of Thoracic Cardiovascular Surgery 100: 817.

68. Shenberger JS (1989) Left subclavian flap aortplasty for coarctation: Effects on the forearm, vascular function and growth. Journal American College of Cardiology 14: 953.

69. Cooper SG (1989) Treatment of recoarctation: Balloon dilatation angioplasty. Journal American College Cardiology 14: 413.

70. Huhta JC (1989) Angioplasty for recoarctation. Journal of American College of Cardiology 14: 420.

71. Ozturk OY, Cicek S, Demirkilic U et al. (1995) Cor triatriatum. A report of unusual variant —Triatrial heart. A case report. Angiography 46 (12): 1149–52.

72. Kitchiner D, Jackson M, Malaiya N et al. (1994) Incidence and prognosis of obstruction of the left ventricular outflow tract in Liverpool (1960–1991). A study of 313 patients. British Heart Journal 71(6): 588–95.

73. Friedman WF (1994) Aortic stenosis. In Adams FH, Emmanouilides GC, Riemenschneider TA (eds) Moss' heart disease in infants, children and adolescents, including the fetus and young adult. Baltimore: Williams and Wilkins.

74. Daenen W, Jalali H, Eyskens B et al. (1998) Mid-term results of the Ross procedure. European Journal of Cardiothoracic Surgery 13 (6): 673–7.

75. Reddy VM, McElhinney DB, Hanley FL (1996) The Ross procedure in children. IS Journal Med SG 32(10): 888–91.

76. Jaggers J, Harrison JK, Bashore TM et al. (1998) The Ross procedure: A shorter hospital stay, lower morbidity and cost effective. Ann Thoracic Surgery 65(6): 1553–7.

77. Jones TK, Lupinetti FM (1998) Comparison of the Ross procedure and aortic valve allograft. Ann Thorac Surgery 66(6 Supp): s170–73.

78. Bockoven JR, Wernovsky G, Vetter VL et al. (1998) Perioperative conduction guidelines: Humidifications during mechanical ventilation. Ann Thorac Surg 66(4): 1383–8.

79. Jonas RA (1995) Advances in the surgical care of infants and children with congenital heart disease. Current Opinion in Pediatrics 7: 572–9.

80. Allan DL, Apfel HD, Levenbrown et al. (1998) Surgical repair of interrupted aotic arch with VSD. Cardiology in the Young 8: 217–20.

81. Ravnan JB, Chen E, Golabi M et al. (1996) Chromosome 22q112 microdeletion in velocardiofacial syndrome patients with widely variable manifestations. American Journal of Medical Genetics 66(3): 250–6.

82. Serraf A, Belli E, Roux D et al. (1998) Modified superior approach for repair of supracardiac mixed total anomalous venous drainage. Ann Thoracic Surgery 65(5): 1391–3.

83. Schreiber C, Mazzitelli D, Haehnel JC et al. (1997) The interrupted aortic arch: An overview after 20 years of surgical treatment. Eur Journal Cardiothoracic Surgery 12(3): 466–9.

84. Bojers AJ, Contant CM, Hokken RB et al. (1997) Repair of interrupted aortic arch by dirtect anastomosis. European Journal of Cardiothoracic Surgery 11(1): 100–4.

85. Hirooka K, Fraser CD Jr (1997) First stage neonatal repair of complex aortic arch obstruction or interruption – Recent exposure at Texas Children's Hospital. Texas Heart Institute Journal 24(4): 317–21.

86. Luciani GB, Ackerman RJ, Chang AC et al. (1996) First stage repair of interrupted aortic arch, VSD, subaortic obstruction in neonates. Journal Thoracic and Cardiovascular Surgery 111: 348–58.

87 Jonas RA, Quaegebeur JM, Kirklin JW et al. (1994) Outcomes in patients with interrupted aortic arch and ventricular septal defect. A multiinstitutional study. Journal of Thoracic Cardiovascular Surgery 107(4): 1099–109.

88. Sato S, Akiba T, Nakasato M et al. (1996) Percutaneous balloon aortoplasty for restenosis after extended aortic arch anastomosis for Type B interrupted aortic arch. Pediatric Cardiology 17(4): 275–7.

89. Archiniegas E et al. (1979) Surgical management of congenital vascular rings. Journal of Thoracic Cardiovascular Surgery 77: 721.

90. Wu JM, Chen CT, Wang JN et al. (1996) Upper airway obstruction caused by vascular anomalies in children. Chung Hua Min Kuo Hsiao Erh Ko I Hsuch Hui Tsachih 37(2): 122–7.

91. Pickhardt PJ, Siegel MJ, Gutierrez FR (1997) Vascular rings in the symptomatic child. Frequency of chest radiographic findings. Radiology 203(2): 423–6.

92. Anand R, Dooley, Williams WH et al. (1994) Following of surgical correction of vascular anomaly causing tracheobronchial compression. Pediatric Cardiology 15(2): 58–61.

93. Marino B, Digilio ML, Grazioli S et al. (1996) Associated cardiac anomalies in isolated and syndrome patients with tetralogy of Fallot. American Journal of Cardiology 77(7): 505–8.

94. Nihill MR, McNamara DG, Vick RI (1976) The effects of increased blood viscosity on pulmonary vascular resistance. American Heart Journal 92: 65.

95. Choudary SK, Bhan A, Sharma R et al. (1997) Severe hypoxic biventricular dysfunction in tetralogy of Fallot: Is Blalock shunt the answer? International Journal of Cardiology 61(2): 119–21.

96. Abramov D, Barak J, Raanani E et al. (1997) Early definitive repair of tetralogy of Fallot: Review of 74 cases. Cardiology in the Young 7: 254–7.

97. Gladman G, McCrindle BW, Williams WG et al. (1997) The modified Blalock–Taussig shunt: Clinical impact and morbidity in Fallots tetralogy in the current era. Journal of Thoracic Cardiovascular Surgery 114(1): 25–30.

98. Kaushall SK, Iyer KS, Sharma R et al. (1996) Surgical experience with total correction of Fallots in infancy. Int Journal Cardiology 56(1): 35–40.

99. Knott-Craig, CJ, Elkins EC, Lane MM et al. (1998) 26 year experience with surgical management of tetralogy of Fallot: Risk analysis for mortality or late reintervention. Ann Thorac Surgery 56(1): 35–40.

100. Reddy VM, Liddicoat JR, McElhinney DB et al. (1995) Routine primary repair of tetralogy of Fallot in neonates and infants below three months. Ann Thorac Surgery 60(6 Supp 1): s592–6.

101. Shah MJ, Rome JJ, Rychik T et al. (1997) Outcome of primary repair of tetralogy of Fallot in the newborn period. Unpublished. The Children's Hospital of Philadelphia.

102. Seleim MA, Wu YT, Glenwright K (1995) Relationship between age at surgery and repression of right ventricular hypertrophy in tetralogy of Fallot. Pediatric Cardiology 15(2): 53–5.

103. Jonnson H, IvertT, Brodin LA (1995) Late sudden deaths after repair of tetralogy of Fallot. Electrocardiographic finding associated with survival. Scandinavian Journal Cardiovascular Surgery 29(3): 131–9.

104. Singh GK, Greenberg SB, Yap YS et al. (1998) Right ventricular function and exercise performance late after primary repair of Fallot with transannular patch in infancy. American Journal Cardiology 81(11): 1378–82.

105. Tchervenkov CI, Salasidis G, Cecere R et al. (1997) One stage unifocalization and complete repair in infancy versus multiple stage unifocalization followed by repair for complex heart disease with major aortopulmonary collaterals. Journal of Thoracic Cardiovascular Surgery 114(5): 727–35.

106. Reddy VM, Petrossian E, McElhinney DB et al. (1997) One stage complete unifocalization in infants — When should the VSD be closed? Journal of Thoracic Cardiovascular Surgery 113(5): 858–66.

107. Marvin WJ, Mattoney LH (1994) Pulmonary atresia with intact ventricular septum. In Adams FH, Emmanouilides GI, Riemenschneider TA (eds) Moss' heart disease in infants, children and adolescents, including the fetus and young adult. Baltimore: Williams and Wilkins.

108. Bull C, de Leval MR, Mercanti C (1982) Pulmonary atresia with intact venticular septum. A revised classification. Circulation 66: 266–72.

109. Choi YH, Seo JW, Choi JY et al. (1998) Morphology of the tricuspid valve in pulmonary atresia with intact ventricular septum. Pediatric Cardiology 19(5): 381–9.

110. Hausforf G, Gravinghoff L, Keck EW (1987) Effects of persisting myocardial sinusoids of left ventricular performance in pulmonary atresia with intact ventricular septum. European Heart Journal 8(2): 291.

111. Calder AL, Co EE, Sage MD (1987) Coronary arterial abnormalities in pulmonary atresia with intact ventricular septum. American Journal of Cardiology 59: 436.

112. Deshpande J, Vaideewar P, Sivaraman A (1996) Coronary artery — Intra myocardial sinosoid communication in a case of pulmonary atresia with intact ventricular septum. Indian Journal of Pathology and Microbiology 39(2): 143–5.

113. Hanley FL, Sade RM, Blackstone EH (1997) Pulmonary atresia with intact ventricular septum. Journal of Thoracic Cardiovascular Surgery 105: 406–26.

114. Dyamenahalli G, Hanna BD, Sharratt GP (1997) Pulmonary atresia in intact ventricular septum. Management of coronary artery abnormalities. Cardiology in the Young 7: 80–7.

115. Gibbs JL, Blackburn ME, Uzun O et al. (1997) Laser valvotomy with balloon valvoplasty for pulmonary atresia with intact ventricular septum. Heart 77(3): 225–8.

116. Ovaert C, Qureshi SA, Rosenthal E et al. (1998) Growth of the right ventricle after successful transcatheter pulmonary valvotomy in neonates and infants with pulmonary atresia and intact ventricular septum. Journal of Thoracic Cardiovascular Surgery 115(5): 1055–62.

117. Joshi SV, Brown WI, Mee RBBB (1986) Pulmonary atresia with intact ventricular septum. Journal of Thoracic Cardiovascular Surgery 91: 192.

118. Mair DD, Seward JB, Driscoll DJ et al. (1985) Surgical repair of Ebstein's anomaly: Selection of patients and early and late postoperative results. Circulation 72(Supp 11): 70–6.

119. Najm HK, Williams WG, Coles JG (1997) Pulmonary atresia with intact ventricular septum: Results of Fontan. Ann Thorac Surgery 63(3): 669–75.

120. Planche C, Lacour-Gayet F, Serraf A (1998) Arterial switch. Ped Cardiology 19(4): 297–307.

121. Van Praagh R, Van Praagh S (1966) Isolated ventricular inversion. A consideration of the morphogenesis, definition and diagnosis of nontransposed and transposed great vessels. American Journal Cardiology 17: 395.

122. Nakajima Y, Momma K, Seguchi M et al. (1996) Pulmonary hypertension in patients with complex transposition of the great arteries: Midterm results after surgery. Ped Cardiology 17(2): 104–7.

123. Berry IM, Padbury J, Novoatakara L et al. (1998) Premature closing of foramen ovale in TGA with intact ventricular septum: Rare cause of sudden death. Pediatric Cardiology 19(3): 246–8.

124. Jamjureeruk V, Sangtawesin C, Layangool T (1997) Balloon atrial septostomy under 2D echocardiographic control: A new look. Pediatric Cardiology 18(3): 197–200.

125. Karl TR, Weintraub RG, Brizard CP et al. (1997) Senning plus arterial switch for discordant transpostion. Ann Thorac Surgery 64(2): 495–502.

126. Losay J, Hougen TJ (1997) Treatment of TGA. Current Opinion Cardiology 12(1): 84–90.

127. Testolin L, Stellin G, Bianco R et al. (1997) Supravalvular pulmonary stenosis following arterial switch for complex transposition: Aetiological and surgical considerations. Cardiology in the Young 7: 31–36.

128. Luciani GB, Mazzucco A (1997) Rastelli procedure for repair of TGA complex. Ann Thorac Surg 63(4): 1152–5.

129. Bryant RM, Shirley RL, Ott DA et al. (1998) Left ventricular performance following arterial switch operation: Use of non-invasive wall stress analysis in the posterative period. Critical Care Medicine 26(5): 926–32.

130. BuLock FA, Tometzki AJ, Kitchiner DJ et al. (1998) Balloon expandable stents for systemic venous pathway stenosis late after Mustard's operation. Heart 79(3): 225–9.

131. Saxena A, Fong LV, Ogilvie BC et al. (1990) Use of balloon dilatation to treat supravalvar pulmonary stenosis developing after anatomical correction for complete transposition. British Heart Journal 64: 151.

132. Bonner D, Bonhoeffer P, Piechaud JF et al. (1996) Long term fate of coronary arteries after arterial switch in newborns with TGA. Heart 76(3): 274–9.

133. Lucas RV, Krabell KA (1989) Anomalous venous connection, pulmonary and systemic. In Adams FH, Emmanouilides GC, Riemenschneider TA (eds) Moss' heart disease in infants, children and adolescents (4th ed). Baltimore: Williams and Wilkins.

134. Bharati S, Lev M (1973) Congenital abnormalities of the pulmonary veins. Cardiovascular Clinics 5: 23.

135. Delisle G, Aldo M, Calder AI (1991) Total pulmonary venous pulmonary connection. American Heart Journal 99: 76.

136. VanderVelde M, Parness SA, Colan SO (1991) 2D echo in pre and postoperative management of total anomalous pulmonary venous connection. Journal American College Cardiology 18: 1746.

137. Sando S, Brawn W, Mee RBB (1989) Total anomalous pulmonary venous drainage. Journal of Thoracic Cardiovascular Surgery 97: 886.

138. Van Mierop LHS, Kutsche LM, Victorica BE (1994) Ebstein's anomaly. In Adams FH, Emmanouilides AC, Reimenschneider TA (eds) Moss' heart disease in infants, children and adolescents, including the fetus and young adult. Baltimore: Williams and Wilkins.

139. Augustin N, Schmidt J, Habelmann P et al. (1997) Results after surgical repair of Ebstein's anomaly. Ann Thorac Surg 63(6): 1650–6.

140. Vargas FJ, Mengo G, Granja MA et al. (1998) Tricuspid annuloplasty and ventricular plication for Ebstein's malformation. Ann Thoracic Surgery 65(6): 1755–7.

141. Kaulitz R, Ziemer G (1995) Modified Fontan procedure for Ebstein's anomaly of the tricuspid valve — An alternative approach preserving Ebstein's anomaly. Journal of Thoracic Cardiovascular Surgery 43(5): 275–9.

142. Chauvaud S, Fuzellier JF, Berrebi A et al. (1998) Bidirectional cavopulmonary shunt associated with ventriculo and valvuloplasty in Ebstein's anomaly — Benefits in high risk patients. European Journal of Cardiothoracic Surgery 13(5): 514–19.

143. Endo M, Ohmi M, Sato K et al. (1998) Tricuspid valve closure for the neonate with Ebstein's anomaly. Ann Thorac Surgery 65(2): 540–2.

144. Borsattino-Callow L (1992) Current strategies in the nursing care of infants with hypoplastic left heart syndrome undergoing first stage palliation with the Norwood operation. Heart and Lung 20: 463–70.

145. Charpie JR, Kulik TJ (1996) Preoperative and postoperative management of infants with hypoplastic left heart syndrome. Progress in Pediatric Cardiology 5: 49–56.

146. Cohen DM, Allen MD (1997) New developments in the treatment of hypoplastic left heart syndrome. Current Opinion in Cardiology 12: 44–50.

147. Norwood WI (1991) Hypoplastic left heart sysndrome. Ann Thorac Surgery 52: 688–95.

148. Jonas RA, Lang P, Hansen DD et al. (1986) First stage palliation of hypoplastic left heart syndrome. Journal of Thoracic Cardiovascular Surgery 92: 6–13.

149. Barnea O, Austin EH, Richman B et al. (1994) Balancing the circulation: Theoretical optimization of pulmonary and systemic flow ratio in hypoplastic left heart syndrome. Journal American Coll Cardiology 24(5): 1376–81.

150. Hickey PR, Hansen DD, Wessel DC et al. (1985) Blunting of stress responses in the pulmonary artery of infants by fentanyl. Anesthetics and Analgesia 64: 1137–42.

151. BuLock FA, Stumper O, Jagtap R et al. (1995) Surgery for infants with hypoplastic systemic ventricles and severe outflow obstruction: Early results with the modified Norwood procedure. British Heart Journal 73(5): 456–61.

152. Bartram U, Grunenfelder J, van Praagh R (1997) Causes of death after the modified Norwood procedure: A survey of 122 post mortem cases. Ann Thorac Surg 64(6): 1795–802.

153. Burakovsky VI, Podzoikov VP, Ivanitsky AV et al. (1997) Surgical treatment for DORV. Cardiology in the Young 7: 22–30.

154. Anderson RH, Ho SY, Wilcox BR (1996) The surgical anatomy of VSD Part IV — DORV. Journal of Cardiac Surgery 11(1): 2–11.

155. Serraf A, Jonas RA, Burke RP et al. (1997) Univentricular repair for complex double right ventricle and transposition of the great arteries. Cardiology in the Young 7: 207–14.

156. Sakamoto K, Charpentier A, Popescu S et al. (1997) Transaortic approach in double outlet right ventricle with subaortic VSD. Ann Thorac Surgery 64(3): 856–8.

157. McElhinnay DB, Reddy VM, Rajasinghe HA et al. (1998) Trends in the management of truncal valve insufficiency. Ann Thoracic Surgery 65(2): 517–24.

158. LaCour-Gayet F, Serraf A, Komiya T et al. (1996) Truncus arteriosus repair: Influence of techniques of RVOT reconstruction. Journal of Thoracic Cardiovascular Surgery 111(4): 849–56.

159. Black MD, Adatia I, Freedom RM (1998) Truncal valve repair: Initial experience in neonates. Ann Thoracic Surgery 65(6): 1737–40.

160. Rajasinghe HA, McElhinney DB, Reddy VM et al. (1997) Longterm follow up of truncus arteriosus repaired in infancy — A 20 year experience. Journal of Cardiothoracic Surgery 113(5): 869–78.

161. Anderson RH, Becker AE, Arnold R et al. (1974) The conducting tissues in congenitally corrected transposition. Circulation 50: 911.

162. Prieto LR, Hordof AJ, Secic M et al. (1998) Progressive tricuspid valve disease in patients with congenitally corrected transposition of the great arteries. Circulation 98(10): 997–1005.

163. Stumper O, Wright JG, DeGiovanni JV et al. (1995) Combined atrial and arterial switch procedure for congenital transposition with VSD. British Heart Journal 73(5): 479–82.

164. Van Praagh R, Papagiannis J, Grunenfelder J et al. (1998) Pathologic anatomy of corrected TGA: Medical and surgical implications. American Heart Journal 135 (5 pt 1): 772–85.

165. Reddy VM, McElhinney DB, Silverman NA et al. (1997) The double switch procedure for anatomical repair of congenitally corrected transposition of the great arteries in infants and children. Eur Heart Journal 18(9): 1470–77.

166. Presbitero P, Somerville J, Rabajoli F et al. (1995) Corrected transposition of the great arteries without associated defects in adult patients: Clinical profile and follow up. British Heart Journal 74(1): 5–59.

167. DeLeon SY (1986) Fontan type operation for complex heart lesions. Surgical considerations to improve survival. Journal of Thoracic Cardiovascular Surgery 92: 1029.

168. Gale AW et al. (1979) Modified Fontan operation for univentricular heart and complicated congenital lesions. Journal of Thoracic Cardiovascular Surgery 78: 831.

169. Matsuda H et al. (1987) Problems in modified Fontan operation of univentricular heart of the right ventricular type. Circulation 76(Supp II): 11–45.

170. Ahmadi A, Rein J, Hellberg K et al. (1995) Percutaneously adjustable pulmonary artery bands. Ann Thorac Surg 60(6 Supp): s520–2.

171. Schlensak C, Sarai K, Gildein HP et al. (1997) Pulmonary artery banding with a novel percutaneously bidirectionally adjustable device. Eur Journal Cardiothoracic Surgery 12(6): 931–3.

172. Bojar RM (1989) Manual of perioperative care in cardiac and thoracic surgery. Boston: Blackwell Scientific.

173. Tometzki A, Houston AB, Redington AN et al. (1995) Closure of BT shunt using a new detachable coil device. British Heart Journal 73(4): 383–4.

174. Godart F, Qureshi SA, Simha A (1998) Effects of modified and classic Blalock–Taussig shunts on the pulmonary artery tree. Ann Thoracic Surgery 66(2): 512–17.

175. Lemes V, Ritter SB, Messina J et al. (1995) Enhancement of ventilation mechanics following bidirectional superior cavopulmonary anastomosis in patients with single ventricle. Journal Card Surg 10(2): 119–24.

176. Donofrio MT, Jacobs ML, Spray TL et al. (1998) Acute changes in preload, afterload and systolic function after superior cavopulmonary connection. Ann Thorac Surg 65(2): 503–8.

177. Angelini A, Frescura C, Stellin G et al. (1998) Cavopulmonary anastomosis in staging towards Fontan operation: Pathologic substrates. Ann Thorac Surg 66(2): 659–63.

178. Podzolkov VP, Zaets SB, Chiaureli MC et al. (1997) Comparative assessment of Fontan operation in modifications of atriopulmonary and total cavopulmonary anastomosis. Eur Journal of Cardiothoracic Surgery 11(3): 458–65.

179. Choussat A, Fontan F, Berse P et al. (1977) Selection criteria for Fontan's procedure. In Anderson RH, Shinebourne EA (eds) Paediatric Cardiology. Edinburgh: Churchill Livingstone.

180. Kaulitz R, Ziemer G (1995) Modified Fontan procedure for Ebstein's anomaly of the tricuspid valve — An alternative approach preserving Ebstein's anomaly. Journal of Thoracic Cardiovascular Surgery 43(5): 275–9.

181. Kruetzer GO et al. (1982) Atriopulmonary anastomosis. Journal of Thoracic Cardiovascular Surgery 83: 427.

182. Zellers TM, Brown K (1996) Protein losing enteropathy after modified Fontan operation: Oral prednisolone treatment with biopsy and laboratory proved improvement. Ped Cardiology 17(2): 115–17.

183. Cecchin F, Johnstude CL, Perry JC et al. (1995) Effect of age and surgical technique on symptomatic arrhythmias after Fontan procedure. American Journal of Cardiology 76(5): 386–91.

184. Sommer RJ, Recto M, Golinko RJ et al. (1996) Transcatheter coil occlusion of surgical fenestration after Fontan circulation 94(3): 249–52.

185. Del Pont JM, De Cicco LT, Vastalitis C et al. (1995) Infective endocarditis in children: Clinical analysis and evaluation of two diagnostic criteria. Pediatric Infective Diseases Journal 14(12): 1079–86.

186. Sable CA, Rome JJ, Martin GR et al. (1995) Indications for echocardiogram in the diagnosis of infective endocarditis in children. American Journal Cardiology 75(12): 810–4.

187. Delahage F, Goulet V, Lacassin F et al. (1995) Characteristics of infective endocarditis in France in 1991 — A one year survey. European Heart Journal 16(3): 394–401.

188. Erbal R, Liu F, Ge J et al. (1995) Infection of high-risk subgroups in infectious endocarditis and the role of echocardiography. European Heart Journal 16(5): 588–602.

189. Martin JM, Neches WH, Wald ER (1997) Infective endocarditis: 35 year experience at a children's hospital. Clin Infect Disease 24(4): 669–75.

190. Kaplan EL, Schulman SR (1994) Bacterial endocarditis. In Adams FH, Emmanouilides GC, Riemenschneider TA (eds) Moss' heart disease in infants, children and adolescents, including the fetus and young adult. Baltimore: Williams and Wilkins.

191. Newberger JW, Nadas AJ (1982) Infective endocarditis. Ped Review 3(7): 226–30.

192. Suddaby EC (1996) Viral myocarditis in children. Critical Care Nurse 16(4): 73–82.

193. Fairley CK, Ryan M, Wall PG et al. (1996) The organisms reported to cause infectious myocarditis and pericarditis in England and Wales. Journal of Infection 32(3): 223–5.

194. Caforio AC, McKenna WJ (1996) Recognition and optimum management of myocarditis. Drugs 52(4): 515–25.

195. Kleinert S, Weintraub RG, Wilkinson JC et al. (1997) Myocarditis in children with dilated cardiomyopathy: Incidence and outcome after dual treatement of immunosuppression. Journal of Heart and Lung Transplant 16(12): 1248–54.

196. Mason JW, O'Connell JB, Heiskowitz A (1995) A clinical trial of immunosuppression treatment for myocarditis. The myocarditis treatment trial investigators. New England Journal of Medicine 333(5): 269–75.

197. Finkelstein Y, Adler J et al. (1997) A new classification for pericarditis associated with meningococcal infection. European Journal Pediatrics 156(8): 585–8.

198. Yazigi A, Abou Charof LC (1998) Colchicine for recurrent pericarditis in children. Acta Paediatrics 87(5): 603–4.

199. Marcolongo R, Russo R, Laveder F et al. (1995) Immunosuppressive therapy prevents recurrent pericarditis. Journal Am Cp Cardop 26(5): 1276–9.

200. Luppi P, Rudert WA, Zanone MM et al. (1998) Idiopathic dilated cardiomyopathy: A superantigen-driven autoimmune disease. Circulation 98(8): 777–89.

201. Keeling PJ, Gang Y, Smith G et al. (1995) Familial dilated cardiomyopathy in the UK. British Heart Journal 73(5): 417–21.

202. Marion B (1994) Cardiomyopathies. In Adams FH, Emmanouilides GI, Riemenschneider TA (eds) Moss' heart disease in infants, children and adolescents, including the fetus and young adult. Baltimore: Williams and Wilkins.

203. Muller G, Ulmer HE, Hoger KJ, Wolf D (1995) Cardiac dysrrhythmias in children with idiopathic dilated or hypertrophic cardiomyopathy. Pediatric Cardiology 16(2): 56–60.

204. Waagstein F (1995) The role of beta blockers in dilated cardiomyopathy. Current Opinions in Cardiology 10(3): 322–31.

205. Gojarski RJ, Towbin JA (1995) Recent advances in etiology, diagnosis and treatment of myocarditis and cardiomyopathies in children. Current Opinions in Pediatrics 7(5): 587–94.

206. Ni J, Bowles NG, Kim YH et al. (1997) Viral infection of the myocardium in endocardial fibroelastosis — Molecular evidence for the role of mumps virus as an etiologic agent. Circulation 95(1): 133–9.

207. Bonne G, Carrier L, Richard P et al. (1998) Familial hypertrophic cardiomyopathy: From mutations to functional defects. Circulation Research 83(6): 580–93.

208. Maki S, Ikeda H, Muro A et al. (1998) Predictors of sudden cardiac death in hypertrophic cardiomyopathy. American Journal of Cardiology 82(6): 774–8.

209. Futterman LG, Lemberg L (1995) Sudden deaths in athletes. American Journal of Critical Care 4(3): 239–43.

210. Valgaeren G, Conraads V, Colpaert C et al. (1998) Sudden death in hypertrophic cardiomyopathy: Risk stratification and prevention. Acta Cardiology 53(1): 23–9.

211. Denfield SW, Rosenthal G, Gajarski RJ et al. (1997) Restrictive cardiomyopathies in childhood. Etiologies and natural history. Texas Heart Inst Journal 24(1): 38–44.

212. Andersson B, Caidahl K, di Lenarda A et al. (1996) Changes in early and late diastolic filling patterns induced by longterm adrenergic beta-blockage in patients with idiopathic cardiomyopathy. Circulation 94(4): 673–82.

213. Cetta F, O'Leary PW, Seward JB et al. (1995) Idiopathic restrictive cardiomyopathy in childhood: Diagnostic features and clinical course. Mayo Clin Prac 70(7): 634–40.

214. Burns JC, Shike J, Gordon JB et al. (1996) Sequelae of Kawasaki disease in adolescence and young adults. Journal American College Cardiology 28(1): 253–7.

215. Shulman ST, De Inocencio J, Hirsch R (1995) Kawasaki disease. Pediatric Clinics of North America 42(5): 1205–22.

216. Takahashi M, Lurie PR (1994) Abnormalities and diseases of coronary vessels. In Adams FH, Emmanouilides AC, Riemenschnieder TA (eds) Moss' heart disease in infants, children and adolescents including the fetus and young adult. Baltimore: Williams and Wilkins.

217. Rosenfield EA, Corydon KE, Shulman ST (1995) Kawasaki disease in infants less than one year of age. Journal of Pediatrics 126(4): 524–9.

218. Kato H, Sugimura T, Akagi T et al. (1996) Longterm consequences of Kawasaki disease. A 10–12 year follow-up study of 594 patients. Circulation 94(6): 1379–85.

219. Jonas RA, Elliot MJ (1994) Cardiopulmonary bypass in neonates, infants and young children. Oxford: Butterworth-Heinmann.

220. Lake C (1998) Pediatric cardiac anesthesia. (3rd ed). New Jersey: Appleton and Lange Prentice Hall.

221. VanOerveren W, Kazatchkins MD, Descampshatscha B et al. (1985) Deleterious effects of cardiopulmonary bypass. A prospective study of bubble versus membrane oxygenators. Journal Thoracic Cardiovascular Surgery 89: 888–99.

222. Pearson DT, McArdle B, Poslad SJ et al. (1986) A clinical evaluation of the perfusion characteristics of the membrane and 5 bubble oxygenators: Haemocompatability studies. Perfusion 1: 81–98.

223. Treasure T (1989) Interventions to reduce cerebral injury during cardiac surgery — The effect of arterial line filtration. Perfusion 4: 147–52.

224. William ED, Seifen AB, Lawson NW et al. (1979) Pulsatile perfusion versus conventional high flow non pulsatile perfusion for rapid core cooling and rewarming of infants for circulatory arrest in cardiac operations. Journal Thoracic Cardiovascular Surgery 78: 667–77.

225. Dunn J, Kirsch MM, Harness J et al. (1974) Hemodynamic metabolic and hematological effects of pulsatile cardiopulmonary bypass. Journal of Thoracic Cardiovascular Surgery 63: 138–47.

226. Swanson DK, Dufek JH, Khan DR et al. (1980) Left ventricular function after preserving the heart for 24 hours at 15°C. Journal of Thoracic Cardiovascular Surgery 79: 755–60.

227. Wesselink RM, de Boer A, Morshuis WJ et al. (1997) Cardiopulmonary bypass time has important influence on morbidity and mortality. European Journal Cardiovascular Surgery 11(6): 1141–45.

228. Allen SM, Bonser RS (1993) The cerebral sequelae of cardiopulmonary bypass. Current Anaesthesia and Critical Care 4: 141–46.

229. Kupst MJ (1976) Improving physician–parent communication. Clinical Paediatrics 15(1): 27–30.

230. Erikson EH (1963) Childhood and society (2nd ed). New York: Norton and Co.

231. Perrin EC, Gerrity PS (1984) Development of children with chronic illness. Pediatric Clinics of North America 31(1): 19–31.

232. Crummer MB, Carter V (1993) Critical pathways — The pivotal tool. Journal Cardiovascular Nursing 7(4): 30–7.

233. Evers C, Odom S Latulip-Gardner J et al. (1994) Developing a critical pathway for orientation. American Journal of Critical Care 3(3): 217–23.

234. Coffey RJ, Richards JS, Remment CS et al. (1992) An introduction to critical paths. Quality Management in Health Care 1(1): 45–54.

235. Kitchiner D, Bundred P (1996) Integrated care pathways. Archives of Disease in Childhood 75: 166–8.

236. Robin I, Donohoe E, Dennison ST (1990) Understanding determinants of cardiac output. Nursing 20(7): 36–41.

237. Slota MC (1987) Assessing systemic perfusion in the child. Critical Care Nurse 7(4): 68–73.

238. Stephenson G (1995) Low cardiac output — A nursing challenge in cardiac ICU. Journal of Neonatal and Paediatric Critical Care 1(2): 10–24.

239. Terry N, Murphy G, Bennett EJ (1992) Low technique high touch perfusion assessment. AJN 92(5): 36–46.

240. Moat NE, Lamb RK, Edwards JC et al. (1992) Induced hypothermia in the management of refractory low cardiac output states following cardiac surgery in infants and children. European Journal of Cardiothoracic Surgery 6(11): 579–84.

241. Shattock MJ, Bers DM (1987) Inotropic response to hypothermia and the temperature dependence of ryanodine action in isolated rabbit and rat ventricular muscle. Circulation 61: 761–71.

242. Engle MA (1975) Immunologic and virologic studies in post pericardiotomy syndrome. Journal of Pediatrics 87: 1103.

243. Engle MA, Zabriskic JB, Senterfit LB et al. (1980) Viral illness and post pericardiotomy syndrome. A prospective study in children. Circulation 62: 1151–8.

244. Hakimi M, Walters HL, Pinsky WW et al. (1994) Delayed sternal closure after neonatal cardiac operations. Journal of Thoracic Cardiovascular Surgery 107(3): 935–43.

245. Odim JNR, Tchervenkov CI, Dobell ARC (1989) Delayed sternal closure: A life saving maneuver after early operation for complex congenital heart disease in the neonate. Journal of Thoracic Cardiovascular Surgery 98: 413–6.

246. Fanning WJ, Vasko JS, Kilman JW (1987) Delayed sternal closure after cardiac surgery. Ann Thorac Surgery 44: 169–72.

247. Mestres CA, Pomar JL, Acosta M et al. (1991) Delayed sternal closure for life threatening complications in cardiac operations. Ann Thorac Surg 51: 773–6.

248. Tabbutt S, Duncan BW, McLaughlin D et al. (1997) Delayed sternal closure after cardiac operation in the pediatric population. Journal of Thoracic Cardiovascular Surgery 113(5): 886–93.

249. British Medical Journal (1997) Advanced paediatric life support. London: BMJ Publishing Group.

250. Watson JE (1979) Medical-surgical nursing and related physiology. Philadelphia: WB Saunders.

251. Gillis J (1986) Results in patient pediatric resuscitation. Critical Care Medicine 14: 469.

252. Dickenson D, Johnson M (1983) Death dying and bereavement. London: Age Publications.

253. Gregory C (1995) I should have been with Lisa when she died. Accident and Emergency Nursing 3(3): 136–8.

254. Hector W, Whitefield S (1982) Nursing care for the dying patient and family. London: William Heineman.

255. Hanson K, Strawser D (1992) Family presence during cardiopulmonary resuscitation: Foote Hospital Emergency Department's 9 year perspective. Journal of Emergency Nursing 18(2): 104–6.

256. Farrell M (1988) Dying and bereavement: The role of critical care nurses. Intensive and Critical Care Nursing 5(1): 39–45.

257. Osuagwu C (1993) ED codes: Keep the family out. Journal of Emergency Nursing 17(6): 363.

258. Jenkins A (1994) Nurses attitudes to the teaching and training of cardiopulmonary resuscitation. Journal of Clinical Nursing 3(3): 193–4.

259. Chellel A (1993) Cardiopulmonary resuscitation: The problems and solutions. Nursing Standard 10(7): 33–6.

260. Suddaby EC (1996) Viral myocarditis in children. Critical Care Nurse 16(4): 73–82.

261. Hewlett-Packard (1997) Guide to physiology of pressure monitoring. Massachusetts: Hewlett-Packard.

262. Windsor J (1998) Haematology management. Care of Critically Ill 14(2): 44–9.

263. Paster SB, Middleton P (1975) Roentgenographic evaluation of umbilical arteries and veins catheters. JAMA 231: 742–6.

264. Kantrowitz A, Wastie T (1986) Intra-aortic balloon pumping 1967 through 1982. Analysis of complication in 733 patients. American Journal of Cardiology 57: 976–83.

265. Pollock JC, Charlton MD, Williams WG et al. (1980) Intra-aortic balloon pumping in children. Ann Thoracic Surgery 29: 522.

266. Anella J, McClosky A, Vieweg C (1988) Nursing dynamics of pediatric intra-aortic balloon pumping. Critical Care Nurse 10(4): 24–37.

267. Booker PD (1997) Intra-aortic balloon pumping in younger children. Paediatric Anaesthesia 7: 501–7.

268. Akoma-Agyin C, Kejriwal NK, Franks R et al. (1999) Intra aortic balloon pumping. Ann Thorac Surg 67: 1415–20.

269. Heath D, Edwards JE (1958) The pathology of hypertensive vascular disease. A description of 6 grades of structural changes in pulmonary arteries with special reference to congenital cardiac septal defects. Circulation 18: 533.

270. Beghetti M, La Scala G, Belli D et al. (2000) Etiology and management of pediatric chylothorax. Journal of Pediatrics 136(5): 653–8.

271. Bessone LN, Ferguson TB, Burford TH (1971) Chylothorax. Ann Thoracic Surgery 12: 527.

272. Pierce LMB (1995) Guide to mechanical ventilation and intensive respiratory care. Philadelphia: WB Saunders.

273. Rivera R, Tibballs J (1992) Complications of endotracheal intubation and mechanical ventilation in infants and children. Critical Care Medicine 20(2): 193–9.

274. Mecca RS (1986) Complications of therapy. In Kirby RR, Taylor RW (eds) Respiratory failure. Chicago: Year Book Med Publishers.

275. Orlowski JP, Ellis NG, Amin NP et al. (1980) Complications of airway intrusion in 100 consecutive cases in a PICU. Critical Care Medicine 8: 324–31.

276. Boothroyd AE, Murthy BVS, Darbyshire A, Petros AJ (1996) Right upper lobe collapse in intubated children. Acta Paediatrics 85: 1422–5.

277. Knox A (1993) Performing endotracheal suction on children: A literature review and the implications for nursing practice. Intensive and Critical Care Nursing 9: 48–54.

278. Czernik RE, Stone KS, Everhart CC et al. (1997) Differential effects of continuous versus intermittent suction on tracheal tissue. Heart and Lung 20: 141–51.

279. Stone KS, Talaganis SAT, Preusser B et al. (1991) The effects of lung hyperinflation and endotracheal suctioning on heart rate and rhythm in patients post cardiopulmonary bypass. Heart and Lung 20: 443–50.

280. Ackerman M (1985) Use of bolus normal saline instillations in artificial airways: Is it useful or necessary? Heart and Lung 14: 505–6.

281. Young CS (1984) A review of the adverse effects of airway suction. Physiotherapy 70(3): 104–8.

282. Link WJ, Spaeth EE, Wahle WM et al. (1976) The influence of the suction catheter tip design on tracheobronchial trauma and fluid aspiration efficiency. Anaesthetics and Analgesia 55: 290–7.

283. Branson RD (1991) Humidification of inspired gases during mechanical ventilation. Chest 3: 55–60.

284. Fisher and Paykell (1995) Why humidification is vital. Auckland New Zealand: Fisher and Paykell.

285. Misset B, Escudier B, Rivara D et al. (1991) Heat and moisture exchanger vs heated humidifier during longterm ventilation. Chest 100: 160–3.

286. Branson RD, Campbell RS, Chatburn RL et al. (1992) Clinical practice guidelines: Humidification during mechanical ventilation. Respiratory Care 37: 887–90.

287. Craven DE, Coularte TA, Make BJ (1984) Contamination condensate in mechanical ventilator circuits. American Rev Resp Dis 129: 625–8.

288. Nellcor Incorporated (1991) Principles of pulse oximetry. California: Nellcor.

289. Higgenbottam T, Pepke-Zaba J, Scott J et al. (1988) Inhaled EDRF in primary hypertension. American Rev Resp Disease 137(Supp): 4.

290. Mulnier C, Evans T (1995) Acute RDS. Care of the Critically Ill 11(5): 182–6.

291. Jacobs BR, Smith DJ, Zingarelli B et al. (2000) Soluble nitric oxide donor and surfactant improve oxygenation and pulmonary hypertension in porcine lung injury. Nitric Oxide 4(4): 412–22.

292. Furchgott RF, Zawadski JV (1980) The obligatory role of endothelial cells in the relaxation of arterial smooth muscle by acetylcholine. Nature 288: 373–6.

293. Power D, Boyle M (1995) Nitric oxide: A positive poison. Australian Critical Care 8(1): 11–15.

294. Ignarro IS, Buga JM, Wood KS (1987) Endothelium derived relaxing factor produced and released from the artery and vein is nitric oxide. Proc Natl Acad Sci USA 84: 9265–9.

295. Kam PCA, Govender G (1994) Nitric oxide: Basic science and clinical applications. Anaesthesia 49: 515–21.

296. Woodrow P (1997) Nitric oxide: Some nursing implications. Intensive and Critical Care Nursing 13: 87–92.

297. Nathan C (1992) Nitric oxide is a secretory product of mammalian cells. FASEB Journal 6: 3051–64.

298. Warner TD, DeNucci G, Vane JR (1989) Comparison of the survival of EDRF and nitric oxide within the isolated perfused mesenteric arterial bed of the rat. British Journal Pharmacology 97: 777–82.

299. Holden K (1994) Nitric oxide — From exhaust fumes to medical revolution. Pharmaceutical Journal 252: 402–7.

300. Jones C (1998) Inhaled nitric oxide: Are the safety issues being addressed? Intensive and Critical Care Nursing 14: 271–5.

301. Ismail-Zade I, Oduro-Dominah A (1997) Nitric oxide: Update on basic science and clinical implications. Care of the Critically Ill 13(4): 130–4.

302. Rykerson S, Thompson J, Wessel DL (1995) Inhalation of nitric oxide. Nursing Clinics of North America 30(2): 381–90.

303. Petros A, Lamb G, Leone A et al. (1994) Effects of a nitric oxide synthase inhibitor in humans with septic shock. Cardiovascular Research 28(1): 34–9.

304. Frosteil C, Fratacci M, Wain J et al. (1998) Inhaled nitric oxide: A selective vasodilator, reversing hypoxic pulmonary vasoconstriction. Circulation 83(6): 2038–47.

305. Young J (1994) A universal nitric oxide delivery system. British Journal Anaesthesia 73(5): 700–2.

306. Foubert L, Latimer R, Oduro A (1993) Vasodilators. Current Opinions in Anaesthesiology 6: 152–7.

307. du Plessis AJ (1998) Neurological care. In Chang (ed) Pediatric cardiac intensive care. Baltimore: Williams and Wilkins.

308. Benson D (1989) Changing profile of congenital heart disease. Pediatrics 83(5): 790–1.

309. Cucchiara RF, Noback CR, Faust RJ (1982) Protection of the brain from ischaemic and embolic phenomena. In Tarhan S (ed) Cardiovascular anesthesia and postoperative care. Chicago: Year Book Medical Publishers.

310. van Houten J, Rothman A, Bejar R (1993) Echoencephalographic findings in infants with congenital heart disease. Pediatric Research 33(4): 376a.

311. Glauser T, Rorke L, Weinberg P et al. (1990) Acquired neuropathologic lesions associated with hypoplastic left heart syndrome. Pediatrics 85(6): 991–1000.

312. Volpe JJ (1994) Intracranial haemorrhage. In Volpe JJ (ed) Neurology of the newborn (3rd ed). Philadelphia: WB Saunders.

313. Roberton NRC (1991) A manual of neonatal intensive care (2nd ed). London: Arnold.

314. Newberger J, Jonas R, Wernovsky G et al. (1993) A comparison of the neurologic effects of hypothermic circulatory arrest versus low flow coronary pulmonary bypass in infant heart surgery. New England Journal of Medicine 329: 1057–64.

315. McCaffery M (1997) Pain relief for the child: Problem areas and selected non pharmacological methods. Pediatric Nursing 3: 11–16.

316. Rushforth JA, Levene MI (1994) Behavioural responses to pain in healthy neonates. Archives of Disease in Childhood 70: F174–6.

317. Carter B (1993) Care of the child in pain. In Carter B (ed) Manual of paediatric intensive care nursing. London: Chapman and Hall.

318. Craig KD, Whitefield MF, Grunau RVE et al. (1993) Pain in the preterm neonate. Pain 52: 287–99.

319. Johnson CC (1994) Development of psychological responses to pain in infants and toddlers. In Schechler NL, Berde CB, Yaster M (eds) Pain in infants, children and adolescents. Baltimore: Williams and Wilkins.

320. Krechel SW, Bildner J (1995) Cries: A new neonatal post-operative pain management score. Paediatric Anaesthesia 5: 53–61.

321. Porter F (1994) Pain assessment in children: Infant. In Schechler NL, Berde CB, Yaster M (eds) Pain in infants, children and adolescents. Baltimore: Williams and Wilkins.

322. Dick MJ (1993) Preterm infants in pain. Clinical Nursing Research 2(2): 176–87.

323. Hamers JPH, Abu-Saad HH, Halijens RJG et al. (1994) Factors influencing nurses' pain assessment and interventions in children. Journal of Advanced Nursing 20: 853–60.

324. Gay J (1992) A painful experience. Nursing Times 88(25): 32–5.

325. Beyer J (1988) The Oucher: User's manual and technical report. Denver Colorado: University Colorado Health Sciences Centre.

326. Hurley A, Whelan EG (1988) Cognitive development and children's perception of pain. Pediatric Nursing 14(1): 21–4.

327. LeBaron S, Zeltzer L (1984) Assessment of acute pain and anxiety in children and adolescents by self reports, observational reports and behavioural check list. Journal Consultant Clinical Psychology 52(5): 729–38.

328. Melzak R (1975) The McGill pain questionnaire: Major properties and scoring methods. Pain 1: 277–99.

329. Mannheimer JS, Lampe GN (1984) Clinical transcutaneous electrical nerve stimulation. Philadelphia: FA Davis Co.

330. Gardener GG, Oldnes K (1981) Hypnosis and hypnotherapy in children. Orlando: Grune and Stratten.

331. Hilgard JR, LeBaron S (1984) Hypnotherapy of pain in children with cancer. Los Altos: William Kaufman.

332. Rutherford I (1996) Haemotasis and DIC. Intensive and Critical Care Nursing 12(2): 161–7.

333. Maxon JH (2000) Management of disseminated intravascular coagulation. Critical Care Nursing Clinics of North America 12(3): 341–52.

334. Baker WF (1989) Clinical aspects of DIC. Seminars in Thrombosis and Hemostasis 15(1): 25.

335. Baglin T (1996) DIC — The diagnosis and treatment. British Medical Journal 312: 683–7.

336. Kalter RD, Saul CM, Wetstein L et al. (1979) Cardiopulmonary bypass: Associated hemostatic abnormalities. Journal of Thoracic Cardiovascular Surgery 77: 427–35.

337. Elliott MT, Delius RE (1998) Renal issues. In Chang A (ed) Pediatric cardiac intensive care. Baltimore: Williams and Wilkins.

338. Kron IL, Joob AW, Van Meter C (1985) Acute renal failure in the cardiovascular surgical patient. Ann Thorac Surgery 39: 590–8.

339. Asquith J, Hicklin M, Griffiths C (1993) Care of the child with acute renal failure. In Carter B (ed) Manual of paediatric intensive care nursing. London: Chapman and Hall.

340. Schwarz SM, Gewitz MH See CC et al. (1990) Enteral nutrition in infants with congenital heart disease and growth failure. Pediatrics 86(3): 368–373.

341. Kudsk KA, Minard G (1994) Management of nutrition in the critically ill patient. Seminars Respir Infect 9(4): 228–31.

342. Ronnto LA (1995) Early admission of enteral nutrients in critically ill patients. AACN Clin Issues 6(2): 242–256.

343. Heyland DK, Cook DJ, Guyatt GH (1993) Enteral nutrition in the critically ill patient. A critical review of the evidence. Intensive Care Medicine 19(8): 435–42.

344. Shuster MH (1994) Enteral feeding of the critically ill. AACN Clinical Issues Critical Care Nursing 5 (4): 459–75.
345. Ricketts R (1990) Necrotizing enterocolitis. In Raffenspergen JD (ed) Swensons pediatric surgery. Connecticut: Appleton Lange.
346. Dolgin SE, Shlasko E, Levitt MA (1998) Alterations in respiratory status: Early signs of severe necrotizing enterocolitis. Journal of Pediatric Surgery 33(6): 856–8.
347. Israel EJ (1994) NEC — A disease of the immature intestinal mucosal barrier. Acta Paediatric Supp 396: 27–32.
348. Kleigman RM (1990) Models of pathogenesis of necrotising enterocolitis. Journal Pediatrics 5(2): 117.
349. Andrews JD, Krowchuk HV (1997) Stool patterns of infants diagnosed with necrotising enterocolitis. Neonatal Network 16(6): 51–7.
350. Lindermann E (1944) Symptomatology and management of acute grief. American Journal of Psychiatry 101–41.
351. Kubler-Ross E (1973) On death and dying. London: Tavistock.
352. Fulton R, Gottesman DJ (1980) Anticipatory grief: A psychosocial concept reconsidered. British Journal of Psychiatry 45: 137.
353. Browne J, Waddington P (1993) Care of the dying child. In Carter B (ed) Manual of paediatric intensive care nursing. London: Chapman and Hall.
354. Miles MS (1985) Emotional symptoms and physical health in bereaved parents. Nursing Research 34(2): 76–81.
355. Miles MS, Perry K (1985) Parental responses to sudden accidental death of a child. Critical Care Quarterly 8(1): 73–84.
356. Alder Hey Book of Children's Doses (1994) Available from the Pharmacy Department, Royal Liverpool Children's NHS Trust (Alder Hey), Liverpool.
357. British National Formulary (2001) British Medical Association and the Royal Pharmaceutical Society of Great Britain.

Appendix 1
Blood results

Clotting profile

Prothrombin time (PT)	10–16 seconds
Activated partial prothrombin time (APPT)	23–49 seconds
Fibrinogen	2–4 g/l
Thrombin	15–27 seconds

Full blood count (FBC)

Haemoglobin	12–18 g/l
White cell count (WCC)	5–10 10^9/l
Haematocrit (HCT)	0.35
Platelets	150–400 10^9/l

Urea and electrolytes (U & E)

Creatinine	20–40 mmol/l
Urea	1–5 mmol/l
Sodium	132–142 mmol/l
Potassium	3.5–5.3 mmol/l
Chloride	95–105 mmol/l
Bicarbonate	22–28 mmol/l
Glucose	3–6 mmol/l
Magnesium	0.78–1.02 mmol/l
Albumin	30–45 g/l
Calcium	2.20–2.79 mmol/l
Ionised calcium	1.13–1.32 mmol/l
Protein	54–75 g/l
Lactate	0.5–2 mmol/l
CRP	0–8 mg/l

Liver function tests (LFT)

Total bilirubin	0–15 micromol/l
Conjugated bilirubin	0–5 micromol/l
Alkaline phosphatase	0–1600 iu/l
ALT	9–44 iu/l
AST	23–73 iu/l

Appendix 2
Blood group compatibility

Blood and platelet group compatibility

	Patient group							
Donor group	AB positive	AB negative	A positive	A negative	B positive	B negative	O positive	O negative
AB positive	Yes	No	No	No	No	No	No	No
AB negative	Yes	Yes	No	No	No	No	No	No
A positive	Yes	No	Yes	No	No	No	No	No
A negative	Yes	Yes	Yes	Yes	No	No	No	No
B positive	Yes	No	No	No	Yes	No	No	No
B negative	Yes	Yes	No	No	Yes	Yes	No	No
O positive	Yes	No	Yes	No	Yes	No	Yes	No
O negative	Yes	Yes	Yes	Yes	Yes	Yes	Yes	Yes

Notes:

- Blood and platelets which are issued for a patient and are not the same ABO group as the patient, should have Neg for HT (negative for high titre haemolysis) on the donor bag. Red cells should also be packed cells or plasma reduced blood, for example, SAGM
- Patients under 1 month of age should receive CMV negative and leukocyte depleted blood products
- Patients under 1 year of age should receive leucocyte depleted products

(Helen Hill, PICU and Jenny Minards, Haematology Department, Royal Liverpool Children's NHS Trust, reproduced with permission)

Fresh frozen plasma (FFP) and cryoprecipitate

	Patient group							
Donor group	AB positive	AB negative	A positive	A negative	B positive	B negative	O positive	O negative
AB positive	Yes	No	Yes	No	Yes	No	Yes	No
AB negative	Yes	Yes	Yes	Yes	Yes	Yes	Yes	Yes
A positive	No	No	Yes	No	No	No	Yes	No
A negative	No	No	Yes	Yes	No	No	Yes	Yes
B positive	No	No	No	No	Yes	No	Yes	No
B negative	No	No	No	No	Yes	Yes	Yes	Yes
O positive	No	No	No	No	No	No	Yes	No
O negative	No	No	No	No	No	No	Yes	Yes

Notes:

- In most cases the patient's own group of FFP will be issued or the universal donor for plasma which is AB negative
- In some cases cryoprecipitate of various groups will be issued depending on availability from the blood transfusion service

(Helen Hill, PICU and Jenny Minards, Haematology Department, Royal Liverpool Children's NHS Trust, reproduced with permission)

Appendix 3
Integrated care pathway for cardiac catheterisation

Modified integrated care pathway for cardiac catheterisation — Nursing assessment and care

Nursing staff answer the following questions and perform the following care

☑ Patient details and nursing assessment

☑ Attended preadmission clinic
- Yes or no

☑ Comments — preadmission clinic
- Family understand procedure/plan of care
- Referral to cardiac liaison nurse
- Other referrals, e.g., social worker, school nurse, health visitor, interpreting service
- Local anaesthetic cream applied for bloods
- Weighed
- Height measured
- Oxygen saturations recorded
- Referred to dietitian if less than 3rd centile, recent weight loss, on special feeds

☑ Pre-catheter check list:
- Family given nil by mouth instructions and understand reasons why
- Last food 6 hours pre-catheter at ...
- Last milk 4 hours pre-catheter at ...
- Last breast milk 3 hours pre-catheter at ...

- Last clear fluids 2 hours pre-catheter at ...
- Seen by doctor
- Jewellery and nail polish removed
- Dress in theatre gown
- Weight, height, oxygen saturations, BP and results in case notes
- Consented
- ID band
- Local anaesthetic cream to both groins if catheter under local anaesthetic
- Local anaesthetic cream to IV sites
- Premedication
- Last food at ....
- Last drink at ...
- Infants under 1 year/cyanosed children who are nil by mouth for more than 4 hours require IV fluids
- Parents must be told to stay within the hospital grounds during their child's catheter
- Pathway, notes and x-rays to catheter

Section to be completed by catheter nurse:

Time patient sent for ....
Time patient arrived in catheter laboratory ....
Reason for delay in patient arriving in catheter laboratory ....
Time patient anaesthetised ....
Time procedure started ....
Reason for delay in starting cardiac catheterisation............
Time procedure finished, including echocardiogram ....
Other comments ....

Post catheter:

☑ Potential for cardiac arrhythmias
☑ Potential for sudden haemorrhage from catheter site
☑ Pressure dressing overnight
☑ To lie flat for 6 hours and thereafter accompanied when out of bed

☑ Inadequate circulation to limb — may need urgent thrombolytic treatment

Observations as below:

Limb pulse and circulation —
- Palpation and Doppler   – Quarter hourly × 1 hour
        – Hourly × 6 hours
- Catheter site for bleeding   – Quarter hourly × 1 hour
        – Hourly × 6 hours
- Pulse and respiratory rate   – Hourly × 6 hours
- BP and temperature   – On return to the ward
- Thereafter monitor as   – 4 hourly at least
  condition indicates

Check catheter sheet in case notes for additional care:

☑ Continuous ECG monitoring if patient had general anaesthetic
☑ Apnoea monitoring
☑ Oxygen via face mask/headbox at ....%/............ l/min to keep SaO$_2$ above .....
☑ SaO$_2$ monitoring × .... hours

Expected patient outcomes:

☑ TPR, BP within acceptable range. No arrhythmias
☑ Patient's colour good
☑ SaO$_2$ above acceptable limit of ......%
☑ Limbs warm, pink, pulses palpable. If not, inform doctor to start antithrombolytic therapy
☑ No oozing from catheter sites — dressing in situ overnight
☑ Family understand patient requires bedrest overnight
☑ Patient's needs addressed, e.g., toileting/play
☑ Pain controlled with paracetamol — yes or no
☑ IV fluids as prescribed
☑ No swelling/redness at IV site monitored hourly
☑ Cautious re-introduction of fluids
☑ Tolerating fluids within 4–6 hours and cannula capped off
☑ Family seen by consultant/registrar. Understand results/plan of care

Discharge assessment — Day 1 post-catheter/day of catheter:

☑ Wound checked — no haematoma/bleeding
☑ If discharged on the day of catheter, parents to be told to keep
      dressing in place until the next day
☑ Limbs well perfused — warm, pink, pulses present
☑ 4 hourly observations within acceptable range. Abnormalities reported
      to doctor
☑ Patient tolerating fluids/solids
☑ IV therapy discontinued
☑ Discharged by doctor
☑ Give post-catheter advice sheet to parents
☑ Give prescribed take home drugs to parents
☑ Ensure parents understand the above
☑ Address any other concerns the parents may have
☑ Additional information
☑ Outpatient appointment made
☑ Patient remaining an inpatient? If so perform a full nursing assessment
      and care plan

Integrated care pathway for cardiac catheterisation — Medical record

☑ Patient details
☑ Full cardiac diagnosis
☑ Type of procedure   – diagnostic or interventional
☑ Type of anaesthetic   – local or general
☑ Proposed intervention   – Balloon dilatation of ....
                                             – Stent of ....
                                             – Occlusion of ....
                                             – RF Ablation ....
                                             – EP study ....
                                             – Other ....

☑ Pre-catheter assessment   – Current symptoms
                                             – Relevant past medical history
                                             – Previous cardiac catheterisations and
                                                operations
                                             – Blocked venous access?
                                             – Current medication — stop warfarin the
                                                night before

– Allergies
– Female: Date of LMP. If >10 days ago
  and possible pregnancy, get permission
  to do a pregnancy test
– Other information ....

Examination:

☑ Weight
☑ Height
☑ Centile
☑ Saturations
☑ CVS: Clubbing?
☑   Cyanosis?
☑   Femoral pulses?
☑   Heart rate regularity
☑   Blood pressure
☑   Heart palpation and auscultation
☑ Respiratory: Rate
☑   Recession?
☑   Chest clear?
☑ Abdominal   Liver .... cm
☑   Spleen palpable?
☑ CNS   Development milestones appropriate for age?
☑ Dental caries?
☑ FBC taken and results obtained?
☑ U&E taken and results obtained
☑ Sickel cell?
☑ Group and save for diagnostic catheter
☑ Cross match for 1 unit if intervention planned
☑ Chest x-ray and result
☑ ECG and result
☑ Consent obtained?
☑ Premedication and local anaesthetic cream prescribed
☑ Post-catheter analgesia prescribed

Cardiac catheter:

☑ Procedure undertaken
☑ Anaesthetic details

☑ Drugs given during procedure
☑ Entry sites and size of sheath
☑ Routes and catheters used
☑ Results of blood gases
☑ Complications since catheter
☑ State observations required post-catheter for nursing staff — see cardiac catheter pathways for nursing staff
☑ Indications for thrombolytic therapy: Peripheral pulse absent to palpation, after removal of dressing which may be obstructing flow; an impalpable pulse which is detectable on Doppler is a borderline indication for therapy; the leg may appear white and cold but this is not a prerequisite for heparin or thrombolytic therapy

Medical discharge assessment:

☑ Clinical findings
☑ Puncture sites
☑ Foot pulses palpable?
☑ Results of predischarge investigations — FBC, CXR, Echo
☑ For discharge
☑ Medication
☑ Catheter results discussed with parents

Both nursing and medical integrated care pathways for cardiac catheterisation are reproduced with permission from the Cardiac Unit, Royal Liverpool Children's NHS Trust

Index